The
Foot
in
Diabetes

The
Foot
in
Diabetes

G. James Sammarco, M.D., F.A.C.S.

Department of Orthopaedic Surgery
University of Cincinnati Medical Center
Cincinnati, Ohio

LEA & FEBIGER
Philadelphia   London   1991

Lea & Febiger
200 Chester Field Parkway
Malvern, Pennsylvania 19355
U.S.A.
(215) 251-2230
1-800-444-1785

Library of Congress Cataloging-in-Publication Data

The Foot in diabetes / (edited by) G. James Sammarco.
    p.   cm.
    Includes index.
    ISBN 0-8121-1358-6
    1. Foot—Diseases. 2. Diabetes—Complications and sequelae.
    3. Foot manifestations of general diseases. I. Sammarco, G. James.
        (DNLM: 1. Diabetes Mellitus—complications. 2. Foot Diseases—
    etiology. 3. Foot Diseases—therapy.   WK 835 F687)
    RD563.F66 1991
    616.4'62—dc20
    DNLM/DLC   90-13338
    for Library of Congress   CIP

Reprints of chapters may be purchased from Lea & Febiger in quantities of 100 or more.

PRINTED IN THE UNITED STATES OF AMERICA

Print number: 5   4   3   2   1

Dedication

To my wife, Frisk, and children;

Alissa
Jim
Alex
Annie
Miss Nat

Foreword

Quality of life is a human attribute that is sometimes overlooked in the treatment of patients with diseases such as diabetes mellitus. In standard medical care, it is usually assumed that curing the basic pathologic process will allow function to recover spontaneously. Unfortunately, there is no cure for diabetes since the basic etiology still eludes us. In treating the multiple complications of diabetes mellitus, we are continuously playing catch up.

The monetary impact is staggering. Direct medical and surgical costs are now estimated in the billions of dollars per year. When the cost of time lost from employment is added, the amounts are even more shocking. Loss of function from a major amputation and finally loss of years of life detract further from the quality of life.

Diabetic patients represent approximately 5% of the population of the United States. However, they compose nearly 50% of the patients that undergo lower extremity amputation. Since the basic disease cannot be cured, the emphasis must be directed toward rehabilitation and prophylaxis.

Rehabilitation medicine is both multispecialty and multidisciplinary as exemplified by the list of contributors to this important text. It is obvious that team effort is represented with a blending of medical, surgical, and allied health personnel. The combined effort is aimed toward rehabilitation of the diabetic patient who started with a foot problem.

I challenge the readers to learn and to apply the valuable information provided for them. They will not be obliged to pioneer again the procedures that now allow amputations to be performed at below knee, ankle, and foot levels, rather than above the knee. The quality of life of their patients will be improved by their diligence in applying these techniques.

F. William Wagner, Jr., M.D.

Preface

Diabetes mellitus is one of the most debilitating diseases that man faces. Throughout the ages it has plagued him with clinical manifestations affecting every body organ. The foot and ankle have recently become areas of particular concern. In the past, concern for control of blood glucose, hypertension, and kidney disease was so great that diabetic foot problems, such as neuropathic ulcers, recurrent infection, and deformity were overshadowed. Thus were problems of the foot and ankle relegated to those familiar with proprietary appliances and home remedies.

Diabetes is a disease of the whole body. To treat one organ system without training and knowledge of the entire body as well as the disease process is poor medicine. We need to continually update our treatment of the diabetic lower extremity. New information is continually being published and physicians and surgeons must be aware of this material. Since it is impossible to review the hundreds of current articles in medical specialty journals to have a working knowledge of contemporary thought about diabetes, this book answers that need.

The discovery and synthesis of insulin has changed the medical treatment of diabetes dramatically. Since then, patients have lived longer, healthier lives. The morbidity of the disease has been significantly reduced.

In recent years, advances in endocrinology, specifically diabetology, nephrology, ophthalmology, neurology, general, orthopaedic and vascular surgery, rehabilitation, orthotics, pedorthotics, and prosthetics have all made tremendous advances in the ultimate care of the diabetic.

Once the above-the-knee amputation was standard procedure for the patient with lower extremity neurovascular disease; it is now performed less often. The differentiation between ulcers caused by vascular insufficiency and neurotrophic ulcers has led to increased salvage rates in treating the foot. All infections of the foot are not osteomyelitis. Amputation is now considered a last resort, not a first line treatment. Stabilizing a collapsing Charcot foot yields satisfactory results, lessening the chance of recurrent ulcers and often permitting the use of regular or extra-depth shoes.

New combinations of special materials also aid in the protection of the foot. Total contact casts and intensified patient education are considered of equal importance in controlling ulcers and saving the Charcot foot.

This book is written for the student interested in understanding the nature and treatment of diabetes in the foot and ankle. Students will find an overview of the important aspects of the disease. Residents and fellows in both surgical and nonsurgical specialities will have a reference to current information in his or her specialty. At the same time, it is a ready reference to associated systems involved in the disease so that it is not necessary to refer to several texts. Practicing physicians and surgeons will use the text as a reference volume to expand their expertise in foot disease. Orthotists, pedorthists, prosthetists, physical therapists, and podiatrists will gain understanding by referring to sections other than the regional problems with which they are familiar.

This text is not to be considered a highly sophisticated technical treatise on the disease of diabetes mellitus in the lower extremities. It is, rather, a current view of the disease, with biomechanics and pathomechanics of the foot. It offers a discussion of the forces within and beneath the foot so the reader can understand the nature of the neuropathic process. It offers specific treatment using medical and surgical rehabilitation techniques as well as recommendations for prevention of recurrence. It is my hope that this book will pull together in one volume the current thought and treatment of the foot in diabetes.

G. James Sammarco, M.D., F.A.C.S.

Acknowledgments

This book is the idea but not the product of one person. It would be impossible for me alone to gather material from all the relevant specialities needed. The contributors have written excellent chapters. Each is a specialist in his own area and has a special interest in the problems caused by diabetes. I thank each of them for their contribution. It is important to recognize those of my staff who have helped so much in organizing and preparing the manuscripts: especially Kathy Hoh, office manager, and Kay Dickerson. A special thanks goes to Mark Myerson who, in addition to being a contributor, was a sounding board for certain surgical approaches included here.

I also wish to thank those who helped me realize the need to share information with other physicians and surgeons: W.W. Ballard (the Beard) of Dartmouth College; R.F. Ryan (Bob) of Tulane University (retired); Uncle Charlie Abbott Sr., Past Chief of Surgery, St. Baranabus Hospital, Livingston, New Jersey; Victor H. Frankel, Chief of Orthopaedic Surgery, Hospital for Joint Diseases, New York; Charles H. Herndon, Chief of Orthopedics, Case Western University; and Nicholas J. Giannestras, Cincinnati. Some of these teachers and friends are now dead, others retired, and others are still actively teaching. No matter; the impression they have left on me is indelible. I also wish to thank my Fellows whose enquiring minds have kept me going.

Lastly, I owe a great debt of gratitude to Ruthann (Frisk) and all my children. It is to them that the book is dedicated. Their love and patience over the last two years has made it all possible.

Contributors

E. DOUGLAS BALDRIDGE, M.D.
Director of Peripheral Vascular Training
Department of Surgery
Good Samaritan Hospital
Cincinnati, Ohio

MICHAEL A. BERK, M.D., F.A.C.P.
Clinical Instructor in Medicine
Washington University Medical School
St. Louis, Missouri

MICHAEL D. BRNCICK, C.P.O.
Director of Prosthetics and Orthotics
Northwestern University
Chicago, Illinois

PETER R. CAVANAGH, Ph.D.
Director
The Center for Locomotion Studies
Pennsylvania State University
Professor
Pennsylvania State University
University Park, Pennsylvania

ALVIN H. CRAWFORD, M.D., F.A.C.S.
Director
Pediatric Orthopaedics
Children's Hospital Medical Center
Cincinnati, Ohio
Professor
Orthopaedic Surgery
University of Cincinnati College of Medicine
Cincinnati, Ohio

JOHN H. FEIBEL, M.D.
Clinical Neurologist
Mayfield Neurological Institute
Cincinnati, Ohio

R. TERRELL FREY, M.D.
Staff Radiologist
Department of Radiology
Good Samaritan Hospital
Cincinnati, Ohio

ARTHUR C. HUNTLEY, M.D.
Associate Professor
Department of Dermatology
University of California, Davis
Sacramento, California

MARK S. MYERSON, M.D.
Director
Foot and Ankle Center
Union Memorial Hospital
Baltimore, Maryland

ISRAEL PENN, M.D.
Professor Surgery
University of Cincinnati Medical Center
Chief of Surgery
Cincinnati Veterans Administration Center
Cincinnati, Ohio

JOEL M. PRESS, M.D.
Clinical Associate of Rehabilitation Medicine
Northwestern University Medical School
Chicago, Illinois

G. JAMES SAMMARCO, M.D., F.A.C.S.
Volunteer Professor
Department of Orthopaedics
University of Cincinnati Medical Center
Cincinnati, Ohio

MARK W. SCIOLI, M.D.
Associate Clinical Professor
Texas Tech University Health
    Sciences Center
School of Medicine, Department
    of Orthopaedics
Lubbock, Texas

MICHAEL M. STEPHENS, MSC.
    (BIOENG), FRCSC(I)
Orthopaedic Consultant
Mater Private Hospital
Dublin, Ireland

JAN S. ULBRECHT, M.D.
The Center for Locomotion Studies
Pennsylvania State University
University Park, Pennsylvania

BARRY C. ULLMAN, C. PED.
Lecturer-Consultant in Biomechanics
    and Pedorthics
Northwestern University Medical School
Chicago, Illinois

RICHARD E. WELLING, M.D.
Chief
Department of Surgery
Good Samaritan Hospital
Assistant Clinical Professor
University of Cincinnati Medical Center
Cincinnati, Ohio

KELLY WILSON, P.T.
Registered Physical Therapist
Union Memorial Hospital
Foot and Ankle Center
Baltimore, Maryland

YEONGCHI WU, M.D.
Director of Amputee Program
Director of Academic Affairs
Rehabilitation Institute of Chicago
Associate Professor
Department of Rehabilitation Medicine
Northwestern University Medical School
Chicago, Illinois

Contents

Diabetes Mellitus: The Disease

MICHAEL A. BERK, M.D.

Diabetes mellitus is a common disease affecting over 10 million people in the United States.[1] It is a leading cause of blindness,[2] end-stage renal disease,[3] heart,[4] and peripheral vascular disease.[5] This chapter provides an overview of the pathophysiology of diabetes and its complications, as well as a general outline of the principles of diabetic management. By understanding pathophysiologic concepts and treatment goals based on both pathophysiology and the natural history of the disease, it may be possible to control not only the acute metabolic complications of diabetes such as diabetic ketoacidosis, but also chronic vascular and neuropathic complications. Long-term care with emphasis on prevention is especially important because, in spite of promising research and new treatment interventions, there is no cure for diabetes.

Diabetes mellitus can be defined as a syndrome of abnormal carbohydrate metabolism with acute metabolic complications and chronic vascular, neurologic, and orthopedic complications affecting most organ systems. While this definition conveys neither the pathophysiologic nor epidemiologic characteristics of the disease, it provides a useful framework for understanding consequences of the disease.

HISTORICAL BACKGROUND

Diabetes mellitus was described as early as 200 A.D. by Chang Chung-ching in China. It was not yet recognized as a separate entity at that time.[6] Aretaeos of Kappadokia, Greece, was the first European to give a complete description of diabetes and to name the syndrome—diabetes ("διαβαινω = I pass through.")[7] He described the natural course of untreated insulin-dependent diabetes as follows:[8]

> Diabetes is a wonder affliction, not very frequent among men, being a melting down of the flesh and limbs into the urine. The patients never stop making water, but the flow is incessant, as if the opening of the aqueducts. Life is short, disgusting and painful; thirst unquenchable; excessive drinking, which, however, is disproportionate to the large quantity of urine, for more urine is passed; and one cannot stop them from drinking or making water; or, if for a time they abstain from drinking, their mouth becomes parched and their body dry; the viscera seems as if scorched up; they are affected with nausea, restlessness and burning thirst; and at no distant term they expire.

This was the natural history of insulin-dependent diabetes until the discovery of insulin by Banting (the only orthopedist to win the Nobel Prize) and Best in 1922. As the use of insulin became routine and longevity of insulin-dependent diabetic patients increased, the chronic complications of diabetes became evident. But insulin was not the panacea for all types of diabetes. Eliot Joslin was one of the first to note that insulin replacement was not the answer for patients with non-insulin dependent diabetes.[9] The importance of diabetes as an inspiration to research is evident from other discoveries relating to it. Radioimmunoassay, a technique that has revolutionized medical research, in general, and endocrinology in particular, was developed by Berson and Yalow to measure insulin, for which they received the Nobel Prize. Sanger received the Nobel Prize for being the first to sequence a peptide—insulin. The first biologic agent to be commercially produced by recombinant DNA technology was also insulin.

CLINICAL FEATURES

In 1979, an international conference sponsored by the National Diabetes Data Group, National Institute of Health, devised a classification scheme for diabetes taking into account pathophysiologic mechanisms of disease and epidemiologic data that would more clearly separate the types of diabetes as well as identify populations at risk for the development of diabetes.[10] This scheme has been generally accepted and provides a framework for classification, epidemiologic research, and treatment. The major classifications are shown in Table 1-1. The contrasts in clinical characteristics between insulin-dependent and noninsulin-dependent diabetes are shown in Table 1-2.

Type I (IDDM)

The sine qua non of insulin-dependent diabetes is absolute insulinopenia. Patients are totally dependent on insulin to prevent ketoacidosis and survive. The disease may occur at any age but generally presents before age 40, hence the older term juvenile-onset diabetes. Patients are usually thin and present with an abrupt onset of polyuria, polydypsia, polyphagia, and weight loss. At presentation hyperglycemia, glycosuria, ketonemia, and ketonuria are usually evident.

Type II (NIDDM)

Patients with Type II diabetes are usually older than 40 years of age, though the disease does occur in younger age groups. Patients are often obese and may be free of the classic symptoms described above. They rarely experience ketoacidosis except during periods of stress, trauma, surgery, or infection. These patients do not require exogenous insulin for survival but may need insulin during periods of stress or to control hyperglycemia when other modalities have failed.

Gestational

Patients with gestational diabetes have diabetes discovered during pregnancy with no antecedent history of diabetes in the nonpregnant state. They are at increased risk for the development of diabetes later in life.[11]

Other

The other types of diabetes listed in Table 1-1 are generally associated with other endocrine disorders or other pancreatic diseases. In the case of other endocrine disor-

TABLE 1-1 ■ Classification of Diabetes and Other Types of Glucose Intolerance

Clinical Class
Type I—Insulin-dependent diabetes mellitus (IDDM)
Type II—Noninsulin-dependent diabetes mellitus (NIDDM)
Other types:
Secondary to pancreatic disease: pancreatectomy, pancreatitis, hemachromatosis, cystic fibrosis
Secondary to endocrinopathies: acromegaly, pheochromocytoma, Cushing's syndrome, glucagonoma
Secondary to drugs and chemical agents: streptozotocin, certain antihypertensive agents, thiazide diuretic, glucocorticoids, estrogens, catecholamines
Associated with insulin receptor abnormalities: acanthosis nigricans
Associated with genetic syndromes: hyperlipidemia, muscular dystrophies, Huntington's disease
Miscellaneous: malnutrition.
Impaired glucose tolerance (IGT)
Gestational diabetes mellitus

From National Diabetes Data Group: Classification of diabetes mellitus and other categories of glucose intolerance. Diabetes, 28: 1039–1057, 1979.

TABLE 1–2 ■ Differences Between Insulin-Dependent and Noninsulin-Dependent Diabetes Mellitus

Clinical Feature	Insulin-dependent	Noninsulin-dependent
Age	Usually <40 years	Usually >40 years
Body type	Usually thin	Usually obese
Onset	Abrupt	Insidious
Hyperglycemia, glycosuria	Yes	Yes
Ketonemia, ketonuria	Yes	No
Exogenous insulin	Required to sustain life	Not required to sustain life

ders, the hormones listed in the table will cause hyperglycemia when present in excess. In acromegaly, for example, growth hormone is present at supraphysiologic plasma concentrations. At these levels hyperglycemia can result even though pancreatic β-cell function is preserved. Hyperglycemia is usually ameliorated when the growth hormone concentration is reduced to normal levels. Patients with such syndromes usually do not have the vascular or neuropathic complications that are seen with diabetes mellitus possibly indicating that the complications of diabetes are not solely related to hyperglycemia. Diseases of the pancreas, such as cystic fibrosis or chronic pancreatitis, generally lead to the destruction of insulin-producing cells so that these patients have a clinical picture more consistent with insulin-dependent diabetes. Drugs causing glucose intolerance may affect the β-cell directly (streptozotocin), impair peripheral utilization of glucose (thiazide diuretics), or both (catecholamines).

PATHOPHYSIOLOGY

The pathophysiology of the diabetic syndrome is different for the component diseases that the syndrome describes. Because of this, hyperglycemia may require different therapeutic approaches based on its underlying cause. The multifactorial origin of diabetes also implies that different modes of inheritance and/or environmental factors contribute to its development, indicating that different populations are at risk for developing the disease and some of its chronic complications. Hyperglycemia may play a role in the development of diabetic complications, but recent evidence suggests diabetic complications may be related to en-

vironmental and genetic factors as well. These components, then, have important implications for screening populations for the disease, therapy, and prevention of complications.

Type I (IDDM)

PATHOGENESIS

Insulin-dependent diabetes is now known to be an autoimmune endocrinopathy. Antibodies directed against pancreatic islet β-cells lead to their progressive destruction with development of insulinopenia and eventually frank diabetes.[12] The origin of these antibodies is unclear. Viral illness prior to the development of disease has raised the possibility that islet cell antibodies may be directed against viral antigens that cross-react with antigenic markers on islet cells. It is also possible that a viral infection of the islet cells themselves may result in alteration of cell surface antigens, leading to a host-immune response resulting in islet cell destruction. In support of the viral theory are epidemiologic studies showing that diabetes has a seasonal variation in its appearance, occurring more commonly in the winter. The fact that islet cell antibodies may be present in patients many years prior to the onset of disease argues against, but does not exclude, an acute viral cause of the disease.[13]

Genetic factors play a critical role in the development of IDDM as shown by studies in identical twins (monozygotic). In the large study by Pyke et al. of 200 pairs of identical twins, it was shown that twin pairs in which both members had diabetes had the same type of diabetes. That study also showed that only 54% of twin pairs were concordant for insulin-dependent diabetes indicating that the disease does not occur entirely on a genetic basis.[14] Leukocyte histocompatibility antigen (HLA) typing has shown a relationship between HLA types that influence the immune response and the development of diabetes. Ninety-five percent of patients with insulin-dependent diabetes possess either HLA DR3, DR4, or both, compared to nondiabetic individuals or noninsulin-dependent diabetic patients, whose rate is approximately 40%.[15,16] Individuals who are heterozygous for DR3/DR4 antigens appear to be at a greater risk for development of diabetes than those homozygous for either one.

Autoimmunity, environmental factors, and genetic factors are not mutually exclusive as potential pathogenic mechanisms for insulin-dependent diabetes. For example, islet cell antibodies have been detected in first-degree relatives of persons with Type I diabetes, implying either a genetic component and/or a common exposure to some environmental pattern.[17] Additionally, some patients with insulin-dependent diabetes also have antibodies to other endocrine organs, including the adrenal gland, thyroid gland, and ovary, with some individuals manifesting failure of these organs as well.[18] This fact does not totally mitigate against an environmental factor in pathogenesis. While the exact pathogenic mechanism of insulin-dependent diabetes is unknown, it is speculated that a genetic predisposition in combination with environmental factors may produce the disease.

PATHOPHYSIOLOGY OF INSULIN-DEPENDENT DIABETES

Lack of insulin affects all metabolites including carbohydrates, fats, and protein homeostasis. In general, insulinopenia results in lack of glucose utilization in insulin sensitive target organs. This may be considered pseudo-starvation because the fuels are available but their path of entry into target tissues is blocked by lack of insulin. This results in the activation of homeostatic mechanisms designed to increase nutrient delivery to target tissues but because of lack of insulin, they fail to solve and may compound the problem. The interaction of these systems is shown in Figure 1-1. Normal physiologic events, such as the switch from the fed to the fasting state late after a meal,

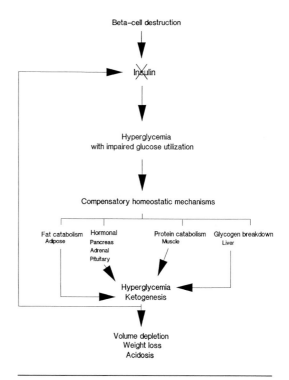

FIGURE 1-1 ■ Schematic representation of the events leading to the acute metabolic consequences of insulin-dependent diabetes. Insulinopenia results in a repetitive cycle of hyperglycemia, ketosis, acidosis, volume depletion, and weight loss.

invoke physiologic mechanisms that, in the absence of insulin, contribute to hyperglycemia and may also affect glycemic control in diabetic patients.[19]

In the absence of insulin, compensatory homeostatic mechanisms act to release glucose stores and to mobilize other fuel sources to provide energy for metabolic processes. This is especially important in the central nervous system, as the brain neither synthesizes nor stores glucose, its primary energy source.

The liver is the primary site of both direct release of stored glucose and the conversion of other metabolites into usable fuels. The liver is also the primary source of glucose stored in the form of glycogen. Glycogen breakdown is stimulated by pancreatic glucogen, which is present in high concentrations in poorly controlled diabetes, and is inhibited by insulin. The production of glucose by the liver increases the plasma glucose pool, resulting in more pronounced hyperglycemia. Amino acids resulting from breakdown of muscle protein are also converted to glucose by gluconeogenic pathways (Cori cycle). The breakdown of muscle protein results in the clinical picture of muscle wasting and weight loss. Plasma glucose is filtered by the kidney with a portion being reabsorbed. When the plasma glucose exceeds the renal tubular reabsorption maximum, glucose is excreted in the urine. Since glucose is osmotically active, water and electrolytes are also excreted in excess, resulting clinically in polyuria, polydypsia, and volume depletion. Laboratory findings show hyperglycemia with increased BUN and creatinine secondary to volume depletion.

Fuel is also stored in adipose tissue in the form of triglycerides. In the absence of insulin, lipolysis occurs at an increased rate. Free fatty acids from stored triglycerides are converted to ketone bodies by the liver. The rate-limiting step of this conversion is the delivery of free fatty acids to the liver, so that if the lipolytic process is not halted, ketogenesis continues unabated. Ketone bodies, mainly acetoacetate and β-hydroxybutyrate, are weakly acidic compounds and must have a neutral charge to be excreted by the kidney. This process requires use of physiologic buffer systems including bicarbonate and ammonia buffers. This physiologic response results in metabolic acidosis. Pulmonary compensation to correct the acidosis by expiring carbon dioxide results in respiratory alkalosis. In addition, hydrogen ions in circulation are buffered by transport from the extracellular to the intracellular space, with potassium ions being transported in the opposite direction. Potassium is then excreted by the kidney, resulting in total body potassium deficit but normal or increased serum potassium measurements. Thus, one sees a picture of ketonemia and ketonuria, hyperkalemia (usually), and metabolic acidosis (serum bicarbonate less than 15 mEq/L) with compensatory respiratory alkalosis. Hypokalemia in the presence of acidosis is an ominous prognostic sign, as it implies large whole-body potassium deficit and a significant risk for arrhythmia. Ketoacidosis also results in nausea and vomiting, promoting further volume depletion and electrolyte loss. Other effects include a negative inotropic effect, peripheral vasodilatation, hypotension, and insulin resistance. If the process is not halted, cerebral depression with coma and death can result.

Hormonal compensatory mechanisms active in the insulinopenic state include glucagon secretion by the endocrine pancreas, epinephrine secretion by the adrenal medulla, cortisol by the adrenal cortex, and growth hormone by the pituitary. All of these hormones cause an increase in plasma glucose concentration, even in the presence of insulin, and in fact, are part of the body's defense against hypoglycemia. They are secreted in uncontrolled insulin-dependent diabetes in response to the lack of glucose utilization by target tissues and in response to the stress of hyperglycemia and acidosis. Glucagon and epinephrine are secreted in the nondiabetic state late after glucose ingestion as a physiologic response to maintain euglycemia until the next meal. In the insulin-dependent diabetic state, because of an inability to secrete insulin, plasma glucose may increase during times when there is no exogenous intake of glucose, especially during the night. This fact emphasizes the potential need for insulin delivery at all times. Each of these counterregulatory hormones has specific direct and indirect effects on fuel metabolism. Glucagon promotes glycogenolysis and proteolysis. Epinephrine promotes lypolysis and ketogenesis in addition to increasing glucose production and inhibiting glucose utilization. Growth hormone and cortisol also act to decrease glucose utilization and enhance glucose production.

Type II (NIDDM)

PATHOGENESIS

Noninsulin-dependent diabetes, while having hyperglycemia as its major clinical marker, has a different pathogenesis than insulin-dependent diabetes. In contrast to insulin-dependent diabetes, absolute insulinopenia and destruction of pancreatic β-cells does not occur. In fact, most NIDDM patients do synthesize and secrete insulin, albeit with inability to maintain euglycemia. The genetic pattern is also different. Twins have a greater degree of concordance than in insulin-dependent, and there is no association with HLA type.[20] Obesity has been invoked as a potential etiology for noninsulin-dependent diabetes, yet up to 40% of NIDDM patients are not obese. This suggests an association with obesity but not a cause and effect relationship. The specific cause for the development of noninsulin-dependent diabetes is not known.[21]

PATHOPHYSIOLOGY

The events leading to noninsulin-dependent diabetes are only now becoming clearly understood. While the exact sequence is still controversial, it appears that insulin resistance in insulin-sensitive target tissues, coupled with a defect in the pancreatic β-cell, combine to produce glucose intolerance and eventual clinical diabetes. These events are shown in Figure 1-2.

Patients with noninsulin-dependent diabetes secrete insulin and are by definition not dependent on insulin for survival on a day-to-day basis. In fact, studies in populations of NIDDM patients show that patients may have normal or even elevated serum insulin concentrations early in the course of disease when compared to Type I patients.[22] The difference in NIDDM patients is that they do not maintain glucose concentration in the euglycemic range. This

implies that a normal insulin molecule is not synthesized, regulation of insulin secretion is defective, or that secreted insulin does not act effectively at target tissues to allow glucose entry and maintain euglycemia.

Except in rare cases, insulin made by NIDDM patients is of the same molecular structure as in the normal population.[23] Pancreatic β-cell defects have been identified in NIDDM patients. These defects are seen in response to a challenge that normally stimulates insulin secretion. Usually an oral or intravenous glucose load is administered with repeated sampling for glucose and serum insulin, i.e., glucose tolerance test. Other stimulants of insulin secretion including amino acids (arginine) and isoproterenol have also been employed.[24] Studies using a glucose challenge have shown that individuals without diabetes demonstrate a biphasic insulin response to the glucose load. The first phase is a rapid increase in serum insulin occurring over minutes. This phase probably represents stored insulin that is immediately available. The second phase is more prolonged, lasting hours, and probably represents insulin newly synthesized or processed by the β-cell.[25] Persons with NIDDM may show a diminished or absent first phase response and a delayed, sluggish second phase response. These findings indicate that the β-cell regulation of insulin release and/or synthesis is defective in some patients with NIDDM. Patients who show an abnormal response to a glucose load may have normal responses to other stimuli of insulin secretion, indicating that the β-cell defect may be selective for glucose.[26]

Insulin resistance is now emerging as the major "trigger" for NIDDM. The reason for this mechanism being proposed as the primary lesion in NIDDM is that many noninsulin-dependent patients have increased serum insulin concentrations in the face of hyperglycemia. Studies using the euglycemic clamp technique have substantiated this claim.[27] In this technique, insulin is infused in a dose-response fashion and a measure of its ability to promote glucose utilization in the subject is calculated. Thus, subjects who are resistant to insulin action would dispose of glucose less efficiently. Studies in NIDDM subjects demonstrate a decreased sensitivity to insulin action (more insulin required to

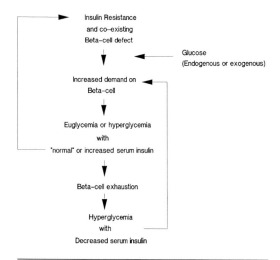

FIGURE 1–2 ■ Schematic representation of the pathogenesis of noninsulin-dependent diabetes. Here insulin resistance coupled with a β-cell defect results in hyperglycemia and β-cell exhaustion.

do the same job), a decreased maximal response to insulin, or both, when compared to lean, nondiabetic subjects.[28] Obese, nondiabetic subjects may also have similar findings without having frank diabetes or glucose intolerance, indicating that the hyperinsulinemia seen in obese subjects may be a normal physiologic response to insulin resistance.[29]

Taken together, insulin resistance combined with β-cell defect can explain the pathogenesis of NIDDM. Subjects, because they are obese or for some other reason, develop insulin resistance. Because they have a coexisting β-cell defect, the physiologic response, i.e., increased insulin secretion, is impaired. Hyperglycemia results, requiring more insulin secretion from an already overtaxed β-cell leading to eventual β-cell exhaustion and clinical diabetes (Figure 1-2).

The clinical picture resulting from the above sequence of events is hyperglycemia without ketoacidosis, polyuria, and polydypsia. Patients may or may not experience weight change. Often patients are totally asymptomatic at presentation because hyperglycemia is not yet profound enough to produce symptoms.

In summary, noninsulin-dependent diabetes is a disease with a multifactorial origin with strong genetic factors. It is not yet definitely established whether insulin resistance is the primary cause or whether a β-cell defect occurs earlier. It does appear that both are necessary to produce clinical disease.

Other Types of Diabetes

GESTATIONAL DIABETES MELLITUS (GDM)

Gestational diabetes mellitus is defined as diabetes occurring during pregnancy when it had not been present in the nonpregnant state. It usually appears between 24 and 28 weeks of gestation and presents with a clinical picture similar to NIDDM. Both a β-cell defect and insulin resistance have been invoked as possible pathogenic mechanisms though it is not clear what the exact mechanisms are. The diagnosis is important because these individuals experience a higher rate of infant and maternal morbidity compared to those without GDM, and because they have a greater risk of developing diabetes later in life. For these reasons, it is rec-

ommended that all pregnant women be screened for GDM between the 24th and 28th weeks of pregnancy.

STATES OF HORMONE EXCESS

Hormonal mechanisms are involved both in the maintenance of euglycemia and in states in which there is a lack of insulin. In certain disease states when these hormones are present in excess, diabetes results. The hormones and their diseases include growth hormone (acromegaly), cortisol (Cushing's syndrome), catecholamines (pheochromocytoma), glucagon (glucagonoma), and thyroxine (hyperthyroidism). Patients with these diseases often have diabetes or glucose intolerance as a disease component. This problem usually disappears when the underlying condition is removed or controlled. The picture is usually one of NIDDM with insulin resistance, as a result of the hormone present in excess, as the primary cause of hyperglycemia.[30,31] Patients with long-standing hormone excess syndromes and diabetes do not develop the vascular complications that patients with diabetes as their primary disease develop.

RARE TYPES OF DIABETES MELLITUS

Diabetes can also result from other rare conditions including an abnormal insulin molecule secondary to anti-insulin antibodies, anti-insulin receptor antibodies, or associated with acanthosis nigricans.[32-34] In general, these syndromes present with a NIDDM clinical picture and are seen rarely in routine clinical practice.

DIAGNOSIS

The Diabetes Data Group has established a classification scheme for diabetes mellitus. As with any medical condition, it is important that the diagnosis be made correctly, especially in diabetes, in which the long-term as well as short term (in the case of pregnancy) implications are so important. The diagnostic criteria are shown in Table 1-3. The diagnosis of diabetes is relatively simple if the fasting plasma glucose is used as the primary test method. While the random plasma glucose may also be used, the pa-

TABLE 1–3 ■ Diagnosis of Diabetes Mellitus in Nonpregnant Adults

1. Fasting plasma glucose of >140 mg/dl on at least *two* occasions
2. A random plasma glucose of >200 mg/dl *with symptoms* including polyuria, polydypsia, polyphagia, and weight loss
3. A fasting plasma glucose of <140 mg/dl with sustained plasma glucose levels during at least *two* oral glucose tolerance tests: a value of >200 mg/dl at two hours *and* at least one value >200 mg/dl at 30, 60 or 90 minutes

tient must also have clinical symptoms of diabetes. The oral glucose tolerance test is now used less often in the diagnosis of diabetes mellitus in nonpregnant adults. It is cumbersome, costly, and requires prior patient preparation that must be done correctly if the test results are to be interpretable. The diagnosis of diabetes per se does not necessarily dictate the specific treatment regimen. Other patient factors and laboratory data must be used to determine the type of diabetes and severity at presentation to dictate therapy.

Screening for diabetes in asymptomatic patients is indicated when

1. There is a strong family history of diabetes.
2. The patient is markedly obese.
3. The patient has a morbid obstetrical history including a history of an infant over 9 pounds at birth.
4. The patient is pregnant and between 24 and 28 weeks gestation.
5. The patient has a co-existing medical condition (e.g., Cushing's syndrome) that has an increased rate of diabetes associated with it.

In nonpregnant adults, the best screening test is a fasting plasma glucose. If it is greater than 115 mg/ml, a repeat test should be done. If the results remain equivocal an oral glucose tolerance test may be done, keeping in mind the caveats mentioned above. In pregnant women a fasting plasma glucose of greater than 105 mg/ml or plasma glu-

cose of 150 mg/ml or greater one hour after a 50 g glucose load is an indication for an oral glucose tolerance test. Blood glucoses obtained by fingerstick testing and the use of visually read reagent strips should not be used to make the diagnosis of diabetes mellitus (Tables 1-3 & 1-4)

Diagnosis of Diabetes Mellitus in Non-Pregnant Adults

1. Fasting plasma glucose of 140 mg/dl on at least two occasions.
2. A random plasma glucose of 200 mg/dl with symptoms including polyuria, polydypsia, polyphagia, and weight loss.
3. A fasting plasma glucose of 140 mg/dl with sustained plasma glucose levels during at least 2 oral glucose tolerance tests: A value of 200 mg/dl at 2 hours and at least 1 value 200 mg/dl at 30, 60 or 90 minutes.

Treatment

The treatment modalities for both IDDM and NIDDM are shown in Table 1-4. Diet and exercise are important forms of therapy in both types. Insulin is required for IDDM, where an oral hypoglycemic agent and/or insulin therapy may be needed in NIDDM. Proper diabetic education with a team approach to management is paramount and should begin at diagnosis. The team includes the patient, the patient's family, physician, educator, nutritionist, and other health care and allied health personnel as required. Education is best performed by individuals who are experienced in diabetic education including nutrition, monitoring, foot care, insulin injection, and so on. Although there are no long-term studies indicating that diabetic education prevents specific morbid events, education does allow the patient to understand his or her dis-

TABLE 1–4 ■ Treatment Modalities in Diabetes Mellitus

Insulin-Dependent	Noninsulin Dependent
Education	Education
Insulin	Diet
Diet	Exercise
Exercise	Oral hypoglycemic agents
	Insulin

ease and provides the necessary tools to deal with the disease on a daily basis. Education should be aimed at not only providing guidelines for management but also preventative steps to avoid excess morbidity, e.g., foot care. The specific approaches to therapy include

Maintain glycemic control
Maintain ideal body weight and adequate nutrition
Maintain adequate growth (in children)
Prevent acute and chronic diabetic complications

The attainment of these goals requires an individualized approach to each patient. Factors that enter into their development include type and duration of diabetes, the presence of diabetic complications, other medical conditions, patient educational and socioeconomic level, and patient compliance with therapy.

The issue of what degree of glycemic control is necessary to prevent complications has never been studied prospectively in a large number of diabetic individuals, though large-scale studies are now in progress.[35] Retrospective data on large numbers of patients suggests that better glycemic control is an important factor in preventing complications.[36] This type of goal is accomplished in a patient with good diabetes education, frequent home glucose monitoring, and the ability to recognize symptoms of hypoglycemia. It is unrealistic in patients who do not monitor glucose or follow a diet. It is also not feasible for patients with complications of diabetes or other medical illnesses in which hypoglycemia would pose a severe risk to health, and it is especially dangerous to diabetic patients who do not have warning symptoms of hypoglycemia. Suggested guidelines are shown in Table 1-5.

Diet[37]

Many factors are involved in prescribing a proper diet for diabetics, including

1. Type of diabetes
2. Age
3. Daily activity and work schedule
4. Initial weight and percentage of ideal body weight
5. Ethnic or racial diets
6. Insulin or oral hypoglycemic therapy
7. Other medical conditions—renal or hepatic disease, hypertension, heart disease, lipid disorders, and pregnancy
8. Level of education
9. The patient's socioeconomic level

The general goals of diet therapy are to maintain proper nutrition with a diet that provides an adequate number of calories and a proper balance of proteins, fats and carbohydrates.

The average individual expends approximately 35 kcal/kg body weight/day, of which 25 kcal/kg is used to maintain basal metabolic function. The remaining calories are used for energy expenditure from exercise and from the thermal effect of food. In general, a sedentary patient requires approximately 30 kcal/kg/day, while more active individuals require 35 kcal/kg/day. These requirements may be adjusted upwards for other conditions including infection, surgical stress, or wound healing. If calories ingested are greater than calories expended, weight is gained. Diet intake should be distributed evenly throughout the day to prevent large excursions in blood glucose after a meal and should be spaced 4 to 5 hours apart.

Approximately 12 to 20% of the diet should be composed of protein (0.8 g/kg). Carbohydrates should compose 50 to 60% of the total calories with 95% of carbohy-

TABLE 1–5 ■ Target Glucose and Glycohemoglobin Concentrations (Nonpregnant Adults)

Measurement	Normal	Good	Fair	Poor
Fasting glucose (mg/dl)	60–100	70–140	141–200	>200
Postprandial glucose	<140	<180	181–240	>240
Overnight glucose*	>70	>70	>70	>70
Glycosylated hemoglobin (%)**	6	8	10	>10

*Lower limit to prevent hypoglycemia
**Values may be different for individual laboratories.

drates as starches and 5% as sucrose eaten as part of a mixed meal. Fat intake should be limited to 30%, with saturated fat limited to 10% of total fat and cholesterol limited to 300 mg/day because of the increased risk of cardiovascular and peripheral vascular disease in diabetic individuals. Sugar substitutes such as aspartame may be consumed ad lib as long as the other calories in the sweetened product are taken into account.

Diet therapy is one of the most difficult aspects of the medical management of diabetes. It should be performed by a qualified nutritionist and requires frequent reinforcement. Dietary control often requires a change in lifestyle, which is difficult in children, adolescents, and older individuals as well as the economically disadvantaged. In addition to a careful explanation, techniques such as behavior modification may be helpful. Diet should be individualized to the patient's likes and dislikes regarding food and work schedule. It is important that the family member who does the shopping and cooks the meals be present for the educational process.

SPECIAL CONSIDERATIONS

Diet therapy is different for the two major types of diabetes. IDDM patients are generally near or below ideal body weight so that caloric intake should be designed to maintain weight. Since many IDDM patients are young and still growing, caloric intake should be designed to permit adequate growth with insulin therapy adjusted to control glucose. In addition, since all of these patients are on insulin therapy by definition, scheduling of meals and insulin injections should be adjusted so that the peak effect of insulin occurs at the time that it is needed to control plasma glucose excursions from oral intake. Because many patients are also on multiple injections of insulin, additional snacks between meals may be needed to prevent hypoglycemia. Snack calories should be included in the calculation of total caloric requirements.

Diet therapy in NIDDM is the cornerstone of therapy. Hyperglycemia may be controlled by diet alone in these patients. The approach is slightly different, however, than in IDDM. Since many patients are obese the diet should be designed to promote weight loss. Successful weight loss may result in patients not requiring oral hypoglycemic agents or insulin therapy, whereas obesity may promote insulin resistance and difficult diabetes control. Studies in which patients with NIDDM have been placed on prolonged fasts show that glucose tolerance and insulin resitance may improve before significant weight loss takes place. This approach as a routine measure is not recommended unless the person using it has experience with such therapy and its complications. In the non-obese NIDDM, diet should be designed to maintain weight. In the patient taking oral hypoglycemic agents or insulin, the same considerations as in IDDM patients must be followed regarding scheduling of meals.

SPECIAL CASES

Concurrent medical conditions must always be taken into account in the diet prescription. Patients with fluid retention or hypertension may require a low salt diet. Diabetic patients with renal disease may require a reduction in total dietary protein. Pregnant women with insulin-dependent diabetes usually require an increase in total calories to provide for adequate fetal growth.

Exercise

Exercise promotes cardiovascular fitness, increases glucose utilization and lowers plasma glucose, aids in promotion of weight loss, and may contribute to a decrease in serum cholesterol. Recently, there has been some controversy as to whether exercise aids in control of blood glucose over prolonged periods of time, but its acute effects on lowering plasma glucose are well documented.[39]

Special considerations in the diabetic patient must be recognized so that morbidity related to exercise does not occur.

EXERCISE PRESCRIPTION IN DIABETES MELLITUS

Exercise must be individualized. Aerobic exercise is probably most advantageous to the diabetic patient because it builds cardiovascular fitness and can be accomplished in the home. Simple exercises such as walking and jogging can be routine. Before an exercise prescription is made the patient should be assessed for evidence of cardio-vascular disease by exercise testing for peripheral vascular disease. An examination for other complications, including proliferative retinopathy and renal disease, should also be done as exercise may increase their morbidity. Vitreous hemorrhage can occur in patients with proliferative retinopathy during heavy exercise. Patients should wear shoes that fit well and examine their feet before and after exercise for evidence of blisters, ulcers, and fungal infections.

Exercise should be preceded by a warm-up period and followed by a cool-down period. Goals of exercise are obtained in a gradual fashion by using a schedule similar to that used in cardiac rehabilitation programs. Exercise is best done on a regular basis and at the same time of day. The time of day should be based on a time when the patient is at least risk for hypoglycemia. This is usually 1 to 1-1/2 hours after a meal when plasma glucose is usually highest. It is helpful if patients check their blood glucose before and after exercise in the beginning of the program to note effects of exercise. It may be necessary to increase calories or reduce hypoglycemic medication or insulin prior to exercise to prevent hypoglycemia. Patients should carry an oral source of glucose with them in case they experience hypoglycemia while exercising.

COMPLICATIONS OF EXERCISE IN DIABETES MELLITUS

Complications resulting from exercise can be divided into those relating to glucose control, chronic diabetic complications, and other illnesses.

Changes in exercise pattern can have pronounced effects on glycemic control. The usual problem encountered is one of hypoglycemia. This can be remedied by adjustment in medication, caloric intake, or both. Hypoglycemia as a result of exercise may occur hours after exercise. Glycogen mobilized during exercise may prevent hypoglycemia in the immediate post-exercise period. Depletion of stores at that time may result in unavailability of glycogen hours later when glucose may be falling for another reason.

Hyperglycemia may also be precipitated by exercise. It occurs when blood glucose is elevated before the exercise takes place and may be due to activation of compensatory mechanisms that normally serve to maintain euglycemia during exercise (glucagon and epinephrine) which, with decreased insulin, may result in an increase in blood glucose.[40,41]

Another problem related to exercise that generally results from complications of diabetes is neuropathy. Poor sensory perception in the feet may lead to foot ulcers from the combination of ill-fitting shoes and the repetitive trauma of exercise.

Oral Hypoglycemics

The characteristics of oral hypoglycemic agents are outlined in Table 1-6. They are the next step in treating NIDDM patients when diet and exercise therapy have failed to achieve the goals of glucose control. The compounds shown in Table 1-6 are sulfonylurea agents. Gylburide and glipizide are of the newer second generation type and are characterized by greater potency. The other agents are first generation.

MECHANISM OF ACTION

The sulfonylurea agents are thought to act be two mechanisms. All increase insulin secretion by the pancreas early in the course of treatment, but it appears that this action, with the possible exception of glipizide, is short-lived. The proposed primary mechanism of action is the agents acting on the insulin receptor or at the post-receptor level in insulin-sensitive target tissues to enhance insulin action and decrease insulin resistance.[42] Thus, it is reasonable to treat patients with noninsulin-dependent diabetes with these compounds since insulin resistance is a major component of their disease.

The primary side effect of all of the oral agents is hypoglycemia.

Oral agents are indicated when diet and exercise have failed to control hyperglycemia in noninsulin-dependent diabetic patients. They are absolutely contraindicated in insulin-dependent diabetes. If there is some question about the type of diabetes a particular patient has, that patient should be

TABLE 1–6 ■ Properties of Oral Hypoglycemic Agents

Drug	Trade Name	Dose (mg)	Dosage Interval	Duration of Action (hr)	Metab-olism	Metab-olites	Excre-tion
Tolbutamide	Orinase	500–3000	2–3 times per day	6–12	Hepatic	Inactive	Renal
Chlorpropamide	Diabinese	100–750	Once per day	60	Hepatic	Active	Renal
Acetohexamide	Dymelor	250–1500	1–2 times per day	12–18	Hepatic	Active	Renal
Tolazamide	Tolinase	100–1000	1–2 times per day	12–24	Hepatic	Active, inactive	Renal
Glyburide	Micronase Diabeta	2.5–30	Once per day	24	Hepatic	Inert	Renal
Glipizide	Glucotrol	5–40	1–2 times per day	24	Hepatic	Inert	Renal

From Galloway JA, Potvin JH, Shuman GR eds. Diabetes mellitus, 9th Ed. Eli Lilly and Company; Indianapolis, IN 1988; and Rifkin H, ed. The physicians guide to Type II Diabetes (NIDDM), American Diabetes Association, Inc; Alexandria VA. 1984.

treated with insulin. Oral agents are also contraindicated in patients with allergies to sulfonylurea compounds or sulfa drugs and pregnant women.

Second generation oral agents, glipizide and glyburide, may be used when first generation agents have failed. There does not appear to be a significant secondary success rate between second generation agents.

Because these drugs appear to improve insulin resistance, they have been used together with insulin on the assumption that exogenous insulin would have greater efficacy in controlling hyperglycemia. Studies done to date are not conclusive about whether this regimen offers significant improvement over insulin alone.

Insulin

Table 1-7 shows the properties of the most commonly used insulin preparations.

Insulin is synthesized in the pancreatic β-cell as proinsulin, a single chain polypeptide. The molecule is then processed by cleaving off a portion of it, the connecting piece or C-peptide, and secreted as a two-chain, 51 amino-acid polypeptide connected by two disulfide bridges.[43] Insulin and C-peptide are secreted in equimolar amounts. Some proinsulin is secreted as well. C-peptide and proinsulin are biologically inactive at physiologic concentrations.

Until recently, insulin was extracted from either beef or pork pancreases and purified for human use. Recent use of recombinant DNA technology has made possible the manufacture of human insulin from Escherichia coli. Both human and animal insulins are commercially available. They differ in cost and purity, with human insulin being the most highly purified and generally the most expensive.

Animal insulins are foreign proteins and therefore provoke an immune response with formation of anti-insulin antibodies in almost all diabetic patients taking insulin. Beef insulin is different from human insulin by 3 amino acids, whereas pork insulin differs by only 1. In general, antibody formation is not a clinical problem and there is no evidence that it has any long-term consequences. Patients also develop low titers of anti-insulin

TABLE 1–7 ■ Properties of Insulin

Insulin Type	Species	Onset of Action	Peak Action	Duration of Action
Short-acting (Regular)	Beef-pork, pork, human	15–30 min	2–4 hr	4–7 hr
Intermediate-acting (NPH, Lente)	Beef-pork, pork, human	1–2 hr	6–12 hr	14–24 hr
Long-acting (Ultralente)	Beef, human	4–6 hr	18–24 hr	28–36 hr

antibodies to manufactured human insulin as well, even though it is identical to native human insulin. Thus, there is no reason to change a patient to human insulin from an animal type unless the patient has demonstrated an allergy to animal insulins. In general, it is probably reasonable to start newly diagnosed insulin-dependent diabetic patients on human insulin because there is a virtually unlimited supply for the future. There is, however, no contraindication to the use of animal insulins either.

DOSAGE REGIMEN

Insulin-dependent diabetes. In general, good glycemic control can only be achieved by multiple injections of insulin. Using this regimen, glycemic excursions after a meal and overnight euglycemia are accomplished with flexibility and without untoward hypoglycemia. In order for such therapeutic plans to work, patients must follow a diet and test their blood glucose on a regular basis, often several times per day. A common dosage schedule is shown in Figure 1-3. In this plan, regular plus intermediate acting insulin (NPH or Lente) is given twice a day, before breakfast and before supper. To determine a reasonable starting dosage, the following formula may be used.

Total daily dose
= patient's weight in kg × 0.6

Amount of intermediate acting insulin equals 2/3 of the total dose, with 2/3 given in the morning and 1/3 before supper.

Amount of short-acting insulin equals 1/3 of the total dose, with 2/3 given in the morning and 1/3 before supper.

These formulae can then be adjusted based on the glucose readings obtained by the patient. In the beginning, patients should monitor blood glucose before each meal and at bedtime. The dose can then be changed based on the particular insulin that affects the glucose level requiring adjustment. For example, in Figure 1-3, the prebreakfast blood glucose (closed circle) is affected primarily by the presupper NPH, so that if it is unacceptably high (or low), that dose of insulin should be adjusted. After a stable dose of insulin with good glycemic levels is achieved, the frequency of testing may be decreased. This type of schedule, with proper patient education, may be manipulated by the patient to maintain daily control.

When adjustments in insulin are made, it is best to adjust the dose based on a percentage increase (or decrease) over the previous dose rather than increasing or decreasing by a specific number of units of insulin. Insulin is a potent hormone and changes of 1 or 2 units may have a profound effect on blood glucose, especially in a patient who is already well-controlled.

Other insulin schedules can be used successfully in IDDM patients. These may involve 3 to 4 injections per day or the use of

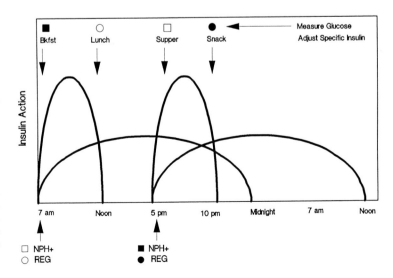

FIGURE 1-3 ■ Schematic diagram of a common insulin regimen using two injections of intermediate and short-acting insulin. The particular dose of insulin and the glucose measurement that it affects are indicated by the same symbol. See text for an example of adjusting insulin with this regimen.

continuous subcutaneous insulin infusion devices (insulin pumps).

Non-insulin Dependent Patients. The use of insulin in NIDDM requires a different strategy than in IDDM. Insulin therapy should be started when diet, exercise, and oral agents have been successful in controlling blood glucose. Since these patients make varying amounts of insulin and may also be insulin-resistant, the initial dose and schedule of insulin injection are difficult to predict. Some patients may have increased fasting blood glucose concentrations but are able to make insulin in response to meals, so that if the fasting glucose is controlled, glucose throughout the day may be acceptable. In such patients, a dose of intermediate-acting insulin before supper or bed may be all that is necessary. In other patients, a single injection of intermediate-acting insulin may be all that is required for good glycemic control over a 24-hour period. Other patients may require a regimen similar to that shown in Figure 1-3.

Insulin may be used in combination with oral agents in some carefully selected patients. The use of oral agents may improve insulin resistance and allow a decrease in insulin dose in NIDDM. This may be especially helpful in severely insulin-resistant patients who may require greater than 100 units of insulin per day.

Adjustment of insulin dose in NIDDM patients should be based on glucose monitoring results; doses should be adjusted based on a percentage increase or decrease of the previous dose. In general, one has more time to adjust insulin dose in NIDDM, as patients are usually not subject to the wide swings in blood glucose as in IDDM.

MONITORING

Modern technology has enabled diabetic patients to monitor blood glucose at home. Strips impregnated with glucose-sensitive reagents give a color response based on blood glucose concentration that can be read visually or by a reflectance meter. Newer technology employs the use of film with a reagent that is read by special meters. Home blood glucose monitoring allows daily adjustment of insulin and may decrease the number of physician visits required to achieve control. Newer devices have built-in memory and data can be uploaded into microcomputers for analysis of daily blood glucose patterns eliminating much of the guesswork in adjusting insulin dose. Monitoring is especially useful during acute illness when adjustment in insulin dose may be required frequently. Some patients do not record or alter their home records. The results of home monitoring can be validated with glycosylated hemoglobin measurements.

The patient is selected for home monitoring based on his ability to learn the technique and to afford the cost of the necessary equipment. All patients do not need reflectance meters though they are usually necessary in patients wishing to achieve near-normal glycemia. The physican should insure that the patient is not color-blind and has sufficient visual acuity to read the strips accurately. He should also be familiar with the technique. With so many reagent strips and meters available, it is probably best to select one or two to use routinely.

Urine

GLUCOSE

Urine glucose testing provides a gross indication of blood glucose concentration. Double-voided urines provide the most accurate measurements. Unfortunately, as the duration of diabetes increases, the renal threshold for glucose reabsorption may change and urine measurements may not be an accurate reflection of blood glucose. Urine testing is a markedly inferior method of monitoring glycemic control in most diabetic patients and is advised only for patients who can neither perform or afford home blood glucose monitoring.

KETONES

Urine monitoring for ketones should be done by insulin-dependent diabetic patients when blood glucose is elevated or when the patient is ill. It should also be done in the face of weight loss or after trauma or surgery. It should be done in noninsulin-dependent patients suffering from marked hyperglycemia or severe illness.

Glycosylated Hemoglobin

Many proteins have carbohydrate moieties as part of their final active forms. These groups are attached after synthesis of the molecule and are reactions dependent on ambient glucose concentration. Thus, when circulating carbohydrate concentration is elevated, the percentage of protein glycosylation is higher. Hemoglobin is such a protein. When glucose concentration is high, a greater percentage of hemoglobin is glycosylated. The percentage of glycosylated hemoglobin in the blood can be measured by chromatographic methods and gives an indication of the integrated blood glucose measurement over the average life of the red blood cell, approximately 120 days. In diabetic patients, this measurement gives an excellent reflection of chronic glycemic control and best indicates glycemic control over the 60 days prior to measurement. It serves as a confirming test of the patient's home monitoring records and provides important information about patients who do no monitoring since it gives a more integrated picture than a laboratory glucose done at single office visit. It is now a routine part of diabetic care.

Glycosylated hemoglobin measurements can be affected by hemoglobinopathies, especially those that increase or decrease red cell turnover. These include sickle cell anemia (decrease measurement value) and thallesemia (increase measurement value). Acute increases in blood glucose immediately prior to measurement, for example, a prior episode of diabetic ketoacidosis will increase measurement. Other tests are now available using proteins that have shorter half-lives (e.g. fructosamine), which give a more accurate picture of glycemic control over a period of 1 to 2 weeks prior to measurement. Glycosylated hemoglobin is unreliable as a screening test and should not be used to make the diagnosis of diabetes mellitus.

OTHER ROUTINE CARE

Patients with diabetes require other routine monitoring to maintain good health. Routine physical examination should include supine and erect blood pressure and heart rate, ophthalmoscopy to search for diabetic retinal disease, careful examination of the feet and ankles and peripheral pulses, and testing for neuropathy. Laboratory studies should include measurement of blood urea nitrogen and creatine and urinalysis. In addition, 24-hour urine collections should be done periodically for creatine and protein excretion to monitor for kidney disease. Because diabetes is associated with hyperlipidemias and these conditions contribute to the risk of cardiovascular and peripheral vascular disease, patients with diabetes should have routine testing for fasting total cholesterol, HDL cholesterol, LDL cholesterol, and triglycerides. In addition, because diabetes is a debilitating illness, pneumococcal and influenza vaccines are recommended.

COMPLICATIONS OF DIABETES MELLITUS AND THEIR THERAPY

The complications of diabetes can be conveniently divided into those that are acute and those that are a result of longstanding disease. Acute problems can usually be managed using well-proven modes of therapy. Chronic complications occur for several reasons. The final common pathway originally ascribed to chronic complications was poor glycemic control. It appears now that after a certain point correction of poor glycemic control may not prevent worsening of certain complications. Prevention of chronic complications may occur with good glycemic control, though the degree of control necessary and its time of initiation are still controversial. The case for good glycemic control has been substantiated in some retrospective studies; until the results of ongoing prospective trials are known, it is probably the more prudent course to take.

Acute Metabolic Complications of Diabetes

DIABETIC KETOACIDOSIS

Diabetic ketoacidosis is a state of hyperglycemia, metabolic acidosis, and ketonemia. Its pathogenesis has been discussed above. The condition remains a serious one with mortality reported to be 10% or higher in older patients.[47,48] Management includes taking a careful history and performing a physical examination to determine the possible precipitating event. Such causes as infection, either bacterial or viral and present in over 50% of patients with ketoacidosis, should be considered.[49] In addition, noncompliance with insulin therapy or surgery, trauma, and pregnancy should also be considered. A careful medication history for such drugs as steroids is important. Medical causes other than infection include myocardial infarction, acute cholecystitis, and acute neurologic events including stroke and seizure.

Treatment of diabetic ketoacidosis involves restoration of intravascular volume, replacement of electrolytes, especially potassium and bicarbonate, and reversal of hyperglycemia and ketogenesis with insulin therapy. Insulin therapy is best done with low-dose intravenous insulin infusion at a starting rate of 0.1 U/kg/hr with frequent laboratory glucose measurements and adjustment of the dose. Intramuscular insulin may be used but is uncomfortable and cannot be adjusted as quickly. Subcutaneous insulin should not be used for the treatment of ketoacidosis, as its absorption from tissue that may be poorly perfused in the volume depleted state is erratic. Therapy should monitor vital signs, input and output, insulin dose, and should include fluid therapy as well as laboratory results recorded on a flow sheet. Potential underlying causes should be treated aggressively and the patient reassessed frequently. An experienced physician will be needed to avoid such complications as hypotension, hypokalemia with cardiac arrhythmia, and hypoglycemia.

NONKETOTIC HYPEROSMOLAR COMA

This problem generally occurs in patients with a history of noninsulin dependent diabetes mellitus, but may also occur in the initial presentation in patients with no previous history of diabetes. Patients are usually profoundly dehydrated and volume depleted, markedly hyperglycemic, and have increased serum osmolality. They often have an underlying illness or condition in which they are unable to maintain adequate oral intake, especially of fluids. As in diabetic ketoacidosis underlying medical conditions should be sought, including infection, myo-

cardial infarction, and acute neurologic events.

Treatment of this condition is slightly different than that of diabetic ketoacidosis. In these patients, the loss of electrolytes and intravascular volume may be so profound that hyperglycemia maintains intravascular osmotic pressure and thus supports systemic blood pressure. Insulin therapy may drive glucose intracellularly so rapidly that vascular collapse may result. Treatment, then, should begin with aggressive volume expansion with normal saline, and insulin should be added when adequate urine output and blood pressure are achieved. In general this process occurs fairly rapidly, so that insulin therapy need not be delayed for long periods. After successful acute therapy with volume replacement, insulin, electrolyte replacement, and treatment of underlying problems, patients may not require exogenous insulin to control blood glucose. Unfortunately, because this condition generally occurs in elderly, debilitated patients, morbidity and mortality are high.

HYPOGLYCEMIA

Hypoglycemia can result in altered mentation and may progress to coma and even death. Mild hypoglycemia, that is, low blood glucose without altered mentation, is common in patients whose goals are to maintain near euglycemia. Warning symptoms include sweating, hunger, and palpitations. Some patients have no warning symptoms at all, however. Treatment of mild hypoglycemia involves oral intake of glucose in the form of fruit juice, glucose in water, or glucose tablets, which elevate glucose quickly, and some source of complex carbohydrate and protein to maintain glucose until the next meal. If possible, patients should measure blood glucose before therapy to make sure that the symptoms they are having are hypoglycemia. Nocturnal hypoglycemia may occur without the patient awakening from sleep. Historic clues include frequent nightmares, diaphoresis, and restless sleep. In some cases, it may be necessary to have the patient awaken at 3:00 a.m. to test blood glucose to determine nocturnal hypoglycemia.

Treatment of hypoglycemic coma involves either injection of glucagon subcutaneously or intravenous glucose in the form of 50% dextrose in water. Intravenous glucose should be administered to any patient who presents with coma of unknown cause, since it provides diagnostic and therapeutic information, if successful. If the patient is in a coma from other causes, it will do no harm. If the patient is in hyperglycemic coma, the increment in plasma glucose is small enough that the benefit of potential information and therapeutic results outweighs the risks.

Chronic Complications

OPHTHALMOLOGIC COMPLICATIONS

Diabetes is the leading cause of blindness in adults in the United States.[50] Ocular complications of diabetes include retinal disease, cataracts, and glaucoma. Great strides have been made in the last 20 years in prevention and treatment of ocular complications so that their early diagnosis can result in significant preservation of vision.

RETINOPATHY

Diabetic retinopathy is clinically divided into two types—background diabetic retinopathy, and proliferative diabetic retinopathy. Both are related to duration of disease. Background retinopathy is present in 80% of patients with diabetes of 20 years duration.[51-53] In insulin-dependent Type I diabetic patients, it is rarely seen until the disease has been present for five years.[54] In noninsulin dependent patients, it may be present at diagnosis, because diabetes in this group may not be clinically evident for years before diagnosis so that complications may have already begun at the time of initial presentation. Background retinopathy includes such conditions as microaneurysms, cotton wool spots, and hard exudates. These can be diagnosed by direct opthalmoscopy, color fundus photography, and fluorescein angiography, which demonstrates leakage from intraretinal blood vessels into the retina. The exact pathophysiologic mechanism for background retinopathy is not clear. Such causes as retinal hypoxia, venous dilatation, and abnormal glycosylation of vessel pro-

tein and collagen matrix have been proposed.[55] The cause is probably a combination of several of these factors. It is not clear whether tight glycemic control prevents background retinopathy. In some studies, rapid institution of glycemic control results in a worsening of diabetic retinopathy.[56-58] Longer term follow-up of these patients shows that this effect is probably transitory.

Proliferative diabetic retinopathy involves the growth of new vessels out of the retina into the vitreous. These vessels do not have the normal supporting tissues and are, therefore, very fragile. They can hemorrhage into the vitreous causing loss of vision. A clot may then form that may dissolve or attach to the retina, resulting in traction on the retina and subsequent retinal detachment. Individuals with proliferative retinopathy usually have a history of background retinopathy, though not all with background retinopathy progress to proliferative disease. After proliferative retinopathy occurs, improvement in glycemic control will not alter its course. However, laser photocoagulation surgery has been found to prevent progression of proliferative disease and preserve sight in 50% of patients when used early.[59] This fact underscores the need for routine ophthalmologic examination in patients with longstanding diabetes. After hemorrhage has occurred, vitrectomy may restore useful vision in selected patients.

There is some controversy over whether nonsteroidal anti-inflammatory drugs such as aspirin can be used safely in patients with proliferative retinopathy. Their use, at present, should probably be avoided until ophthalmologic consultation is obtained. Other conditions such as uncontrolled hypertension or therapy with heparin or warfarin may cause intraocular hemorrhage as well.

Cataracts occur more frequently in patients with diabetes, especially noninsulin dependent diabetes, and appear to be related to chronic poor glycemic control.[60] Treatment is surgical excision.

Patients with poorly controlled diabetes may experience blurred vision as a result of osmotic shifts in the vitreous and a change in the shape of the lens. They should not be fitted with glasses or contact lenses until blood glucose control is stabilized.

RENAL COMPLICATIONS

Diabetes is a leading cause of end-stage renal disease resulting in dialysis, transplantation, or both in the United States.[2] Like ocular disease it is related to duration of diabetes.[61] Patients with renal disease usually have diabetic retinopathy, though the converse is not always true.[2]

Diabetic renal disease usually begins with a silent phase in which glomerular filtration is actually increased.[62] This is followed by a phase in which protein excretion by the kidney is increased and glomerular filtration may be normal or slightly decreased.[63] The next phase involves overt proteinurea into the nephrotic range greater than 1.5 g protein/24 hours, and finally a development of overt end-stage renal disease with steady decline in glomerular filtration until dialysis or transplantation becomes necessary. Once the disease progresses to the point where the patient has nephrotic syndrome, end-stage renal disease is predictable.[64] At this point, improvement in glycemic control does not help.[65] Evidence is emerging that control of blood glucose in the early stages may prevent or delay progression to end-stage renal disease.[66,67] Control of hypertension may also delay progression.[68] Dietary therapy with low protein diets has also been advocated but long-term results are not known.[69]

The most sensitive indicator of diabetic renal disease currently available is measurement of 24-hour urine protein excretion. Abnormalities in this parameter develop long before other indicators such as serum creatinine show a change.[70-72] New techniques of measuring μg quantities of albumin in urine specimens have made the early diagnosis possible.

Renal disease can be aggravated by problems such as volume depletion and drugs such as diuretics and x-ray contrast material. Diabetic patients undergoing radiologic procedures such as angiography must be well hydrated before and after the procedure with a prior assessment of renal function. Evidence also indicates that nonsteroidal anti-inflammatory drugs may aggravate renal disease. They should be used with caution in patients with known renal disease and in those with long-standing diabetes and unknown renal status.

NEUROPATHIC COMPLICATIONS

Neurologic complications of diabetes can include sensory, motor, and autonomic nerves. The pathophysiologic mechanism for neuropathy is multifactorial. The factors include increased sorbitol content in nerve cells resulting in swelling and osmotic lysis,[73] decreased myoinositol content resulting in poor nerve conduction,[74] and poor nutrient supply to nerves as a result of diabetic microangiopathy.[75] More recent studies seem to indicate that the abnormalities in polyol metabolism (sorbitol) may have a more primary role, as some improvement in nerve conduction studies and clinical findings are seen when patients are treated with drugs, such as aldose reductase inhibitors, that decrease nerve cell sorbitol content.[76] The difficulty in studying diabetic neuropathy has been that there is no reliable test that correlates clinical improvement with objective measurements. Nerve conduction studies may improve with worsening of clinical symptoms and vice versa. Physical findings may remain unchanged or worsen while patients report subjective symptomatic improvement. This situation has also made it difficult to evaluate the efficacy of pharmacologic therapy for diabetic neuropathy. Thus, there are many drugs that are efficacious in some patients but none that, at present, qualify as first-line agents.

AUTONOMIC NEUROPATHY

Diabetes also results in autonomic neuropathy that can include abnormal regulation of heart rate and blood pressure, the ability to recover from hypoglycemia, gastric emptying, and sexual function.

Cardiovascular manifestations of autonomic neuropathy include the loss of vagal inhibition of heart rate (parasympathetic), resulting in tachycardia and orthostatic hypotension with the inability to augment heart rate in response to standing (parasympathetic and sympathetic).[77] Studies have shown that the development of orthostatic hypotension is an ominous prognostic sign with an increased risk of sudden death.[78] Diagnosis of orthostatic hypotension is made by measuring blood pressure and heart rate supine and then in the erect position after 5 minutes. A fall in mean arterial pressure of greater than 30 mmHg without a compensatory increase in heart rate is strongly suggestive of autonomic orthostatic hypotension.[79] There is no real treatment of orthostatic hypotension beyond preventing exacerbating problems, including volume depletion and the use of drugs that may cause hypotension such as beta blockers and other sympatholytic agents. Mineralocorticoid therapy with fluodrocortisone has met with variable success.

Problems with gastric motility can make patient management most difficult. Patients usually complain of excess belching, bloating, and nausea. They may develop intactable vomiting as well, expecially if a concurrent viral gastroenteritis is present. Because their stomachs do not empty predictably, glycemic control can be difficult, with wide swings in blood glucose measurements resulting. If vomiting is severe, volume depletion and dehydration may result. Diagnosis is based primarily on clinical symptoms. Use of radiolabeled meals to measure gastric emptying time is helpful. Treatment includes the use of nasogastric suction, anti-emetics, and the antidopaminergic agent, metachlopromide.

Impotence occurs at a greater rate in diabetic men. The cause is usually autonomic neuropathy or vascular insufficiency, or both. The picture is often complicated by the use of medication that also causes impotence, including antihypertensive agents such as alpha-methyldopa, propranolol, and clonidine. Additionally, some patients suffer from retrograde ejaculation. Impotence does not appear to be a poor prognostic sign for other neurologic or vascular events, but should alert one to the possible presence of other autonomic or vascular disease.

Other manifestations of autonomic neuropathy include abnormal sweating, neurogenic bladder, diabetic diarrhea, and abnormal pupillary light reflexes.

HYPOGLYCEMIC UNAWARENESS

Hypoglycemia, defined as a plasma glucose of less than 55 mg/dl, is a major side effect in patients with diabetes who are treated with either oral hypoglycemic agents or insulin and occurs at a greater rate in patients who are more strictly controlled. It is a critical problem because the central nervous system neither synthesizes nor stores glucose, with the result that glucose deprivation may cause altered mental status, seizure, or coma. The body has evolved hormonal defense mechanisms to maintain euglycemia in the face of insulin-induced hypoglycemia. These include the secretion of glucagon and epinephrine to increase plasma glucose within minutes, and growth hormone and cortisol that act hours later. Epinephrine is responsible for the warning symptoms of hypoglycemia—palpitations, nervousness, and tremor.

Studies have shown that patients with insulin-dependent diabetes lose their ability to secrete glucagon after several years' duration of diabetes. They are left with epinephrine secretion as their only immediate defense against hypoglycemia. After a greater duration of disease, usually 10 to 20 years, epinephrine secretion is also impaired as a result of autonomic neuropathy.[80] This problem is important in several ways. First, in patients who have virtually no glucagon secretion and are dependent on epinephrine for recovery from hypoglycemia, any drug that blocks epinephrine action, such as beta-adrenergic antagonists, places these patients at increased risk for hypoglycemia without warning. Second, patients who have no acute hormonal defenses are at increased risk for severe hypoglycemia because they have no endogenous epinephrine secretion. Both groups are at greater risk when they are placed on a treatment regimen aimed at achieving euglycemia.[81] Recent studies have demonstrated a diminished adrenergic response in patients after a period of strict control, suggesting an adaptive response of defense mechanisms as control improves.[82] Studies also suggest that the glucose concentration triggering epinephrine secretion is higher in patients who are poorly controlled compared to those who are well controlled.[83] The physician must assess individual patients carefully for evidence of autonomic neuropathy and be careful in selecting patients to receive β-adrenergic antagonist therapy for hypertension or coronary artery disease, excluding those patients with long duration of diabetes. These patients are also at greater risk for severe hypoglycemia if placed on a strict glycemic control treatment regimen. It is also possible that poorly controlled patients may experience adrenergic warning symptoms at blood glucose concentrations that are higher than previously thought.

Another complication that may be related to the recovery from hypoglycemia is the Somogyi phenomenon. This is described as hyperglycemia, on awakening, due to a hypoglycemic episode during sleep with activation of counterregulatory hormones resulting in hyperglycemia the next morning. All of the counterregulatory hormones have been implicated but none has proven to be the causative agent. In fact there is now some controversy as to whether the Somogyi phenomenon occurs as frequently as previously thought.[84] The Somogyi phenomenon should not be confused with the "dawn phenomenon." In this case, patients have early morning hyperglycemia with no antecedent hypoglycemia. They simply require more insulin in the dawn hours. Again, controversy exists over the exact cause of the dawn phenomenon though counterregulatory hormones have been implicated. These two disorders can be differentiated by having the patient measure blood glucose before bed, at 3:00 a.m., and upon awakening to determine if the blood glucose falls into the hypoglycemic range during the night. The Somogyi phenomenon may respond to decreasing the dose of intermediate acting insulin at night or giving it at bedtime rather than before supper, so that its peak effect occurs in the morning rather than the middle of the night. The latter approach will also control fasting hyperglycemia due to the dawn phenomenon.

VASCULAR DISEASE OF LARGE VESSELS

In addition to the complications of retinopathy and nephropathy that are caused mainly by microvascular disease, diabetic patients are also prone to large vessel vascular disease, including coronary artery disease and peripheral vascular disease such as stroke. Diabetes is an independent risk factor for myocardial infarction and stroke and is a leading cause of amputation secondary to large vessel disease. Myocardial infarction is a major cause of death in patients with diabetes. Individuals with diabetes may have silent coronary artery disease. This means that they may suffer angina pectoris or even myocardial infarction without the typical symptom of chest pain. They may instead have chest pain of an atypical nature, congestive heart failure due to ischemic disease, or hypotension without pain. The physician should be suspicious of patients developing such problems acutely and take aggressive diagnostic and therapeutic measures.

HYPERTENSION

Hypertension is relatively common in diabetic individuals. It may be of the essential type or secondary to renal disease. Treatment should be instituted to prevent long-term complications including myocardial infarction, stroke, and end-stage renal disease. The use of antihypertensive medication is somewhat different. Beta adrenergic antagonists may mask hypoglycemic symptoms in some patients while these and other drugs may produce impotence in diabetic men. Recent data suggests that angiotensin-converting enzyme inhibitors may be of benefit in slowing the progress of renal disease in some patients but may exacerbate it in others. Thus, the approach to therapy must be individualized with duration of diabetes and presence of complications taken into account. Renal function, especially, should be assessed. Frequent follow-up with measurement of serum potassium, BUN, and creatinine should be done. Urine collections for creatinine clearance and urine protein excretion should also be monitored.

CONTROL DURING SURGERY

Diabetic patients undergoing surgical and diagnostic procedures often require special preparation in order to prevent excess hyper- or hypoglycemia during or after the procedure. This is especially important in patients undergoing general anesthesia or who cannot eat before or after the procedure. In general, the goals of glucose control during these periods should be to maintain the plasma glucose under 250 mg/dl and to avoid hypoglycemia. Procedures should be scheduled in the morning, when possible. Patients who take insulin should be given half of their total morning dose in the form of intermediate acting insulin and should have 5% glucose in water given intravenously during surgery and after surgery until they are tolerating oral intake. Blood glucose should be measured every 3 to 4 hours and subcutaneous insulin given as needed to maintain plasma glucose under 250 mg/dl. Intravenous or continuous subcutaneous insulin infusion may be required in some cases. In insulin-dependent patients, ketoacidosis may develop due to the stress of surgery so that urine and/or serum ketones should be monitored postoperatively. Noninsulin dependent patients controlled with diet or taking oral agents may require insulin postoperatively as hyperglycemia may be excessive because of the stress of the surgical procedure. Insulin may later be discontinued as glycemic control is achieved and the patient is more temporally removed from the acute stress of surgery. In patients undergoing outpatient studies in which they must fast prior to the procedure, the same rules apply. Phone contact with the physician to adjust insulin based on home measurements may be necessary for the immediate post procedure period.

PREGNANCY

Pregnancy in the insulin-dependent diabetic patient requires a team approach by perinatologists, diabetologists and neonatologists. Pregnant insulin-dependent women are at increased risk for spontaneous abortion, premature labor, and preeclampsia. Infants of diabetic mothers are at risk for macrosomia,[85] respiratory distress syndrome,[86] congenital malformations,[87] polycythemia,[88] hyperbilirubinemia, hypocalcemia[89] and hypomagnesemia.[90] The rate of most of these complications can be reduced if patients are under good glycemic control prior to conception and maintained at near euglycemia during gestation. Frequent fetal monitoring has reduced the rate of maternal complications. Diabetic women should be urged to report any menstrual abnormality as early as possible so that pregnancy can be diagnosed at an early stage. In female patients presenting with unaccounted changes in glycemic control, pregnancy should be considered as a possible cause. Women with noninsulin, dependent diabetes may require insulin therapy during pregnancy as oral hypoglycemic agents are contraindicated. All nondiabetic pregnant women should be screened for gestational diabetes between the weeks 24 and 28 of gestation.

THE FUTURE

The diagnosis and management of diabetes mellitus is a challenge to all areas of medicine. Management of acute complications and prevention of the sometimes devastating long-term complications requires not only the science but the art of medicine.

Research efforts towards a cure for diabetes and treatment of its complications are promising. Treatment with immunosuppressive agents has resulted in halting destruction of β-cells and preventing insulin-dependent diabetes. Unfortunately, the beneficial effects of this therapy are currently outweighed by the risk of long-term immunosuppression. New modes of insulin delivery including implantable insulin pumps may make the delivery of insulin more physiologic and control of hyperglycemia less complicated. Insulin delivery via nasal and conjunctival routes may spare patients the inconvenience of injections. Promising research toward understanding the factors involved in the chronic complications of diabetes may make them preventable while new drugs may improve their prognosis. The enthusiasm that occurred with the discovery of insulin might now be replaced with cautious optimism for individuals with diabetes mellitus and its complications.

Recommended Reading

1. Bliss M: The discovery of insulin. Chicago: University of Chicago Press; 1982.
2. Galloway JA, Potvin JH, Shuman CR eds. Diabetes mellitus, 9th ed. Indianapolis: Eli Lilly and Company; 1988.
3. Shafir E, Bergman M, Felig P. The endocrine pancreas: diabetes mellitus. In: Felig P, Baxter JD, Broadus AE, Frohman LA, eds. *Endocrinology and metabolism, 2nd ed.* New York: McGraw-Hill Book Co; 1987.
4. Schade DS, Santiago JV, Skyler JS, Rizza RA. Intensive insulin therapy. Amsterdam: Excerpta Medica; 1983.
5. Long term complications of diabetes. Clin Endocrin Metab. London: WB Saunders; 1986; 15:4.
6. Benson WE, Brown GC, Tasman W. Diabetes and its ocular complications. Philadelphia: WB Saunders Company; 1988.
7. Sperling MA ed. Physician's guide to insulin dependent (Type I). Alexandria, Virginia: American Diabetes Association, Inc.; 1988.

8. Rifkin H ed. The physician's guide type II diabetes (NIDDM) Alexandria, Virginia: American Diabetes Association, Inc.; 1984.

References

1. US Dept. of Health, Education and Welfare. Diabetes data publication No. 78-1468, 1978.
2. Kahn HA, Hiller R. Blindness caused by diabetic retinopathy. Am J Ophthalmol. 1974; 78:58–67.
3. Grenfell A, Watkins PJ. Clinical diabetic nephropathy: natural history and complications. Philadelphia: Clinics in Endocrinology and Metabolism. 1986; 15(4):783–805.
4. Barrett-Connor E, Orchard T. Diabetes and heart disease. In: Harris MI, Hamman RF eds. Diabetes in America. US Dept. Health and Human Services, 1985; National Diabetes Data Group, publication 85-1468.
5. Keen H, Jarrett RJ, Fuller JH et al. Hyperglycemia and arterial disease. Diabetes. 1981; 30 (suppl. 2):49–53.
6. Medvei VC. A history of endocrinology. Lancaster, United Kingdom: MTP Press, Ltd; 1984; 16.
7. Medvei VC. A history of endocrinology. Lancaster, United Kingdom: MTP Press, Ltd; 1984; 16.
8. Adams F. Araetaeos of Kappadokian: the extant works. London, 1856. In: Medvei VC. A history of endocrinology. Lancaster, United Kingdom: MTP Press, Ltd; 1984; 16.
9. Bliss M: The discovery of insulin. Chicago: University of Chicago Press; 1982.
10. National Diabetes Data Group. Classification of diabetes mellitus and other categories of glucose intolerance. Diabetes, 1979; 28:1039–1057.
11. Rifkin H ed. The physician's guide to type II diabetes. 1984; American Diabetes Association.
12. Cahill GF Jr, McDevitt HO. Insulin-dependent diabetes: The initial lesion. N Engl J Med. 1981; 304:1454–1465.
13. Srikanta S, Ganda OP, Eisenbarth GS, et al. Islet cell antibodies and beta-cell function in monozygotic triplets and twins initially discordant for Type I diabetes mellitus. N Engl J Med. 1983; 308:322–325.
14. Barnett AH, Eff C, Leslie RDG, Pyke DA: Diabetes in identical twins: A study of 200 pairs. Diabetologia. 1981; 20:87.
15. Wolf E, Spencer KM, Cudworth AG. The genetic susceptibility to Type I (insulin-dependent) diabetes: analysis of the HLA association. Diabetologia. 1983; 24:224.
16. Owerbach D, Lernmark A, Platz P, et al. HLA-D region B-chain RNA endonuclease fragments differ between HLA-DR identical healthy and insulin-dependent diabetic individuals. Nature. 1983; 303:851.
17. Eisenbarth GS. Type I diabetes: a chronic autoimmune disease. N Engl J Med. 1986; 314:1360–1368.
18. Turkington RW, Labovitz HE. Extra-adrenal endocrine deficiencies in Addison's disease. Am J Med. 1967; 43:449–457.
19. Tse TF, Clutter WE, Shad SD, et al. The mechanisms of postprandial glucose counterregulation in man: physiologic roles in glucagon and epinephrine vis-a-vis insulin the prevention of hypoglycemia late after glucose ingestion. J Clin Invest. 1986: 77:212–218.
20. Galloway JA, Potvin JH, Shuman CR eds. Diabetes Mellitus, 9th ed. Indianapolis: Eli Lilly Company; 1988.
21. Horton ES. Role of environmental factors in the development of noninsulin-dependent diabetes mellitus. Am J Med. 1983: 75 (suppl 5B):32–40.
22. DeFronzo R, Ferrannini E, Koivisto V. New concepts in the pathogenesis and treatment of noninsulin dependent diabetes mellitus. Am J Med. 1983: 74 (suppl 1A) 52.
23. Given B, Make M, Tager H, et al. Diabetes due to secretion of an abnormal insulin. N Engl J Med. 1983: 302:129.
24. Gerich J, Charles M, Grodsky G. Regulation of pancreatic insulin and glucagon secretion. Annu Rev Physiol. 1983: 38:353.
25. Ward WK, Beard JC, Porte D Jr. Clinical aspects of islet β-cell function in non-insulin-dependent diabetes mellitus. In: DeFronzo RA ed. Diabetes Metab Rev. 1986: 2:297–313.
26. Olefsky JM. Etiology and pathogenesis of noninsulin dependent diabetes (type II). In Degroot LJ ed. Endocrinology, 2nd ed. Orlando: Grune and Stratton; 1988.
27. Gerich J. Assessment of insulin resistance and its role in noninsulin-dependent diabetes. J Lab Clin Med. 1984: 103:497.
28. Kolterman O, Gray R, Griffen J, et al. Receptor and post-receptor defects contribute to insulin resistence in noninsulin dependent diabetes mellitus. J Clin Invest. 1981: 68:957.
29. Kolterman O, Insel J, Saekow M, et al. Mechanism of insulin resistance in human obesity: evidence for receptor and post-receptor defects. J Clin Invest. 1980: 65:1272.
30. Rizza R, Mandarino L, Gerich J: Effects of growth hormone on insulin action in man: mechanisms of insulin resistance, impaired suppression of glucose production and impaired stimulation of glucose utilization. Diabetes. 1982: 31:633.
31. Riza R, Mandarino L, Gerich J. Cortisol-induced insulin resistance in man: impaired suppression of glucose production and stimulation of glucose utilization due to a postreceptor defect of insulin action. J Clin Endocrinol Metab. 1982: 54:131.
32. Davidson J, DeBra D. Immunologic insulin resistance. Diabetes. 1978: 27:307.
33. Flier J, Kahn C, Roth J. Receptors antireceptor antibodies and mechanisms of insulin resistance. N Engl J Med. 1979: 300:413.
34. Kahn C, Podskalny J. Demonstration of a primary genetic defect in insulin receptors in fibroblasts from a patient with the syndrome of insulin resistance and acanthosis nigricans type A. J Clin Endocrinol and Metab. 1980: 50:1139.
35. DCCT Research Group. Results of feasibility study. Diabetes Care. 1987: 10:1–19.
36. Pirart J. Diabetes mellitus and its degenerative complications: a prospective study of 4,400 patients observed between 1947 and 1973. Diabetes Care. 1978: 1:168–188, 252–263.
37. Shuman CR. Dietary management of diabetes

mellitus. In: Galloway JA, Potvin JH, Shuman CR eds. Diabetes Mellitus 9th ed. Indianapolis: Eli Lilly and Co.; 1988.

38. Ruderman NB, Ganda OP, Johnson K. The effect of physical training on glucose tolerance and plasma lipids in maturity-onset diabetes. Diabetes. 1979: 28 (suppl 1):89–92.

39. Caron D, Poussier P, Marliss EB, et al. The effect of post-prandial exercise on meal-related glucose intolerance in insulin-dependent diabetic individuals. Diabetes Care. 1982: 5:364–369.

40. Zinman B. Exercise in the patient with diabetes mellitus. In: Galloway JA, Potvin JH, Shuman CR eds. Diabetes Mellitus 9th ed. Indianapolis: Eli Lilly and Co.; 1988; 216–223.

41. Hoelzer DR, Dalsky GP, Clutter WE, et al: Glucoregulation during exercise: hypoglycemia is prevented by redundant glucoregulatory systems, sympathocromaffin activation and changes in islet hormone secretion. J Clin Invest. 1986: 77:212.

42. Reaven GM. Theraputic approaches to reducing insulin resistance in patients with non-insulin dependent diabetes mellitus. Am J Med. 1983: 109–112.

43. Hodgkin DC. The structure of insulin. Diabetes. 1972: 21:1131–1150.

44. Mazze RS, Shamoon H, Pasmantier R, et al. Reliability of blood glucose monitoring by patients with diabetes mellitus. Am J Med. 1984: 77:211–217.

45. Tattersall RB, Gale E. Patient self-monitoring of blood glucose and refinements of conventional insulin treatment. Am J Med. 1981: 70:177–182.

46. Skyler JS, Reeves ML. Intensive treatment of Type I diabetes mellitus. In: Olefsky JM, Sherwin RS eds. Diabetes mellitus: management and complications. New York: Churchill Livingstone; 1985: 2:31–79.

47. Carroll P, Matz R: Uncontrolled diabetes mellitus in adults: experience in treating diabetic ketoacidosis and hyperosmolar nonketotic coma with low-dose insulin and a uniform treatment regimen. Diabetes Care. 1983: 6:579–585.

48. Gale EM, Dornan TL, Tattersall RB. Severely uncontrolled diabetes in the over-fifties. Diabetologia. 1981: 21:25–28.

49. Hockaday TDR, Alberti KGMM. Diabetic coma. Clin Endocrinol Metab. 1972: 1:751.

50. Dwyer MS, Melton LJ, Ballard DJ, et al: Incidence of diabetic retinopathy and blindness, a population based study in Rochester, Minnesota. Diabetes Care. 1985: 8:316–322.

51. Palmberg P, Smith M, Waltman, S, et al: The natural history of retinopathy in insulin-dependent juvenile onset diabetes. Ophthalmology. 1981: 88:613–618.

52. Klein R, Klein BEK, Moss SE, et al. The Wisconsin epidemiologic study of diabetic retinopathy. II. Prevalance and risk of diabetic retinopathy when age at diagnosis is less than 30 years. Archives of Ophthalmology 102:520–526, 1984.

53. Klein R, Klein BEK, Moss SE et al: The Wisconsin Epidemiologic Study of Diabetic Retinopathy. II. Prevalance and risk of diabetic retinopathy when age at diagnosis is 30 or more years. Arch Ophthalmol. 1984: 102:527–532.

54. Frank RN, Hoffman WH, Podgor MJ, et al. Ret-

inopathy in juvenile onset type I diabetes of short duration. Diabetes. 1982: 31:874–882.

55. Benson WE, Brown GC, Tasman W. Diabetes and its ocular complications. Philadelphia: WB Saunders; 1988.

56. Lauritzen T, Larsen HW, Frost-Laresen K, Deckert T. The Steno study group: effect of 1 year of near normal glucose levels on retinopathy in insulin-dependent diabetics. Lancet. 1983: 1:200–204.

57. Dahl-Jorgensen K, Brinchmann-Hansen O, Hanssen KF, et al: Rapid tightening of blood glucose leads to transient deterioration of retinopathy in insulin-dependent diabetes mellitus: The Oslo study. Br Med J. 1985: 290:811–815.

58. Helve E, Laatikainen L, Merenmies L, et al. Continuous insulin infusion therapy and retinopathy in patients with Type I diabetes. Acta Endocrinol (Copenh). 1987: 115:313–319.

59. Diabetic Retinopathy Study Research Group. Photocoagulation treatment of proliferative diabetic retinopathy. Clinical application of Diabetic Retinopathy Study (DRS) findings. DRS Report Number 8. Ophthalmology. 1981: 88:583–600.

60. Klein R, Klein BEK, Moss SE. Prevalance of cataracts in a population based study of persons with diabetes mellitus. Ophthalmology. 1985: 92:1191–1196.

61. Andersen AR, Christiansen JS, Andersen JK, et al. Diabetic nephropathy in type I (insulin-dependent) diabetics: an epidemiological study. Diabetologia. 1983: 25:496–501.

62. Ellis EN, Seffes MW, Goetz FC, et al. Relationship of renal size to nephropathy in type I (insulin-dependent) diabetes. Diabetologia. 1985: 28:12–15.

63. Ireland JT, Viberti GC, Watkins PJ. The kidney and the urinary tract. In: Keen H and Jarret J eds. Complications of diabetes. London: Edward Arnold; 1982: 137–178.

64. Jones RH, Hayakawa H, Mackay JD, et al. Progression of diabetic nephropathy. Lancet. 1979: i:1105–1106.

65. Viberti GC, Bilous RW, Mackintosh D, et al. Long term correction of hyperglycaemia and progression of renal failure in insulin-dependent diabetes. Br Med J. 1983: 286:598–602.

66. Christiansen JS, Gammelgaard J, Frandsen M, et al: Kidney function and size in diabetics before and during initial insulin treatment. Kidney Int. 1982: 21:683–688.

67. Viberti GC, Pickup JC, Bilous RW, et al. Effect of control of blood glucose on urinary excretion of albumin and beta$_2$-microglobulin in insulin dependent diabetes. N Engl J Med. 1979: 300:638–641.

68. Mogensen CE. Long term anti-hypertensive treatment inhibiting progression of diabetic nephropathy. Br Med J. 1982: 285:685–688.

69. Maschio G, Oldrizzi R, Tessitore, et al: Effects of dietary protein and phosphorus restriction on the progression of early renal failure. Kidney Int. 1982: 22:371–376.

70. Viberti GC, Hill RD, Jarrett RJ, et al. Microalbuminuria as a predictor of clinical nephropathy in insulin dependent diabetes mellitus. Lancet. 1982: 1:1430–1432.

71. Mathiesen ER, Oxenboll K, Johansen PA, et al. Incipient nephropathy in Type I (insulin-dependent) diabetes. Diabetologia. 1985: 26:406–410.

72. Mogensen CE, Christiansen CK. Predicting diabetic nephropathy in insulin-dependent diabetic patients. N Engl J Med. 1984: 311:89–93.

73. Gabbay K. The sorbitol pathway and the complications of diabetes. N Engl J Med. 1973: 288:831–836.

74. Clements R. Diabetic neuropathy—new concepts of its etiology. Diabetes. 1979: 28:604–611.

75. Greene DA, Lattimer S, Ulbrecht J, et al: Glucose induced alterations in nerve metabolism: Current perspective on the pathogenesis of diabetic neuropathy and future directions for research and therapy. Diabetes Care. 1985: 8:290–299.

76. Anders AFS, Bril V, Nathaniel V, et al. Regeneration and repair of myelinated fibers in sural-nerve biopsy specimens from patients with diabetic neuropathy treated with sorbinil. N Engl J Med. 1988: 319:548–555.

77. Clarke BF, Ewing DJ, Campbell IW. Diabetic autonomic neuropathy. Diabetologia. 1979: 17:195–212.

78. Ewing DJ, Campbell IW, Clarke BF. The natural history of diabetic autonomic neuropathy. Q J Med. 1980: 49:95–108.

79. Ewing DJ, Clarke BF. Autonomic neuropathy: its diagnosis and prognosis. Clin Endocrin Metab. 1986: 15:855–888.

80. Bolli G, DeFeo P, Compagnucci P, et al. Abnormal glucose counterregulation in insulin-dependent diabetes mellitus. Interaction of anti-insulin antibodies and impaired glucagon and epinephrine secretion. Diabetes. 1983: 32:134–141.

81. White NH, Skor DA, Cryer PE, et al. Identification of type I diabetic patients at increased risk from hypoglycemia during intensive therapy. N Engl J Med. 1983: 308:485–491.

82. Simonson DC, Tamborlane WV, DeFronzo RA, et al. Intensive insulin therapy reduces counterregulatory responses to hypoglycemia in patients with type I diabetes. Ann Intern Med. 1985: 103:184–190.

83. Boyle PJ, Schwartz NS, Shar SD, et al. Plasma glucose concentrations at the onset of hypoglycemic symptoms in patients with poorly controlled diabetes and nondiabetics. N Engl J Med. 1988: 318:1481–1486.

84. Tordjman KM, Havlin CE, Levandoski LA, et al. Failure of nocturnal hypoglycemia to cause fasting hyperglycemia in patients with insulin-dependent diabetes mellitus. N Engl J Med. 1987: 317:1552–1559.

85. Berk MA, Mimouni F, Miodovnik M, et al. Factors influencing macrosomia in infants of insulin-dependent diabetic mothers. Pediatrics. (In press).

86. Mimouni F, Miodovnik M, Whitsett JA, Holroyde JC, et al. Respiratory distress syndrome in infants of diabetic mothers in the 1980's: no direct adverse effect of maternal diabetes with modern management. Obstet Gynecol. 1987: 69:191–195.

87. Miodovnik M, Dignan P, Berk MA, et al: Major malformations in insulin-dependent diabetic women: An association with early first trimester poor glycemic control. Diabetes Care. 1988: 11:713–718.

88. Mimouni F, Miodovnik M, Siddiqi TA, Butler JB, et al. Neonatal polycythemia in infants of insulin-dependent diabetic mothers. Obstet Gynecol. 1986: 68:370.

89. Tsang RC, Kleinman L, Sutherland JM, et al: Hypocalcemia in infants of diabetic mothers. Studies in Ca, P and Mg metabolism and in parathormone responsiveness. J Pediatr. 1972: 80:384.

90. Tsang RC, Strub R, Steichen JJ, Brown DR, et al. Hypomagnesemia in infants of diabetic mothers: perinatal studies. J Pediatr. 1976: 89:115.

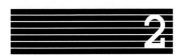

Foot Problems in Children with Diabetes

ALVIN H. CRAWFORD, M.D., F.A.C.S.

Foot lesions, such as non-healing ulcers, a patch of gangrene following minor trauma, or a simple blister, may lead to the diagnosis of diabetes mellitus in a previously undiscovered diabetic patient. The continued increase in the number of diabetic patients and its impact on the United States and the western industrial world is staggering. The cost to the nation in time lost from work, hospitalization costs, medical costs, and decrease in quality of life is enormous and increases each year.[1]

Most of the problems concerned with the diabetic foot occur in adults. In the adult population, 20% of diabetes mellitus admissions involve foot complications; 62,000 lower-extremity amputations per year result from diabetes mellitus or vascular disease; and 45% of all lower-extremity amputations are performed on diabetics.

CHILDREN AND DIABETES

Published statistics concerning the foot and ankle in diabetics are not true for children. Children affected with insulin-dependent diabetes mellitus, Type I diabetes, tend to have few complications when under good control in a well-supervised environment. In general, foot problems associated with diabetes do not affect children until their adult years because the foot problems are largely a consequence of peripheral neuropathy and/or vasculopathy complications that take 10 to 15 years to evolve. These complications seem to appear only after puberty. However, cutaneous manifestations have been described in juvenile and adolescent dia-

betics. The syndrome of restricted joint mobility, growth impairment, delayed maturation and thick, tight, waxy skin was first reported in 3 patients.[1] Up to 30% of young diabetics may be affected including both Type I and Type II patients.[3,4] This may be caused in part by increased glycosylation of tissues.[5] Nevertheless, we simply do not see major problems in childhood.[6] At Children's Hospital Medical Center in Cincinnati, 60 new cases of insulin-dependent diabetes in children are admitted annually for initial stabilization and management, and there has not been a significant foot problem identified in longstanding diabetes in the past 10 years.

Children with diabetes are encouraged not only to live a normal life, but also to participate in exercises and athletics with non-diabetic children.

During the past decade, regimens to control blood glucose have been designed to allow children with diabetes to enjoy normal health and to be generally regarded as normal by their peers. Small glucose meters can now be used for home monitoring, and various insulin preparations and delivery devices are available. Aspiring young athletes with diabetes should have access to these methods in order to attain optimal performance.[7]

PERIPHERAL NEUROPATHY

Peripheral neuropathy is one of the most common and most troubling chronic complications of diabetes. Most notably, neurotrophic loss of sensation in the foot, together with infection and vascular insufficiency, make diabetes the most common cause of nontraumatic lower limb amputations in the United States. The frequency of diabetic neuropathy parallels the duration and severity of hyperglycemia and rarely occurs within the first 5 years after diagnosis. One study in children 6 to 19 revealed changes in vibration and temperature thresholds of sensation.[8] As a result of chronic, unrecognized neuropathy, however, patients may present with foot ulceration, foreign objects embedded in the foot, unrecognized trauma to the extremities, or Charcot's joints.

Patients with longstanding diabetes and neuropathy are also predisposed to chronic venostasis ulcers, as well as ischemic gangrene and vascular ulcers due to macro- and micro-vascular insufficiency. Although difficult to control, euglycemia with insulin therapy has been shown to improve nerve function in the lower extremities of recently diagnosed patients.[9]

Imbalance of extensor and flexor muscles in the feet due to impaired function and atrophy of intrinsic extensor muscles may lead to tendon shortening and chronic toe flexion, the so-called "claw-toed deformity."

FOOTWEAR

Although none of the problems associated with the diabetic foot are found in children, they occur in adolescents. It is important to inform diabetic children approaching adolescence about the potential problems that await them. Adolescent diabetics should pay careful attention to their feet to stop blistering or significant friction problems. The areas of friction will be different from one pair of shoes to another, thus decreasing the likelihood of blisters.

Children with diabetes should be taught to inspect their feet daily for areas of rubbing, fissuring, or blisters. They should also check the inside of their shoes before wear to detect foreign bodies or protruding sole nails. Socks should be chosen to provide an adequate cushion.[10] Athletic socks with a thick cushioning pile are inexpensive and available at all clothing stores. These help broaden and cushion the load-bearing surface in areas of peak forces at the foot/shoe interface. Shoes with an adequate toebox and

a proper fit are vital. They should be selected so that the child's foot can grow and not be forced into the end of the toebox. The shoe break should be at the metatarsal flexion axis with enough room to permit foot growth without a shoe length over which the child can trip. Shoes should also fit activity needs. For day-to-day use, a wellmade shoe with uppers of soft leather and insoles and innerlinings that are soft without rough edges are recommended. Another type is the welted sole shoe with a firm counter worn with a thick athletic sock. The child should be taught to not be active in shoes that have a significant tapering. They should have available shoe changes for different activities.

Tennis shoes are soft, pliable, and have an upper that breathes. They have cushioned heels and soles, and many types have a built-in arch support. Children should be cautious when wearing these shoes since holes and tears in the coarse lining expose the edge of the counter that can rub blisters. Sharp objects can penetrate a rubber sole easily. Excessive wear, natural in children, causes tennis shoes to age more quickly than leather shoes. Shoe styles, height, manufacturer and how the child wears the shoe are all important considerations. Some children put their weight on the counter, collapsing it, and using the shoe as a slipper without a heel support. Tennis shoes often are not tied, permitting the foot to slop and chafe as the child walks. Holes are deliberately cut in the canvas uppers. User acceptance varies so widely that the practitioner is pitted against both the patient and his peer group when advising parents about footwear.

INFECTION

The risk of infection in the young diabetic is real. Abnormal tissue structure secondary to glycosylation as well as early neuropathic and vascular changes predispose the adolescent to significant infection as a result of trauma.

Lack of awareness and immaturity of the patient may lead to denial of a problem until it becomes serious. Even minor foot infections should be cultured and appropriate antibiotics prescribed.

If an abscess is present, x-rays of the foot should be obtained to search for the presence of a metallic foreign body or signs of osteomyelitis. Persistent or recurrent drainage at the same site may indicate the presence of a nonradiopaque foreign body. An MRI of the foot may reveal such an object, as well as a cyst or a deep abscess.

Treatment includes incision and drainage of the abscess, with removal of the foreign body. Intraoperative cultures are obtained as well as a gram stain. The wound is closed loosely over drains and immobilized in a short leg splint or packed open. The postoperative course includes elevation of the foot as well as intravenous antibiotics in appropriate dosage for 5 days. A heparin lock intravenous needle is a convenient home method of antibiotic administration in the older child. Oral antibiotics should be continued for an additional 10 days.

Osteomyelitis in the young diabetic is treated in a manner similar to nondiabetic children. However, close observation of blood sugar levels is necessary since infection often makes the diabetes difficult to control. Antibiotics are continued until clinical manifestations of infection disappear and the sedimentation rate returns to normal limits.

PHYSICAL ACTIVITY AND THE LONG-TERM PERSPECTIVE

The child with poorly controlled diabetes often starts to develop complications after only 5 years.[11] Adolescents may be less careful about monitoring blood sugar and diet and prefer to compete athletically with their peers. The relationship of physical activity to long-term complications was evaluated at the University of Pittsburgh by LaPorte, et al.,[12] who studied 696 individuals with Type I diabetes diagnosed between 1950 and 1964. Preliminary conclusions were that "activity early in life by patients with Type I diabetes does not appear to be associated with an adverse health effect, and may in fact be beneficial." The data suggest a negative association between physical activity and both cardiovascular disease and overall mortality. Therefore, the diabetic child should be encouraged to participate in sports.

Particular attention needs to be directed to adolescents who begin an exercise program with poor control of longstanding diabetes that has caused stunted growth. They may tend to overcompensate, leaving them more susceptible to foot problems. Ulcers, stress fractures, and other overuse syndromes can occur when the unsupervised diabetic starts a conditioning program.

PATIENT COUNSELING

New diabetics at any age require patient education that gives them insight into their disease and the behavior patterns and life style needed to live a long life with reduced complications. Although foot problems are minimal in the child, teaching at this time prepares the patient for foot problems as an adolescent. Rebellion, which is part of the natural development in the adolescent, must be recognized by the practitioner. Patient acceptance of the disease, its manifestations, treatment, and complications are closely related to natural emotional development. Patient rejection of shoe prescription and simple, practical advice is common. The attitude of the adolescent diabetic must be considered since it is a reflection of socio-economic conditions, emotional immaturity, and peer pressure, to name a few factors.

Since none of the problems associated with the diabetic foot are found in children, but do occur in adolescents, it is important to counsel patients to implement new technology for control of Type I diabetes, and to select proper shoes for walking and for exercising. Patients should be aware that the natural history of their disease causes foot problems in adults. Despite the excellent control of glucose in the Type I diabetic, the long-term complications of arthropathy, atherosclerosis, microangiopathy, retinopathy, nephropathy, and neuropathy have not been irradicated. Making the diabetic child and adolescent aware of these potential dangers will allow him to avoid many of the deleterious effects that this disease has historically caused.

References

1. The National Diabetes Data Group. Selected statistics on health and medical care of diabetes. 1980; PA-3.
2. Rosenbloom AL, Frais JH. Diabetes mellitus, short stature and joint stiffness—A new syndrome. Clin Res. 1974: 22:92A.
3. Fitzcharles MA, Duby S, Wadell RW, Banks E, et

al. Limitation of joint mobility (cheiroarthropathy) in adult noninsulin-dependent diabetic patients. Ann Rheum Dis. 1984: 43:251–257.

4. Rosenbloom AL, Silverstein SH, Lezotte DC, Richardson K, et al. Limited joint mobility in childhood diabetes mellitus indicates increased risk for microvascular disease. N Eng J Med. 1981: 305:191–198.

5. Backingham BA, Uitto J, Sandberg C, et al. Scleroderma-like syndrome and the non-enzymatic glucosylation of collagen in children with poorly controlled insulin dependent diabetes (IDDM). Pediatr Res. 1981: 15:626 (Part I).

6. Sperling MA. Children's Hospital Medical Center, Cincinnati, OH, personal communication, 1988.

7. Blackett PR. The child and adolescent athletes with diabetes. Physician & Sports Med. 1988: 16(3):133–149.

8. Heimans JJ, Bertelsmann FW, de Beaufort CE, de Beaufort AJ, et al. Quantitative sensory examination in diabetic children: Assessment of thermal discrimination. Diabetic Medicine. 1987: 4:251–253.

9. Terkildsen AB, Christensen NJ. Reversible nervous abnormalities in juvenile diabetics with recently diagnosed diabetes. Diabetologia. 1971: 7:113–117.

10. Lorver DL. For your diabetic patient, correct shoe and foot care are steps to healthy feet. J Musculoskeletal Med. 1988: 4:10–11.

11. Knowles HC, Jr., Guest GM, Lampe J, et al. The course of juvenile diabetes treated with unmeasured diet. Diabetes. 1965:14:239–273.

12. LaPorte RE, et al. Pittsburgh insulin dependent diabetes mellitus morbidity and mortality study: Physical activity and diabetic complications. Pediatrics. 1986: 78:1027–1033.

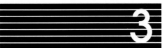

3 Examination of the Foot and Ankle

G. JAMES SAMMARCO, M.D., AND
MARK W. SCIOLI, M.D.

EVALUATION OF THE LOWER LIMB IN THE DIABETIC PATIENT

Successful treatment of the diabetic foot mandates a basic understanding of the disease process and the interplay between the neurologic, vascular, anatomic, and biomechanical changes it produces. Equally important is patient education in order to permit an understanding of the disease, often difficult because of patient denial. The misconception that diabetics are only afflicted with vascular disease can lead to inaccurate diagnoses, misadventures, and failures of treatment. A failure to recognize the subtleties of neuropathy with or without associated vascular compromise can lead to ulceration, secondary infection, and loss of part or all of the limb. The recurrence rate of neuropathic ulceration in a long-term review was 50%.[1] It is incumbent upon the treating physician to assess the patient's level of understanding of diabetes and the complications it can produce.

The purpose of this chapter is to emphasize key aspects in the evaluation of diabetic patients with foot problems. Without an accurate history and physical examination, misdiagnoses are often made. For any treatment plan to succeed, it is imperative to address all components of the pathologic process, and in the case of the dysvascular or insensitive foot, simultaneous patient education is critically important as well.

Obtaining the History

The examiner may use a questionnaire, or choose to ask questions and personally re-cord the responses for an accurate, complete documentation of the history. Standardized history and physical examination forms may save time, and ensure completeness and consistency from patient to patient, but should be supplemented by additional questions from the examiner (Fig. 3-1).

Much information is gathered in the first few minutes of the interview.[2] The patient's occupation, level of education, socioeconomic status, and level of activity help to assess the degree to which a patient will be able to participate in care. How well a patient is able to report past medical and surgical history also allows the treating physician to determine his level of understanding of the disease process. It is helpful for the physician to know the age of onset of the patient's disease and the type of care he has been receiving. Patients with neuropathic foot changes usually had onset of diabetes before age 50, take insulin, and have had their diabetes for at least 10 years.[3]

A review of systems with emphasis on neurologic, ocular, renal, and cardiovascular organs will allow the examiner to grade the patient's general medical status. The degree of systemic involvement correlates well with the prognosis and amount of intervention likely to be required for a patient.

Examination

Patients with lower extremity problems should be evaluated in a gown with both shoes and stockings removed. All too often, only the symptomatic foot is shown to the examiner, and impending or occult pathol-

FOOT AND ANKLE HISTORY

NAME: _____ SEX: M F   DATE:_____

AGE: _____OCCUPATION: _____

Describe the problem with your foot/ankle/leg which brings you to the office today.

_____

_____

How long have you had the problem? _____
Were you referred by another doctor?   Yes   No
By whom? _____

If you were injured, did the injury occur while working?   Yes   No
Please describe how your injury occurred. _____

_____

Have you ever had a similar previous injury?   Yes   No   When? _____

_____

Were you born with any type of physical abnormality?   Yes   No   Please describe

_____

List in order, with appropriate dates, all doctors and/or podiatrists you have seen for
your problem and any medicines, appliances, surgeries, or therapy you received. _____

_____

_____

_____

If you have had foot/ankle surgery have you been satisfied with the results?
Yes   No   If no, why not? _____

Have you ever been given cortisone shots?   Yes   No   How many shots? _____
Where? _____

Have you lost time from work due to your problem?   Yes   No   How much? _____

_____

Have you ever been given a disability rating?   Yes   No _____
If yes, describe: %_____ Limits on work _____

MEDICAL/SURGICAL HISTORY

Do you have any allergies to medicines?   Yes   No   If yes, list the medications
and reaction (hives, itching, etc.). _____

List all medication you take at this time: _____

_____

Have you taken any medicine today? (List) _____

Please list other surgery you have had: _____

_____

Please circle any medical condition you have been treated for: diabetes (use insulin,
use medication only, use diet control, other control), high blood pressure, heart disease,
kidney disease, ulcers, lung disease, cancer, rheumatoid arthritis, paralysis, gout, poor
circulation, neurological disorder. List any other medical problem you have been treated
for: _____

_____

Have you ever had treatment for back trouble?   Yes   No   When and by whom?

Please circle the part(s) of your foot/ankle that give you trouble: ankle, heel, midfoot, arch, ball of the foot, toes.

Have you noticed any of the following changes or deformities in your feet? Please circle all that apply: bunions, hammertoes, corns, calluses, clawing, cocking up toes, deformed or painful toenails, burning or tingling in the leg, foot or toes, ulcers on the feet.
If yes, when did this occur? _____
Did you have flat feet as a child?   Yes   No
Do you limit your activities because of your problem?   Yes   No   If yes, how

---

Do you have any pain in the morning on rising?   Yes   No

Do you have pain at night?   Yes   No   Does it wake you?   Yes   No

Do you notice swelling in your foot/ankle?   Yes   No   What time of day?
Please circle: morning, afternoon, night, all day.

What activity is it related to? _____

Do you have pain with walking?   Yes   No   Standing?   Yes   No   Jogging?   Yes   No   If yes, how far? _____ Number of miles per week. _____

Do you have difficulty wearing certain types of shoes?   Yes   No   What shoes are comfortable? Please circle: pumps, low heels, flats, boots, running shoes, canvas shoes.

If you have used braces or supports in the past did they help ease your symptoms?   Yes   No   Describe: arch support, heel cups, ankle brace, other. _____

Please add any information the doctor should know regarding your case in addition to the above. _____

_____

_____

_____

FIGURE 3–1 ■ History form used in evaluation of foot and ankle problems. It supplements the oral history provided by the patient.

ogy on the other foot is overlooked. Both feet should be evaluated for comparison. The gait pattern should be assessed while the patient walks both toward and away from the examiner. Style and pattern of gait (such as a shuffle) and foot position, including rotation and arch configuration (collapsed or rocker bottom) are noted. Early in the course of neuropathic foot disease, pain may be a prominent finding. Antalgic gait, pelvic tilt, alteration in cadence, abnormal arm swing, as well as foot and leg position both in stance and swing phase are noted. Hip position, varus or valgus at the knee, and tibial alignment are also important. During stance, emphasis is placed on forefoot and hindfoot

position as well as the configuration of the arch. Foot print studies are useful in demonstrating abnormal pressure areas in both early stance and later propulsive phases of gait.

The examiner should inspect the shoes both inside and out for abnormal wear patterns and offending objects within the shoe. If a patient uses orthotics, these should be routinely inspected for durability and repair. It is common to find that the patient has inadvertently placed the orthotic for the right foot in the left shoe and vice versa, not realizing the error because of an insensitive foot. The potential for skin compromise and ulceration is obvious.

Next, the feet are evaluated by palpation and inspection. Examination of femoral, popliteal, posterior tibial, and dorsalis pedis arterial pulses is performed and recorded. Foot temperature is assessed by palpation. Any dermal lesions, particularly in the web spaces, as well as ulcerations on the sole, corns, callosities, and nail abnormalities are noted for depth, size, and location. Each interdigital space is examined for preulcerations as well as macerated skin since lesions, if overlooked, can bring disastrous consequences. The thickness of the plantar skin is also checked by palpation.

The ankle is observed for edema, erythema, and ulceration. Stasis dermatitis, varicosities, and scant hair growth are a few of the changes which help to determine the vascular status of the limb. Evaluation of both acute pitting edema and chronic edema is also important.

The use of Wagner's staging system in evaluating the state of the skin and degree of neuropathic or vascular ulcer involvement is of both diagnostic and therapeutic benefit.[4] A Grade 0 lesion implies no open ulcer, only callus formation or an area of potential breakdown at the site of a bony prominence. Grade I lesions are full-thickness skin, but only go as deep as the skin without involvement of tendon or bone. Grade II ulcers, in addition to skin and subcutaneous tissue, may also involve tendon or joint capsule. Grade III lesions involve bone, often with associated infection. Grade IV lesions have associated wet or dry gangrene. Grade V lesions indicate large, non-salvageable, infected, or necrotic areas necessitating amputation. This grading system helps determine the extent of the lesion, and guides the physician in choosing appropriate treatment.

After the visual inspection of the foot and ankle has been made, a biomechanical examination is performed starting with the ankle. Holding the leg with one hand, grasp the heel with the other hand, pulling the heel forward on the fixed tibia. Laxity of the lateral ankle ligaments is evidenced by anterior sliding of the talus out of the ankle mortise when the heel is pulled forward in the anterior drawer test. It may be difficult to determine the extent of ligament laxity because of edema and lack of sensation secondary to peripheral neuropathy. Laxity here indicates anterior talofibular and capsular laxity.

In the talar tilt test, the leg and heel are held in a similar manner. The heel is then pulled into varus. Laxity is determined by the amount of varus in the heel. A palpable "clunk" may be felt also. Lateral ankle ligament laxity often accompanies subtalar joint instability if neuropathic destruction of the talus has occurred.

Mobility of the hindfoot is tested by holding the ankle fixed in neutral, grasping the heel and rocking it in valgus and varus. The heel is held fast in one hand and the midfoot examined by rotating the metatarsals internally and externally to determine the degree of flexibility at Chopart's joint. Abduction and adduction of the forefoot are examined by holding the heel in the palm with the thumb placed on the talar neck medially. The opposite hand grasps the forefoot moving it in the respective direction. Dorsiflexion and plantarflexion of the intertarsal and tarsometatarsal joints (Lisfranc's joint), are tested by holding the midfoot fixed with one hand and rocking the metatarsals up and down with the other. The first metatarso-cuneiform joint is independent and more flexible than the others. The second metatarsal middle cuneiform joint is the stiffest joint with increasing flexibility in the third, fourth, and fifth joints respectively. The width and general shape of the foot is noted. Stiffness and deformity as well as surgical absence and drifting of the toes are all noted. A depressed longitudinal arch and pronated foot may indicate destruction of the tarsometatarsal joint with spreading metatarsals as the first ray splits away from the lateral rays. A red, swollen, sausage-shaped foot may indicate an early fracture dislocation here consistent with Charcot arthropathy.

Examination of the forefoot includes rotation of the metatarsals. A red, swollen, "sausage shaped" foot may indicate an early fracture dislocation. Metatarsal position is important. Metatarsus elevatus of the first metatarsal along with hallux elevatus caused by relative shortening of the tendons of the great toe are often seen. A large bunion deformity may have formed with hallux valgus with or without metatarsus primus varus. Arthritis of the first metatarsophalangeal joint may be accompanied by hallux rigidus and a grossly deformed and enlarged joint.

Fixed hammertoe deformity may be present caused by several factors that include stiff glycosylated tissue and relative shortening of the long toe flexors and extensors, along with impaired function of the foot intrinsic muscles as a result of polyneuropathy and/or ischemia.

Vascular Exam

Evaluation of vascular status in the diabetic should begin with general inspection for areas of gross discoloration, ischemia, and varicosities. Palpation of the pedal pulses and a routine evaluation of proximal pulses, including the femoral and popliteal arteries, is made. The grading system of Andros, et al, facilitates rapid assessment.[5] An absent pulse is given a Grade 0, if barely palpable 1+, moderately reduced 2+, slightly reduced 3+, and 4+ for a normal bounding pulse. The use of an ultrasonic Doppler both on the major vessels as well as on the digital vessels is a quick and simple means of assessing the quality of the pulses when palpation fails to adequately demonstrate their presence. In using such a device, hold the probe at a right angle to the skin over the vessel being studied, and move it around until the maximum volume of pulse is heard. However, a falsely loud pulse may be heard if the vessel examined has medial sclerosis, since this will permit increased volume of the pulse.

The ankle/brachial ischemic index[4,10] has proved useful in predicting healing of forefoot surgery, as well as forefoot amputations. In general, ankle-arm indices of 0.5 or greater are required in the dysvascular diabetic patient to afford a reasonable chance of healing. It is generally felt that if pedal pulses are palpable, digital amputations will usually heal.[6] It has also been shown that calcification of the vessels, that can lead to arterial incompressibility, has some limitation on the usefulness of the ankle pressure measurements. In some instances, other means of vascular assessment are necessary, including digital photoplethysmography[7] and arterial digital doppler examinations.

Venous filling time is a valuable test of general vascular status. It is measured in seconds and denotes the time it takes dorsal foot veins to distend above the skin level but not become engorged after the elevated foot is placed in a dependent position. Less than 20 to 25 seconds is considered normal. A longer time indicates decreased blood flow. This test is unreliable when varicosities are present.

After evaluating vascular status, further specialized studies, such as evaluation of distal arterial pulses, arteriography, or digital plethysmography can be done. Skin temperature measurement, thermography, and cutaneous oxygen tension can be measured if surgery is contemplated in the presence of questionable circulatory competence.

Neurologic Exam

The neurologic examination includes vibratory testing and pinwheel sensory testing. These are quick and easy tests of neurologic function that indicate the status of the peripheral nerve. Cofield found that the degree of vibratory sensation in the leg is the most consistent finding in estimating the overall amount of sensory deficit and that the absence of deep tendon reflexes, especially the Achilles reflex, is almost always present in diabetic neuropathy.[3] A Tinel's exam over the major cutaneous and motor nerves of the foot should be routinely performed to rule out nerve entrapment. The use of the electromyogram and nerve conduction velocity studies can often help distinguish among the variety and severity of neurologic diagnoses possible in the diabetic.

Radiographic Evaluation

Radiographic assessment of the foot and ankle should consist of weight-bearing views: anteroposterior, lateral, and oblique of the ankle, and anteroposterior and lateral of the foot with the oblique nonweight-bearing. Occasionally nonweight-bearing views and specialty views, such as sesamoid, metatarsal head projections, and axial views of the calcaneus, are included. Ankle x-rays should be included to evaluate all hindfoot problems. It is helpful to place lead markers beneath ulcerations and callosities to better define sites of pathology, especially in the edematous or deformed foot. It may be difficult in these situations to determine where offending bony prominences originate.

Changes in bony contour, periosteal reaction, osteolysis, fracture, and other Charcot changes should be noted. Bony changes should be correlated with cutaneous lesions. Attention to soft tissue changes such as swelling or gas in tissue planes is most important. These changes could represent the presence of gas-forming organisms or communication of the lesion with the outside environment. Three-phase technetium bone scans, Gallium scans, Indium-labeled white cell studies, CT, and MRI studies are all useful adjuncts to diagnosis in determining the extent of bony destruction, fracture, soft tissue destruction, bleeding, and infection.

Laboratory Evaluation

Useful lab tests in the diabetic patient include the CBC, Westergren sedimentation rate, and serum chemistry and enzyme profiles, as well as serum protein electrophoresis. Much information can be obtained from these commonly performed tests with respect to the possibilities of infection as well as the coexistence of other conditions such as gout. The patient's nutritional status and degree of control of the diabetes can also be determined. A total lymphocyte count greater than 1500 and an albumin level of greater than 3.5 gm/dl along with an ischemic index of at least 0.45 have been shown to correlate with higher rates of healing in diabetic and dysvascular patients.[8]

Patient Education

Patient education is the single most important factor in the successful treatment and prevention of progressive or recurrent problems in the insensitive or dysvascular foot.[9] Effective patient education requires repetition of instructions and constant reinforcement. Key points of information include:

1. Poor circulation can produce ulcers that lead to infection and gangrene and loss of part or all of the limb.

2. Loss of sensation can prevent appreciation of minor wounds, lead to repetitive trauma, and culminate in major injury or infection to bones and soft tissues.
3. Daily foot inspection and good foot hygiene are most important as a preventative measure.
4. Appropriately fitted supportive and protective footwear reduces the risk of infection, ulcers, and fracture.
5. Palliative care for corns, calluses and nails, and the dangers of bathroom surgery should be emphasized.
6. The deleterious effects of smoking, excess weight gain, and other environmentally affected conditions that aggravate tissue breakdown or prevent healing.

SUMMARY

A basic understanding of the diabetic disease process, as well as the anatomy and biomechanics of the foot and ankle, allows the physician to devise a diagnostic and therapeutic regimen appropriate for each individual patient. Appropriate consultations in the team approach lead to accurate diagnosis, expedite timely care, and are cost efficient. Patient education nurtured in both the inpatient and outpatient setting is critically important.

References

1. Brindley G, Cofield R. Local treatment for neuropathic foot ulceration and osteoarthropathy. Foot Ankle. 1985: 5:245–250.
2. Miller W. General considerations in the examination of the foot and ankle in your patient in office practice. Foot Ankle. 1982: 2:180–184.
3. Cofield R, Morrison M, and Beabout J. Diabetic neuroarthropathy in the foot: Patient characteristics and patterns of radiographic change. Foot Ankle. 1983: 4:15–21.
4. Wagner F. The dysvascular foot: A system for diagnosis and treatment. Foot Ankle. 1981: 2:64–122.
5. Anros G, Harris R, Leopoldo D, et al. The need for arteriography in diabetic patients with gangrene and palpable foot pulses. Arch Surg. 1984: 119:1260–1263.
6. Sizer J, Wheelock F. Digital amputations in diabetic patients. Surgery. 1972: 72:980–989.
7. Bone G, Pomajzl M. Toe blood pressure by photoplethysmography: An index of healing in fore-

foot amputations. Surgery. 1981: 89:569–574.

8. Pinzure M, Kaminsky M, Sage R, et al. Amputations at the middle level of the foot. A retrospective and prospective review. J Bone Joint Surg. 1986: 68A:1061–1064.

9. Jacobs R, Karmody A. Office care of the insensitive foot. Foot Ankle. 1982: 2:230–237.

10. Winsor T. Influence of arterial disease on the systolic blood pressure gradient of the extremity. Am J Med Sci. 1950: 220:117.

Diabetic Foot Function

G. JAMES SAMMARCO, M.D.,
AND MICHAEL M. STEPHENS, MsC.
(BIOENG), FRCSI

BASIC PRINCIPLES

Introduction

The foot has five basic functions: it is the base of support for the body; it can accommodate by loose adaption to uneven ground; it acts as a shock absorber during gait; its shape and stability give leverage for propulsion; and it has a mechanism to absorb transverse leg rotation. Loss of any part of these functions will allow undesirable forces to be transmitted through the foot. A man weighing 150 pounds (70 kilograms) walking a mile dissipates approximately 60 tons of force through each foot. The foot is a finely tuned organ coordinating efforts through all tissues including the bones, ligaments, muscles, and skin. These load-bearing, stress-absorbing tissues must carry body weight, overcome gravity, and propel it forward on flat or uneven ground. A person takes 10,000 to 15,000 steps every day. It is not surprising that, with repeated stress, the bones and ligaments in the foot over the years become misaligned. This process can easily be hastened if the person wears ill-fitting shoes and has the swollen, insensitive, stiff, and ischemic foot associated with diabetes.

Mobility and Stability

Skeletal architecture is functionally designed for mobility. It could be inherently stable only if all bones were cubes with flat surfaces aligned perpendicularly to gravity and applied stress. The skeleton of the foot possesses abilities that allow it to be rigid when necessary, converting 26 bones into a single solid unit, or quite flexible as when climbing barefoot. This is possible because the bones in the tarsus are shaped to fit closely together, are relatively small in size, and have curved articular surfaces permitting only a small amount of motion. This contrasts with the maximally curved surface of the mobile hip or shoulder joint. Large joint surfaces offer broad areas of contact between the bones to share the large loads, e.g., up to three times body weight when running. This close-fitting arrangement of bones avoids the necessity for the joints to have stabilizing rims.

The mobility of these joints is accentuated by the mechanical qualities of hyaline cartilage covering each joint and the synovial fluid that lubricates them. A thin film of this fluid allows the joints to glide almost friction free, i.e., only 0.2% of the compression load created by body weight and muscular action is required for conversion into a sheer force to overcome resistance to motion.[1] Motion is required for the penetration of synovial fluid solute, but cartilage also requires insulin for glucose uptake and oxidation of carbon dioxide[2] for DNA synthesis through cyclic AMP,[3] and for chondrocyte proliferation.[4] Hyaline cartilage, therefore, both requires and can tolerate repetitive cyclical motion. Abrupt impacts cannot be absorbed by the cartilage and underlying cancellous bone, and lead to subchondral and stress fractures. The altered hyaline cartilage metabolism with the osteopenia of diabetes mellitus[5] lowers the threshold at which these fractures occur.

Thus, abnormal metabolism in part puts the weight-bearing bones and joints of the diabetic foot at risk of fracture.

In contrast to the bones, the surrounding joint capsules and ligaments, muscles, tendons, and fiber sheaths are designed to stabilize the foot. They must allow certain movements to occur within a functional range of motion. They are composed of two basic elements: relatively non-elastic collagen fibers for strength, and a supporting ground substance that is a flexible gel.[6] Since collagen can only elongate by 3% of its length, it must accomodate movement by altering the alignment of fibers. The fibers may be oriented like a mesh, so that the tissue can elongate, with the fibers becoming less angulated to each other and shortening by increasing the obliquity of the fibers. Or they may be wavelike and undulating so that they lengthen by becoming straight (Fig. 4-1).[7] This occurs if the fibers are mobile, which is the function of the ground substance. Ground substance is composed of glycoproteins that, being hydrophillic, have a high water content. Compared to collagen, it is more active metabolically with a half life of 7 days in contrast to the 300 days of collagen.[8] Hyperglycemia causes increased nonenzymatous glycosylation of collagen.[9] This leads to increased cross linking, which alters the structure of collagen and keratin[10] so that they become more rigid, increase their tensile strength, and become resistant to collagenase. The foot becomes stiff and joints less mobile.

FACTORS ALLOWING DEFORMITY IN THE DIABETIC FOOT AFFECTING FOUR BASIC STRUCTURES

FACTORS	BONES	LIGAMENTS	CARTILAGE	MUSCLES
osteoporosis	X			
hyperostosis	X	X		
neuropathy	X			X
previous deformity	X	X		
body weight	X	X	X	
decreased glucose uptake			X	
collagen crosslinking		X		X

FIGURE 4-2 ■ Factors allowing deformity in the diabetic foot affecting four basic structures.

Individual ligaments and capsules provide passive stability to joints by limiting terminal range. Muscles, however, give dynamic stability by providing a selective restraint at lesser joint positions. The range of motion depends on the position of attachment of ligaments relative to the axis of rotation, as well as ligament mechanical adaption such as fiber orientation and mobility. Since ligaments consist of dense bands of collagen, in diabetes they are also subject to inflexibility resulting from cross linking between individual fibers, like other connective tissue. Joint mobility will be reduced[11] as ligaments become taut early in the arc of physiological motion. This subjects the ligament to greater stress, and therefore a higher risk of injury. To compound this structural abnormality in collagen, obese maturity onset diabetic patients are susceptible to hyperostosis of the extremities which constitutes part of the spectrum of diabetic osteoarthropathy.[12] This contrasts with osteoporosis—more commonly seen in the insulin dependent and poorly controlled diabetic. Excessive production of new bone is formed in the region of ligamentous attachment[13] and further contributes to stiffening the foot. (Fig. 4-2).

Muscles provide the dynamic stability for joints through timing, speed of contraction, strength, and resistance to movement. A muscle, however, cannot protect a ligament if it is relaxed when a force is applied because there is no muscle ligament reflex. If a muscle is already tense, it can give some protection to resist movement before ligamentous injury occurs.[14] Proprioceptive and

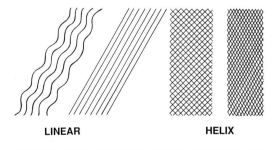

LINEAR   HELIX

FIGURE 4-1 ■ Fibrous tissue flexibility changes with motion. Collagen fibers alter their alignment. Linear orientation (left), helical orientation (right). After Perry J: In Cruess RL and Rennie WRJ eds. Adult orthopaedics. New York, Churchill Livingstone, 76–111, 1985.

sensory responses provide input that influences muscle contraction and the motion in a weight-bearing joint. Agonistic and antagonistic muscles work reciprocally, one to resist a force, and the other to act as a holding force until the desired posture is attained.[15] Joint position sense, plantar skin sensation, timing, and control of these muscle contractions are all altered in diabetic neuropathy[16] and lead to unexpected foot injuries.[17] This neurologic deficit can also affect muscle strength and lead to muscle imbalance and foot deformity, which, in turn, places certain parts of the foot at risk to overuse syndromes and trauma. Various muscle groups have been found to be weak in different series, and reflect the diversity of pathology: ankle dorsiflexors,[18,19] inverters and everters,[20] and the intrinsic muscles of the foot, the most common finding.[21] Muscle strength is further diminished in diabetes since a muscle can contain up to 5% connective tissue,[22] and those with a greater percentage of connective tissue support body weight over the forefoot.[15] This tissue along with tendons, muscle sheaths, and fasciae are all subjected to damage by nonenzymatic glycolysation, resulting in stiffness through the increased cross linking of collagen fibers.

PLANTAR PADS

Force Transmission

To function as an end-weight bearing structure for locomotion, the skeleton of the foot requires the plantar skin to react to the ground. This has adapted structurally to perform 5 functions. As the interface between the ground and the soft tissues and bones of the foot it transmits the reactive force, acts as a shock absorber, accommodates to shear forces, protects the deep structures, and provides friction. The plantar skin is particularly thick due to epidermal hypertrophy which results from stress on the foot at the heel and metatarsal pad. Under this lies the dermis, containing collagen, elastic fibers, blood vessels, and fat. In the heel pad, the fat is contained in chambers formed by well structured fibrous septa. These septa are arranged spirally to resist torsion and are attached to themselves, the calcaneus, and skin.[23] A similar framework is seen over the metatarsal heads. Here the fibrous bands are arranged to allow nerves, vessels, and tendons to pass through the weight bearing area below the metatarsal heads. They are arranged in 3 directions: longitudinal, vertical, and transverse. The longitudinal fibers are the anterior extensions of the plantar aponeurosis, and the superficial parts extend to the skin while the deep fibers are inserted into the flexor sheaths. The vertical fibers run from the skin to the flexor sheath and plantar ligaments while the transverse fibers connect the digitations of the plantar ligament distal to the metatarsal heads.[24] This complex arrangement of septae forms compartments to enclose the fat and serves as a barrier to the rapid migration of fluids from areas of elevated pressure. This anatomical arrangement converts loads to tensile stress and hydrostatic pressure, and makes the plantar skin and subcutaneous tissue efficient in transmitting forces, acting as a shock absorber, protecting the deeper structures, and, combined with skin cleavage lines, affording traction in locomotion.

Impact forces on the heel at heel strike in the gait cycle are commonly obliquely oriented which results from two vectors, the normal force of compression, and a shear force tangential to it. The compartments of fat resist compressive forces and the fibrous septa connecting the skin to bony structures resist shear forces. Shear forces are difficult to measure but can vary from 0 when standing to a third of body weight (mediolateral axis) and body weight (anteroposterior axis).[25] Vertical compression force can vary from body weight in stance to as much as 3 times body weight in running. Considering the magnitude of such forces, it is clear that the plantar pads have a major and important role in foot function.

The loading pressure on the heel pad can be calculated by the vertical compression force divided by heel area, 23 sq cms. This can vary from $3kg/cm^2$ to $9kg/cm^2$. These high pressures have a cumulative daily effect particularly with repetitive high impact activities, such as running. Brand[26] demonstrated the effects of repetitive trauma that led to pain and inflammation. If this was increased and repeated daily, the inflammation increased and culminated in subcutaneous necrosis and later epithelial discontinuity. Under normal circumstances, the pain of inflammation would alter the gait pattern of the athlete to prevent continuing insult and progression. However, in the diabetic patient with a neuropathy, this feedback mechanism may be partially or completely absent. Considering that such a patient may also be obese, have thin plantar skin,[27] poor arterial circulation, abnormal collagen and keratin,[21] and abnormal high pressure areas from Charcot's joints, it is not surprising that the delicate balance of plantar skin function is easily disturbed and results in breakdown and ulceration (Fig. 4-2).

KINEMATICS

Motion of the foot is complex, occurring simultaneously in several planes to allow inversion or eversion, plantar or dorsiflexion, supination or pronation, and adduction or abduction. Gait influences this motion so that the foot may function as a single unit, or a subtle organ, to withstand impact forces and uneven surfaces.

Flexion and extension is seen predominantly in the ankle joint which acts as a hinge joint. The axis of rotation is 20° to 30° externally rotated with respect to the knee, and parallel or up to 20° inverted in relation to the ground (Fig. 4-3). This allows up to 30° of dorsiflexion and 50° of plantar flexion in

the normal subject. The subtalar joint is more complex; it is the articulation between the talus and calcaneous. The talus has no muscle attachments and relies on ligamentous attachments to the tibia, fibula, calcaneous, and navicular for stability. The subtalar joint has 3 parts: the anterior, the medial, and posterior facets. Their orientation is such that this joint moves like a screw, i.e., when the heel is inverted the calcaneous also rotates medially. The right foot acts as a right-handed screw and a left foot as a left screw.[28] The axis of this rotation lies 41° from the ground from the heel upward and forward, and in 23° of internal rotation to the foot axis (calcaneus to second metatarsal) (Fig. 4-4). This allows 20° of inversion and 5° of eversion with a wide normal variation. When the foot is loaded, there is only 6° of movement at this joint.[29]

The talonavicular and calcaneocuboid joints constitute the transverse tarsal (Chopart's) joint. Since the calcaneus and talus are intimately attached to each other at the subtalar joint, any movement of this joint will influence the transverse tarsal joint, where flexion, extension, and mediolateral rotation occurs. The axis of rotation of the subtalar joint is set obliquely, rising from the ground anterodorsally at 52°, and is directed from the midline of the foot anteromedially at 57°. The axis of Chopart's joint is directed from the floor anterodorsally at 15° and from the midline of the foot anter-

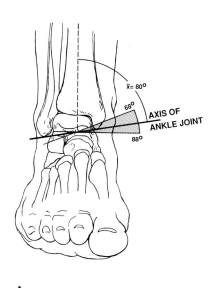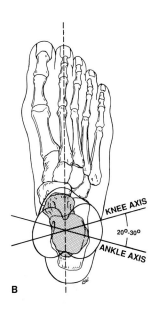

FIGURE 4-3 ■ A, The general axis of the ankle lies beneath the malleoli. B, The ankle axis is 20° to 30° externally orientated with respect to the knee axis. The foot axis (dotted line) is internally oriented with respect to the ankle axis. Adapted from Isman RE, Inman VT. Bull Prosthet Res. 10,11:97, 1969.

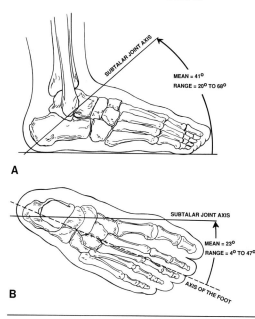

A

B

FIGURE 4–4 ■ A, The subtalar axis is oriented obliquely upward from the heel to provide supination and pronation; B, The axis passes from lateral to medial to provide inversion and eversion. Adapted from Inman VT. The joints of the ankle. Williams & Wilkins, Baltimore, 1976.

omedially at 9°. These axes allow a small amount of flexion and 30° of rotation. Elftman[30] and Mann and Inman[31] noted that motion in the transverse tarsal joint depended more on the relationship of the talonavicular to the calcaneocuboid axis rather than the individual axes of these two joints. When the calcaneus is everted, these axes are parallel to each other, that is, 40° to the ground, directed dorsilatrally. However, when the calcaneus is in a neutral or inverted position, these axes diverge dorsally from each other at 25° and 65° respectively. Therefore, when the heel is everted, the transverse tarsal joint is unlocked, because the axes are parallel (Fig. 4-5). Movement at this joint is then possible and the foot is flexible. When the heel is inverted, (placed in varus) the transverse tarsal joint is locked (the axes are divergent) and the foot becomes rigid. This allows a variation in tarsal mobility with the changing positions of the foot during gait. It also means that, when performing a subtalar fusion, the os calcis should always be in some eversion, or heel

valgus, to allow some flexibility to be maintained in the transverse tarsal joint. The intertarsal and tarsometatarsal joints have many interconnecting ligaments which are much stronger on the plantar surface and, combined with the stable bony architecture, allow minimal gliding movement. About 15° of flexion is possible within the tarsal bones, including the transverse tarsal joint. The relative rigidity in flexion/extension of this part of the foot is mechanically suitable to load-transfer during gait, since it acts as a long lever arm.

The bony architecture of the tarsus and metatarsals forms the proximal transverse arch of the foot (Fig. 4-6). The cuneiform bones and bases of the metatarsals are all wedge shaped and broader dorsally. They can be described as a gothic arch, with the intermediate cuneiform and second metatarsal base acting as the keystones. The medial longitudinal arch has less inherent bony stability but relies on strong intertarsal ligaments, the tibialis posterior muscle, and the plantar fascia. The latter acts as a tether between the calcaneus and metatarsophalangeal joints and as a Spanish windlass when the metatarsophalangeal joints are dorsiflexed. The calcaneus, through the sustentaculum tali to the talus, navicular, medial cuneiform, and first metatarsal, make up the medial border of this arch, and combined, make up the medial pillar of the foot. The calcaneus, cuboid, fourth, and fifth meta-

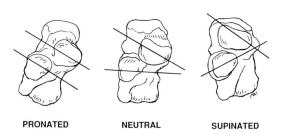

PRONATED   NEUTRAL   SUPINATED

FIGURE 4–5 ■ The orientation of the two axes of Choparts joint. Neutral stance allows the axes to converge, stabilizing the foot. The pronated foot has parallel axes permitting increased motion while the supinated (cavus) foot has axes which approach a right angle, making the foot rigid. After Mann RA, Inman VT. Phasic activity of the intrinsic muscles of the foot. J Bone Joint Surg. 46A: 469–481, 1964.

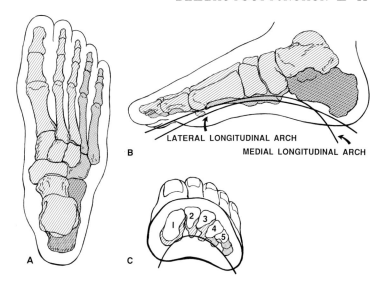

FIGURE 4–6 ■ A, The arches of the foot. The medial arch (lines) is composed of the medial three rays, cuneiforms, navicular talus, and calcaneus. **B,** The proximal transverse arch is rigid. **C,** It is more flexible and concave than the lateral arch (dots). After Mann RA. Biomechanics of the foot. In: Gould JS (ed) The foot book. Baltimore, Williams & Wilkins, 48–63, 1988.

LATERAL LONGITUDINAL ARCH

MEDIAL LONGITUDINAL ARCH

tarsals constitute the lateral pillar of the foot. The transverse arch and both these pillars are important for the normal transmission of forces during gait. If a disease process, such as neuroarthropathy, damages and destabilizes these joints, load transmission during gait will break this lever, resulting in serious consequences. Deformity develops in various patterns depending on the pillar or arch affected.

The relative rigidity of the tarsus contrasts with the mobility of the metatarsophalangeal portion of the forefoot. Over 90° of flexion/extension is possible at the metatarsophalangeal articulations; it is known as the metatarsal break (Fig. 4-7). The break has two axes and the second metatarsal is the longest. The lateral axis passes through the heads of the second to fifth metatarsal bones and is oriented 50° to 70° to the long axis of the foot. It is an amalgamation of the instant axes of rotation of the 4 lateral metatarsophalangeal joints. The first metatarsal is usually a little shorter than the second and longer, or equal to, the third. The second axis of movement runs from the first to the second and is essentially transverse.[24] The interphalangeal joints act in the same plane as their respective metatarsophalangeal joints somewhat like a hinge joint. Extension of the toes is effected, like the hand, by the extensor hood mechanism. Flexion of the metatarsophalangeal joint is done by the intrinsic muscles (interossei and lumbricals), at the proximal interphalangeal joint

by flexor digitorum brevis, and, at the distal interphalangeal joint, by flexor digitorum longus. Movement at these joints is maintained by the coordinated and balanced tone and contractions of these muscles. If, for some reason, these become altered, deformity develops. For example, when the intrinsic muscles become weak, the metatarsophalangeal joint dorsiflexes and the flexor and extensor muscles become overactive in an effort to correct this interphalangeal joint deformity. It flexes the interphalangeal joints and further extends the dorsiflexes and the metatarsophalangeal joint leading to hammertoe and claw toe. This deformity is common in patients with peripheral neuropathy, Charcot's arthropathy.

Gait Cycle

To understand the forces that are transmitted through the foot, it is necessary to examine the gait cycle because these forces are not static in magnitude or direction. They change as the body moves. The walking cycle is divided into stance phase (60%) and swing phase (40%). In the swing phase, the limb is not weight bearing, and relatively minor forces are transmitted through the foot. This phase is divided into initial swing and terminal swing. During these periods, the tibia is in relative internal rotation, the ankle is dorsiflexed, the subtalar joint is everted, Chopart's joint is mobile, with pretibial

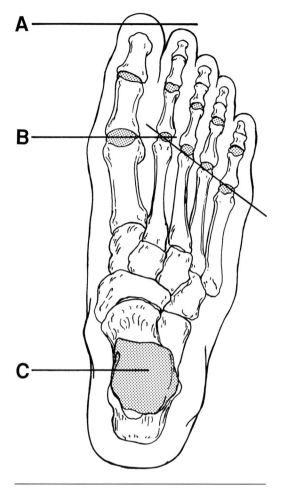

FIGURE 4–7 ■ A, The "advanced axis" is located at the tip of the hallux. B, The metatarsophalangeal joints with two axes divide the forefoot into two segments. C, The ankle axis. Adapted from Bojsen-Moller F. Anatomy of the forefoot—normal and pathologic. Clin Orthop Rel Res. 142:10–18, 1979.

muscles active, and the calf and intrinsic muscles inactive. The stance phase has three periods: the first and third occupy 25% and the middle 50% of stance. The first period begins with heel strike, continues into flat foot, and ends with the toe off of the opposite foot. During this time, both limbs are weight bearing. In the second period, the limb carries all body weight bcause the opposite leg is in the swing phase. The third period starts with the opposite limb heel strike while the foot is still in flat foot and ends with its own toe off.

At heel strike, body weight is dropped on the heel with the tibia internally rotated with active motor activity in the pretibial and peroneal muscles. The floor reaction exceeds body weight by 20% while walking.[32] The point of contact is lateral to the centre of the ankle joint[33] (Fig. 4-8). This creates a valgus thrust on the subtalar joint as the calcaneus everts 10° within the first 8% of stance at average walking velocity.[29] Eversion is accommodated by the anterior calcaneus moving inferiorly and laterally, and thereby transmits an internal upward-rotating force through the limb.[31] After heel strike, this movement slowly reverses to culminate in inversion as the heel rises during terminal stance. Tibialis anterior is the only inverting muscle active during the period of maximum stress, e.g., when body weight is entirely on the heel.[34] When the forefoot hits the ground, the tibialis posterior muscle takes over and soleus becomes active as body weight moves forward of the ankle. Tibialis posterior has the longest lever arm and a larger cross-section gives it an 88% advantage over tibialis anterior. Soleus has a shorter lever arm but a much greater diameter, resulting in an inversion torque twice that of tibialis posterior (Fig. 4-9). While the heel is everted, Chopart's joint is unlocked and the forefoot is flexible which assists the foot in two of its important functions—shock absorbancy at heel strike, and accommodation to uneven surfaces at flat foot. This funciton is passive which contrasts with the later stages of stance. During the last two-thirds of stance, progressive external tibial rotation occurs which, with contraction first of the tibialis posterior and then lateral soleus, produces inversion at the subtalar joint. This locks Chopart's joint to establish a rigid forefoot so that the heel can be elevated. Weight is transferred to the forefoot across this long lever arm without forefoot collapse and prevents the development of a rocker bottom. Chopart's joint is not the only area that gives the forefoot stability. The intrinsic muscles have increased activity through the second and third periods of stance adding support to the longitudinal arch as does the windlass action of the plantar fascia. This happens late in the second period and all of the third period, as dorsiflexion of the metatarsophalangeal joints tightens the plantar fascia. The metatarso-

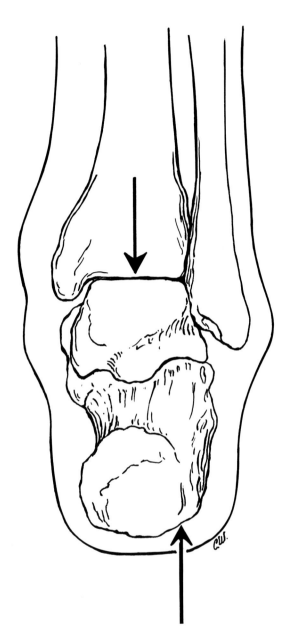

EVERSION LEVER ON LOADING

FIGURE 4-8 ■ The point of contact at heel strike lies lateral to the alignment of body weight creating a valgus thrust on the subtalar joint. Adapted from Perry J. Anatomy and biomechanics of the hindfoot. Clin Orthop Rel Res. 177:9–15, 1983.

phalangeal break acts in unison with inversion of the hind foot at heel off so that body weight is distributed over all the metatarsal heads at the completion of foot flat. Any pathological process that affects the bony structure, ligaments, or intrinsic muscles can lead to abnormal load and force transmission resulting in deformity and gait abnormalities.

Load Distribution and Transmission

While walking, only 7% of a normal gait cycle is occupied by a single foot when it is flat on the ground. Studies of force transmission must assess foot pressures dynamically as well as statically. The forces exerted against the foot by the ground, therefore, do not only compress. Since the centre of gravity alters with gait and does not remain equidistant from the ground at all times, compression forces vary in various stages of gait. As the body is moving, shearing forces occur parallel to the ground. As the heel strikes the ground there is forward shear force and, at heel off, a backwards shear force. Also medial and lateral body sway generate shear forces in those directions. Alterations in tibial rotation are not all accommodated in the subtalar joint, and they exert torque between the foot and ground. A 70 kg man may have normal loading pressures on the heels of 5 kg/cm^2 while walking. This increases with faster velocities and as do shear and torque.[25] It is not surprising that any shift in the load from one part of the foot to another in the presence of abnormal sensation, collagen, and vasculature, easily compromises the foot.

Soon after heel strike, the vertical force is 120% of body weight, 10% forward shear, 5% medial shear, and 20 in/pound of internal torque.[35] In the second stage of stance, forward/backward shear and torque are diminished, vertical compression is less than body weight, and lateral shear is 5% of body weight. In this period, forces are transmitted down the lateral side of the foot beneath the cuboid and then towards the base of the first metatarsal. Toward the end of the second stage of stance, force is transmitted to the second metatarsal head and then to the hallux for toe off.[36] The forefoot sustains

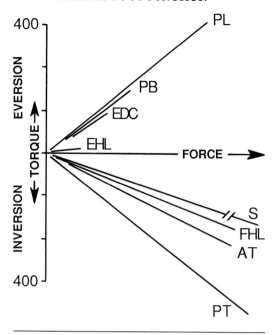

FIGURE 4–9 ■ Relative muscle forces acting on the subtalar joint. The angle of the line indicates the effectiveness of each muscle. Eversion is produced by muscles acting above horizontal force line and inversion is produced by muscles acting below horizontal force line. PL—peroneus longus; PB—peroneus brevis; EDL—extensor digitorum longus; EHL—extensor hallucis longus; S—soleus (actual line is 5 times longer than shown); FHL—flexor hallucis longus; AT—anterior tibialis; PT—posterior tibialis. Adapted from Perry J. Anatomy and biomechanics of the hindfoot. Clin Orthop Rel Res. 177:9–15, 1983.

this force and accelerates it to carry the person forward. Shear and torque forces once again increase after heel off when the metatarsals are carrying the most weight. The heel and metatarsal pads are the structures most subjected to torsional and shear forces. The first metatarsal transmits twice the force of each of the lateral 4 metatarsal heads during quiet standing, but if the first metatarsal is short, the second metatarsal head transmits a greater proportion.[37]

DIABETIC OSTEOARTHROPATHY

The metabolic changes associated with diabetes mellitus affect the tissues of the foot

in various ways, which in turn alter the biomechanical properties and lead to deformity (Fig. 4-10).

Since cartilage requires insulin for glucose uptake, the oxidation of carbon dioxide,[2] and collagen synthesis,[38,39] the articular cartilage in the diabetic patient does not tolerate repetitive trauma, compression, and motion well. McNair et al.[5] and Wiske et al.[40] have confirmed by measuring bone mineral that generalized osteoporosis is a feature in diabetes mellitus. It usually occurs in the first 5 years from onset and is worse in insulin-dependent patients. This puts them at greater risk for fractures.[41] This osteopenia is caused by microangiopathy,[42] sympathetic neuropathy,[43,44] and hyperemia[44A] or infection.[45] However Forgacs et al.[46] believes that it may be caused by gluconeogenesis-induced lesions in the protein matrix, renal components with secondary hyperparathyroidism, increased steroids, or increased osteoclastic activity induced by acidosis. No matter what the cause it ultimately increases susceptibility to fractures and their recurrence. When there is a combination of abnormal articular cartilage with weak underlying bone, the joints are at risk for pathological fractures.

The neuropathy of diabetes affects the autonomic, sensory, and motor systems,[20] and alters joint pain fibers as well as proprioceptive fibers. Minor trauma easily produces injury when there are no surrounding proprioceptive protective responses. Micro fractures can occur in an already weakened bone and cartilage that go unrecognized because of the lack of pain appreciation. A vi-

DIABETIC METABOLIC DISORDERS THAT CHANGE
FOOT FUNCTION AND THEIR SITES OF ACTION

FACTORS	BONES	LIGAMENTS	MUSCLES	SKIN	CARTILAGE
osteoporosis	X				
hyperostosis	X	X			
neuropathy	X		X	X	
collagen crosslinking		X	X	X	
keratin crosslinking				X	
decreased fat				X	
decreased glucose uptake					X

FIGURE 4–10 ■ Diabetic metabolic disorders that change foot function and their sites of action.

cious cycle ensues, leading to further damage, joint destruction, and consequent joint instability.[47]

In a large series of 90 cases of diabetic osteoarthropathy, Clouse and Gramm[48] found 70% had Charcot joint, 72% sclerosis, 73% fragmentation, 60% periosteal new bone formation, 38% resorbtion, 75% subchondral osteoporosis, and 10% had a "sucked candy" appearance. Recent[12,13,46] attention has been drawn to hyperostosis and the calcification of ligaments that occurs in maturity-onset diabetes, especially in obese patients. This phenomenon in association with stiffer collagen caused by nonenzymatic glucosylation[10] makes the foot stiffer. Joints with less movement transmit abnormal forces through the foot to injure already damaged joints, especially during gait, when large moments are placed on the mid tarsal and tarsometatarsal joints. Obesity further increases these forces. If there are any pre-existing gait abnormalities or deformities, additional stress compounds the condition. For example, if the foot is excessively pronated, there is increased shearing on the medial forefoot, excessive supination gives increased lateral pressures, equinus, increased forefoot loading, and intoeing.

Specific Areas Affected

Since the Charcot joint was first described in 1877 when anaesthetic feet were commonly caused by syphillis, multiple causes have been found including leprosy and diabetes mellitus. Diabetic incidence is 2–5% of the population and accounts for the majority of cases. Ten percent have foot disorders[49] and 15% of these have features of diabetic osteoarthropathy. The American Diabetic Association reports 10 million people in the United States suffering from diabetes, 1 million of whom will have foot problems, and 150,000 with osteoarthropathy. Unlike tabes dorsalis and leprosy which commonly affect the hindfoot, the tarsometatarsal joints are involved in 84% of cases, the tarsus in 63% and the phalanges in 62%[48,50] which confirmed the large series of Sinha et al.[51] and Cofield et al.[52] who stated that the majority of cases involved the tarsometatarsal area (Fig. 4-11). More re-

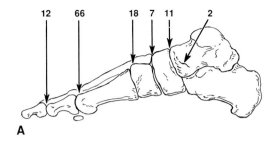

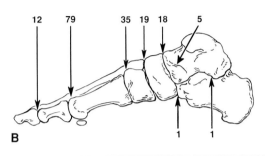

FIGURE 4–11 ■ A, Major areas of joint destruction from diabetes in 116 feet. B, Frequency of involvement of individual joints with respect to severity of changes. Adapted from Cofield RH, Morrison MJ, Beabour J. Diabetic neuropathy in the foot: patient characteristics and patterns of radiographic change. Foot and Ankle. 4:15–22, 1983.

cently Wagner[53] stated that 80% occurred within Lisfranc's joints and those adjoining them.

Harris and Brand[45] described 5 patterns of destruction in the neuropathic foot:

1. posterior pillar—direct compressive forces lead to destruction of the os calcis
2. central destruction of the talus and subsequent subtalar joint damage and valgus hindfoot deformity
3. anterior pillar, medial arch—collapse occurs in and around the navicular
4. anterior pillar, lateral arch—destruction of the lateral pillar of the foot
5. cuneiform/metatarsal base—the Lisfranc joints are involved (Figs. 4-12 and 4-13).

Different diseases give different patterns of joints affected (Fig. 4-14). There is no clear explanation for these patterns. Perhaps the various neurological defects associated with other factors give differing patterns of mo-

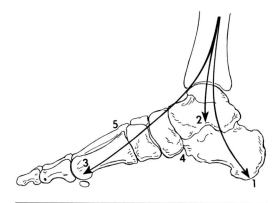

FIGURE 4–12 ■ Patterns of foot collapse in leprotic neurarthropathy. 1. Posterior pillar with calcaneal collapse. 2. Central collapse with talar body fragmentation. 3. Anterior pillar medial arch with collapse of talar head, navicular and medial cuneiform. 4. Anterior pillar, lateral arch with calcaneocuboid subluxation. 5. Destruction of all 3 cuneiforms. Note: Types 3 and 5 are frequently found in diabetic neurarthropathy. Adapted from Harris JR, Brand PW. Patterns of disintegration of the tarsus in the anaesthetic foot. J. Bone Surg. 48B:4–16, 1966.

tor and sensory loss. If certain muscle groups are weak, there will be foot imbalance. This will subject the foot to abnormal stresses and eventual joint breakdown. For this to happen, the individual joint must be insensate. Tabes dorsalis often gives an ankle lesion, but leprosy and diabetes do so less often because in leprosy, as with diabetes, the lesion is usually distal to the articular branch from the tibial nerve.[54] Pattern 4 is common in leprosy with paralyzed peronei.

In diabetes, the sensory neuropathy is of a glove and stocking type.[55] It is distal, and can effect motor, somatic sensory, proprioceptive, and autonomic elements separately or in combination with others.[19] This may explain why the diabetic pattern of Charcot joints is distal at the Lisfranc (pattern 5) and phalangeal joints,[48] and uncommon in leprosy.[45] Patterns 3 and 5 in leprosy are associated with intrinsic muscle weakness. These muscles help maintain the medial arch. In diabetic neuropathy, the intrinsic muscles of the foot are also often involved.[21,53,55–58] Intrinsic muscle weakness in the presence of a distal sensory neuropathy helps explain why diabetics develop Charcot joints at the

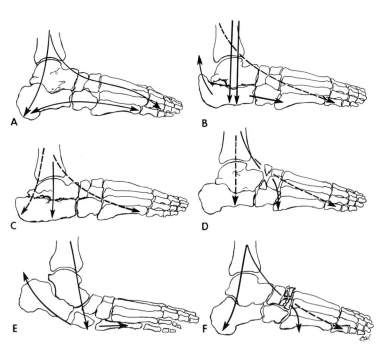

FIGURE 4–13 ■ A, Normal forces passing through the foot. B, Pattern 1: Collapse of posterior pillar, effective thrust on anterior pillar now becomes vertical. C, Pattern 2: Disintegration of the talus from subtalar incongruity. D, Pattern 3: Fracture with displacement of navicular resulting in flat foot and increased pressure beneath the midfoot. E, Pattern 4: Destruction of the lateral ray permits equinus in the calcaneus and talus with dorsiflexion and subluxation of the anterior pillar. F, Pattern 5: Fracture and disintegration of the cuneiforms. Adapted from Harris JR, Brand PW. Patterns of disintegration of the tarsus in the anaesthetic foot. J Bone Surg. 48B:4–16, 1966.

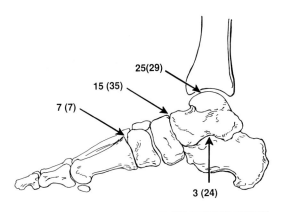

25(29)
15 (35)
7 (7)
3 (24)

FIGURE 4–14 ■ Location of leprotic neuropathic joints in 50 feet. Number indicates number of feet with primary joint involvement. Numbers in parentheses indicate number of joints which eventually become involved. Adapted from Horibe S, Tada K, Nagano J. J Bone Joint Surg. 70B:481–485, 1988.

Lisfranc and mid tarsal joints rather than in the hindfoot. Another factor may be ankle dorsiflexor weakness,[18] occasionally seen in diabetics. This weakness puts stress on the forefoot earlier in the stance phase since these muscles are normally active in the early part of the second stage of stance. Intrinsic muscles normally increase activity in the second and third part of stance and that helps to stabilize the forefoot and the longitudinal arch. Both these abnormalities put greater loads on the Lisfranc's joint and mid tarsal joints as they form part of the links in the lever arm of propulsion.

The etiology of arthropathy in diabetes is multifactorial, caused by insensitive joints, muscle imbalance, soft tissue stiffness, and abnormal biochemistry. The relative distal location of the disease can be explained by distal neuropathy, ankle dorsiflexor, and intrinsic weakness. These ultimately lead to the commonest deformity of pes planus from collapse of the medial longitudinal arch at the tarsometatarsal joint or talonavicular/cuneiform joint,[50,59] forefoot abduction[60] and clawing of the toes.

DIABETIC ULCERATION

The etiology of ulceration is also multifactorial. Vascular insufficiency is now rec-ognized as a relatively minor etiological factor. Proper footwear, foot care, hygiene, failing vision, and poor diabetic control (Fig. 4-15) are important factors. Pressure changes and changes in gait, fat atrophy, sensory neuropathy, and muscle weakness are all mechanical factors that influence the development of plantar skin abnormalities, including ulceration.

The presence of a sensory neuropathy and elevated foot pressures are related to the development of plantar ulcers,[61] and has been confirmed by many other studies.[20,62–64] Diabetic patients with neuropathy tend to have higher plantar pressures under their feet than nondiabetic controls and diabetic patients without neuropathy.[65] The reason for this is uncertain but indicates that other factors must be involved.

Body weight[64] and activity level will increase the force that the foot must transmit, and this may increase pressure, especially if there is an underlying bony prominence or foot imbalance. Shear forces increase and become a factor in skin breakdown.[66] Previously healed ulcers leave scars that transmit force to underlying tissues in a more concentrated manner[66] and tether the fat pad locally so that it cannot function physiologically. This implies that it is unable to transmit shear forces and is easily damaged.[67]

Gait abnormalities increase plantar pressures. For example, equinus and dropfoot deformities will increase forefoot loading and may increase shear forces through abduc-

FACTORS ALLOWING DIABETIC FOOT ULCERS
AFFECTING THREE BASIC STRUCTURES

FACTORS	SKIN	FAT	BONE / LIGAMENT COMPLEX
poor diabetic control	X	X	X
autonomic neuropathy	X		X
sensory neuropathy	X		X
instability and fractures	X		X
deformity (old & new)	X		X
body weight / activity level	X		X
poor vision	X		
previous ulcers	X	X	
vascular insufficiency	X	X	
fat atrophy			X
bad footwear and care	X		

FIGURE 4–15 ■ Factors allowing diabetic foot ulcers affecting 3 basic structures.

tion twist. The deformity of Charcot joints in the midfoot and forefoot leads to an increase in pressure areas; midfoot weight bearing increases after tarsal and longitudinal arch collapse. Associated with forefoot pronation is increased shearing force on the medial forefoot.[68] Fractures and foot instability also load the foot abnormally (Table 4-1). The normal human response is to spare damaged areas because they are painful. In the insensitive foot, this does not occur and the insult continues, culminating in subcutaneous and cutaneous necrosis and skin breakdown (Fig. 4-16). This is compounded by a thinner fat pad[27] and atrophy of fat tissue.[69] The fat pad has moved distally and no longer covers the metatarsal heads.

Autonomic neuropathy is another significant factor that is present in 68% of patients with diabetic ulcers, 19% of diabetics without ulcers, and 3% in nondiabetics.[70] The feet do not sweat and can cause the skin to crack. It contributes to hyperkeratotic plaque, arteriovenus shunting, and edema along with an increased risk of infection.[44]

The skin itself is likely to contribute to ulceration because the collagen and keratin are glycosylated with increased cross linking making skin stiff. Keratin builds up in response to the increased pressure and cannot be removed as readily as normal keratin. It covers the opening of an unhealed ulcer. Collagen is inflexible, so that breakdown occurs more easily with shear forces.[21] Cross-linked collagen is resistant to the normal

process of degradation of collagenases, which also contributes to poor wound-healing.

Specific Areas Affected

The distribution of foot ulcers is variable in the literature. The areas commonly affected are first metatarsal head, second and third metatarsal heads, toes, base of fifth metatarsal, and midfoot.[21,55] Ulceration under the first metatarsal head occurred in 36 to 40%, second 40%, and third metatarsal heads 25%, of 28 patients with diabetic ulcers (Fig. 4-17). The incidence of midfoot ulceration seems small but, with the addition of Charcot feet, the incidence of ulceration beneath the talus and navicular becomes more common. Although these patients did not have lesions on the heels, in clinical practice, ulceration may also be found here.

The majority of ulcers occur at, or distal to, the metatarsal heads. Weakness of the intrinsic muscles results in clawing of the toes and distal migration of the metatarsal fat pad.[69,71] This in turn causes a load reduction on the toes which should normally carry 40% of body weight for a short period at the end of stance,[37] and increases load at the metatarsal area.[20] The functional lever of the foot is shortened[72] and Charcot osteoarthropathy involving the destruction of metatarsophalangeal joints may further shorten the foot.[60] This deformity is rigid and makes normal heel-to-toe gait difficult. It places

TABLE 4–1 ■ Common Gait Problems and Their Relationship to Injury in the Diabetic Foot*

Problems	Relationship to Injury
Excessive pronation	Increased shearing on medial forefoot
Excessive supination	Increased lateral forefoot pressures and lateral instability
Midfoot weight bearing	Neuropathic destruction of tarsal bones
Equinus	Increased forefoot loading and functional lower extremity length discrepancy
Abductory twist	Increased forefoot shear loads
Marked asymmetry in gait	Increased stress on preferred side
Impaired balance and navigation	Increased risk of falling and self injury
Excessive outtoeing or intoeing	Increased stress on medial (lateral) border of the foot
Drop foot deformity	Instability and increased risk of ankle sprains and fractures, toe injuries from inadequate floor clearance, increased forefoot pressures from secondary equinus deformity
Amputations or shortened foot	Increased pressure over distal end of foot from a shoe that is too long, blistering from rubbing on toe fillers in footwear

*Adapted from Sims DS, Cavanagh PR and Ulbrecht JS. Submitted to Phys. Ther. 1988.

increased shear under the metatarsal heads.[57] In patients with a short first metatarsal, there is increased pressure on the second and third metatarsal heads that predisposes these to ulceration.

If the foot is already affected by diabetic osteoarthropathy, the deformity increases pressure to other areas, which depends on the portion of the foot affected. For example, with the collapse of the arch at Lisfranc's joint, the cuneiform and fifth metatarsal base become prominent and ulcers may develop there. Associated with this are forefoot abduction and pronation which increase pressure on the first metatarsal head and hallux.

Diabetic foot ulcers, therefore, are pri-

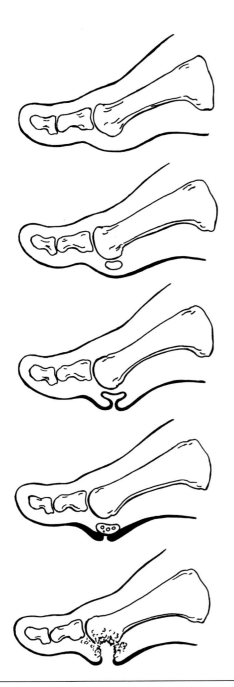

FIGURE 4-16 ■ The development of a neuropathic ulcer. Top figure is that of a normal hallux in sagittal section. In each succeeding diagram below the top, the ulcer beneath the sesamoid is seen to develop, eventually involving the sesamoid, then the metatarsophalangeal joint and finally the metatarsal itself. Adapted from Delridge L, et al. The etiology of diabetic neuropathic ulceration of the foot. Br J Surg. 72:1–6, 1985.

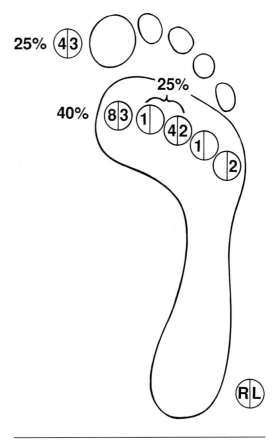

FIGURE 4-17 ■ The distribution of 28 neuropathic foot ulcers: 7 occurred in the toes, 21 beneath the metatarsal heads. R = right, L = left. Adapted from Cterctko et al. Vertical forces acting on the feet of diabetic patients with neuropathic ulceration. Br J Surg. 68:608–614, 1981.

marily caused by local increased areas of pressure on insensitive skin. Many other factors expedite this process both generally and locally. Autonomic neuropathy, body weight, metabolic skin changes, bad footwear, poor vision, and inadequate foot care are important general factors predisposing to skin breakdown. Locally, fat pad atrophy and migration, scarring from previous ulcers, intrinsic muscle weakness, and deformity from Charcot joint degeneration give rise to areas of elevated pressure which are already susceptible to damage from normal or abnormal shear forces.

BIOMECHANICAL APPROACH TO TREATMENT

Individual cases require individual conservative treatment; some require nonoperative approaches, while others require a surgery. It is important that general treatment of the disease process be under control, including diabetic control, medical management of neuropathy, reconstitution of vasculature, improvement of vision, and patient education for hygiene and foot care. Certain structural abnormalities cannot be changed, such as fat atrophy, collagen and keratin cross linking, and previous healed ulcers. However, those areas should be protected so that shear and compression forces are at a minimum. Soles of shoes should have maximal shock absorbency to accommodate for loss of plantar fat pads (Table

4-2). Shear forces may be limited by wearing double socks so that the rigidity of the soft tissues, which prevents movement of the skin over the subcutaneous tissues, can be accommodated at the interface between the two socks. However, this may allow extra movement of the foot over the orthosis or shoe and create other pressure on the foot in the shoe.

Body weight and activity level must be specifically addressed. Each of these modalities increases the loading of the foot; body weight increases compressive forces, and activity increases shear forces. The patient's weight should be kept to a minimum. If there is a previous history of plantar ulceration, the activity level must be controlled to lessen shear forces on these scars.

Diabetic Osteoarthropathy

The Charcot joint constitutes the majority of diabetic osteoarthropathy. Before complete joint destruction, acute episodes from mild injuries develop, and the foot is hot and swollen. No deformity is present at this stage, and immobilization of the offending limb is the most important treatment (Fig. 4-18). This allows the tissues to heal and may permit spontaneous arthrodesis or prevent the development of deformity. Surgery may be necessary later before deformity has developed, in that prophylactic arthrodesis is justified for instability, e.g., at Lisfranc's joints, in view of the likelihood

TABLE 4–2 ■ Summary of Risk Factors in the Diabetic Foot

Risk Factor	Relationship to Injury
Loss of protective sensation	Absent pain warning system
High plantar pressures	Ulcers usually at sites of peak pressure
Autonomic neuropathy	Dry noncompliant skin
Previous ulcer or amputation	Stress concentration in scar or transfer lesions
Foot deformity	Increased local pressures
Neuropathic fractures	Foot instability and dramatically increased plantar pressures
Abnormal foot function	Abnormal load application
High activity level	Increased cumulative stress
Vascular disease	Devitalized tissue more susceptible to injury; healing potential is less
Poor footwear	Decreased protection from environment and increased pressures on sides and top of feet
Poor footcare habits	Barefoot walking, increased pressures from thick callus lesions or foreign objects in shoes, nailbed infections, inadequate shoe break-in period, delayed detection of injuries
Vision loss	Selfcare injuries, delayed detection of injuries and frequent trauma during activity
Inadequate diabetic control	Increased susceptibility to complications

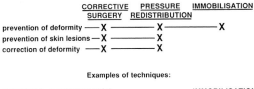

FIGURE 4–18 ■ Goals of treatment for Charcot's joints.

of tarsometatarsal fracture dislocation and arch collapse.[51]

The basic treatment of deformities associated with the diabetic foot is pressure redistribution. This gives greater distribution of the force so that pressure is diminished overall and there are no areas of high pressure generated by the deformity. In this way, skin lesions are prevented. However, since the underlying deformity remains, and may progress, it requires close observation of the foot and its orthosis. If changes in this situation go unnoticed, skin breakdown occurs. Corrective surgery of the deformity to redistribute the pressure to a more physiological state and arthrodesis in such a corrected position prevents progression.

Control of Plantar Skin Breakdown and Bony Deformity

The approach to treatment of plantar ulceration must be aimed at ulcer healing, protection of the scar of the healed ulcer, and prevention of recurrence. Pressure (Fig. 4-19) must be redistributed to the rest of the foot, so that external forces do not inhibit ulcer healing. This can be done by contact casts, orthosis, and special shoes. The healed ulcer is protected from compressive and shear forces by the orthosis. The orthosis should give even distribution of force over the whole weight-bearing area of the foot to equalize pressure and prevent recurrence of the ulcer. This requires special fabrication. This treatment does not alter the underlying physical structure of the foot. A more definitive approach is to correct the abnormality by local pressure relief, such as paring of callosities, condylectomy, metatarsal osteotomy, and excision of bony exostosis. The deformity may be less localized, and the structure of the foot may require corrective osteotomy, triple arthrodesis, midfoot arthrodesis, or flexor to extensor transfer. By these methods, both nonoperative and operative, the ultimate goal of treatment—diminution and redistribution of pressure, and restoration of the balance of the foot so that the patient regains a more normal stance and gait pattern—can be achieved.

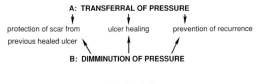

FIGURE 4–19 ■ Goals of treatment for plantar skin abnormality.

References

1. Radin EL, Paul IL. Response of joints to impact loading. Arthritis Rheum. 1971A: 14:356–362.
2. Bernstein DS, Leboeuf B, Cahill GF. Studies on glucose metabolism in cartilage in vitro. Proc Soc Exp Biol Med. 1961: 107:458–461.
3. Tell GPE, Cnatrecases P, Wyk JJ, Hinz RL. Somatomedin: Inhibition of adenylate cyclase activity in subcellular membranes or various tissues. Science. 1973: 180:312–315.
4. Weiss RE, Reddi AH. Influence of experimental diabetes and insulin on matrix induced cartilage and differentiation. Am J Phsiol. 1980: 238:E200–E207.
5. McNair P, Madsbads S, Christiansen C, Faber OK, Transbøl, Binder C. Osteopenia in insulin-treated diabetes mellitus: Its relation to age at onset, sex and duration of disease. Diabetologia. 1978. 15:87–90.
6. Carlstedt CA, Nordin M. Biomechanics of tendons and ligaments. In: Nordin & Frankel eds.,

Basic Biomechanics of the Musculoskeletal System, 2nd ed. Philadelphia, Lea & Febiger, 1989: 59–74.

7. Harkness RD. Mechanical properties of collagenous tissues. In: Gould BS ed, Biology of Collagen, vol. 2. London: Academic, 1968: 248–292.

8. Akeson WT, Savio LYW, Amiel D, Coutts RD, Daniel D. The connective tissue response to immobility. Biomechanical changes in periarticular connective tissues of the immobilized rabbit knee. Clin Orthop. 1973: 93:356–362.

9. Schnider SL, Kohn RR. Effects of age and diabetes mellitus on the solubility and non-enzymatic glycosylation of human skin collagen. J Clin Invest. 1981: 67:1630–1635.

10. Delridge L, Ellis CE, Lequesne LP. Nonenzymatic glycosylation of keratin from the diabetic foot. Br J Surg. 1983: 70:305.

11. Grgic A, Rosenbloom AL, Weber FT, Giordano B, Malone JI, Shuster JJ. Joint contracture—common manifestation of childhood diabetes mellitus. J Pediatr. 1976: 88:584–588.

12. Griffiths HJ. Diabetic osteopathy. Orthopedics. 1985: 8:401–406.

13. Newman JH. Non-infective disease of the diabetic foot. J Bone Joint Surg. 1981: 63B:593–596.

14. Steiner B, Peterson I. Electromyographic investigation of reflex effects upon stretching the partially ruptured medial collateral ligament of the knee joint. Acta Chir Scand. 1962: 124:396–411.

15. Perry J. In: Cruess RL, Rennie WRJ eds. Adult Orthopaedics. New York, Churchill Livingstone, 1984: 1161–1207.

16. Perry J. Normal and pathologic gait. In: American Academy of Orthopaedic Surgeons. Atlas of Orthotics. St. Louis, CV Mosby, 1985: 76–111.

17. Friedman SA, Rakow RB. Osseous lesions of the foot in diabetic neuropathy. Diabetes. 1971: 20:302–307.

18. Jacobs JE. Observations of neuropathic (Charcot) joints occurring in diabetes mellitus. J Bone Joint Surg. 1958: 40A:1043–1057.

19. Mayne N. The short term prognosis in diabetic neuropathy. Diabetes 1968: 17:270–273.

20. Stokes IAF, Faris IB, Hutton WC. The neuropathic ulcer and loads on the foot in diabetic patients. Acta Orthop Scand. 1975: 46:839–847.

21. Delridge L, Ctercteko G, Fowler C, Reeve TS, Lequesne LP. The etiology of diabetic neuropathic ulceration of the foot. Br J Surg. 1985: 72:1–6.

22. Maximow AA, Blomm WA. Textbook of histology. Philadelphia: Saunders, 1942: 166–167.

23. Kuhns JG. Changes in elastic adipose tissue. J Bone Joint Surg. 1949: 31A:541–547.

24. Bojsen-Moller F. Anatomy of the forefoot—normal and pathologic. Clin Orthop. 1979: 142:10–18.

25. Cavanagh PR, Lafortune MA. Ground reaction forces in distance running. J Biomech. 1980: 13:397–406.

26. Brand PW. Pressure sores—the problem. In: Kennedi RM & Cowden JM eds, Bedsore biomechanics. Baltimore: University Press, 1976: 19–23.

27. Gretchen AW, Gooding GAW, Stess RM, Graf PM,

Moss KM, Louie KS, Grunfield C. Sonography of the sole of the foot. Invest Radiol. 1986: 21:401–406.

28. Manter JT. Movements of the subtalar and transverse tarsal joints. Anat Rec. 1941: 80:397–410.

29. Wright DG, Desai SM, Henderson WH. Action of the subtalar and ankle joint complex during the stance phase of walking. J Bone Joint Surg. 1964: 46A:361–382.

30. Elftman H. The transverse tarsal joint and its control. Clin Orthop. 1960: 16:41–45.

31. Mann RA, Inman VT. Phasic activity of the intrinsic muscles of the foot. J Bone Joint Surg. 1964: 46A:469–481.

32. Morris JM. Biomechanics of the foot and ankle. Clin Orthop. 1977: 122:10–17.

33. Perry J. Anatomy and biomechanics of the hindfoot. Clin Orthop. 1983: 177:9–15.

34. Perry J. The mechanics of walking. In: Perry J, Hislop HJ eds, Principles of lower extremity bracing. New York, American Physical Therapy Association. 1967: 9–32.

35. Mann RA. Biomechanics of the foot. In: Gould JS ed, The Foot Book. Baltimore: Williams & Wilkins, 1988: 48–63.

36. Sammarco GJ. Biomechanics of the foot. In: Nordin M, Frankel VH eds. Basic Biomechanics of the Musculoskeletal System. Philadelphia, Lea & Febiger, 1989: 163–181.

37. Stokes IAF, Hutton WC, Stott JRR, Lowe LW. Forces under the hallux valgus foot before and after surgery. Clin Orthop. 1979: 142:64–72.

38. Wittenhall REH, Schwartz PL, Bornstein J. Actions of insulin and growth hormone on collagen and chondroitin sulphate synthesis in bone organ cultures. Diabetes. 1969: 18:280–284.

39. Canalis E. Effect of insulin-like growth factor I on DNA and protein synthesis in cultivated rat calvaria. J Clin Invest. 1980: 66:709–719.

40. Wiske PS, Wentworth SM, Norton SA, Epstein S, Johnston CC. Evaluation of bone mass and growth in young diabetics. Metabolism. 1982: 31:848–854.

41. Weintroub S, Eisenberg D, Tardiman R. Is diabetic osteoporosis due to microangiopathy? Lancet. 1980: 983, November 1.

42. Burkhardt R, Moser W, Bartl R, Mahl G. Is diabetic osteoporosis due to microangiopathy? Lancet. 1981: 844, April 11.

43. Cundy TF, Edmonds ME, Watkins PJ. Osteopenia and metatarsal fractures in diabetic neuropathy. Diabetic Med. 1985: 2:461–464.

44. Watkins PJ, Edmonds ME. Sympathetic nerve failure in diabetes. Diabetologia. 1983: 25:73–77.

44A. Brower AC, Allman RM. Pathogenesis of the neurotrophic joint: Neurotraumatic vs neurovascular. Diag Radiol. 1981: 139:349–354.

45. Harris JR, Brand PW. Patterns of disintegration of the tarsus in the anaesthetic foot. J Bone Joint Surg. 1966: 48B:4–16.

46. Forgacs S, Salamon F. Bone changes in diabetes mellitus. Isr J Med Sci. 1972: 8:782–783.

47. Edmonds ME. The diabetic foot: Patholphysiology and treatment. Clin Endocrinology. 1986: 15:889–916.

48. Clouse ME, Gramm HF, Legg M, Flood T. Dia-

betic osteoarthropathy: Clinical and orentgeno-graphic observations in 90 cases. AJR. 1974: 121:22–24.

49. Staple T. Radiology of the diabetic foot. In: Levin ME ed, The Diabetic Foot. St. Louis, CV Mosby, 1983: 142–168.

50. Bailey CC, Root HF. Neuropathic foot lesions in diabetes mellitus. N Engl J Med. 1947: 236:397–401.

51. Sinha S, Munichoodappa CS, Kozak GP. Neuro-arthropathy (Charcot joints) in diabetic patients. Medicine. 1972: 51:191–209.

52. Cofield RH, Morrison MJ, Beabout J. Diabetic neuropathy in the foot: Patient characteristics and patterns of radiographic change. Foot Ankle. 1983: 4:15–22.

53. Wagner FW. The diabetic foot. Orthopedics. 1987: 10:163–172.

54. Brand PW. Paralysis of nerves in leprosy. Int J Lepr Other Mycobact Dis. 1966: 34:184–186.

55. Ellenberg M. Diabetic neuropathic ulcer. Mt. Sinai J Med. 1968: 35:585–594.

56. Dabezies E, Chuinard RG. The diabetic foot. Orthopedics. 1979: 2:290–295.

57. Catteral RC. The diabetic foot. Br J Hosp Med. 1972: 7:224–227.

58. Klenerman L. The foot and its disorders. Oxford: Blackwell's Scientific Publications. 1976: 180–181.

59. Boehm HJ. Diabetic Charcot joint. N Engl J Med. 1962: 267:185–187.

60. Zlatkin MB, Pathria M, Sartoris DJ, Resnick. The diabetic foot. Radiol Clin North Am. 1987: 25:1095–1105.

61. Boulton AJ, Hardisty CA, Betts RP, Franks CI, Worth RC, Ward JD, Duckworth T. Dynamic foot pressures and other studies as diagnostic and management aids in diabetic neuropathy. Diabetes Care. 1983: 6:26–33.

62. Lang-Stevenson AI, Sharrard WJ, Betts RP, Duck-worth T. Neuropathic ulcers of the foot. J Bone Joint Surg. 1985: 67B:438–442.

63. Cavanagh PR, Henning EM, Rogers MM. The measurement of pressure distribution on the plantar surface of diabetic feet. In: Whittle M and Harris D eds, Biomechanical measurement in orthopaedic practice. Oxford London: Clarendon Press, 1985: 159–168.

64. Ctercteko GC, Dhanendran D, Hutton WC, Lequesne LP. Vertical forces acting on the feet of diabetic patients with neuropathic ulceration. Br J Surg. 1981: 68:608–614.

65. Boulton AJ, Betts RP, Franks CI, Newrick PG, Ward JD, Duckworth T. Abnormalities of foot pressure in early diabetic neuropathy. Diabetic Med. 1987: 4:225–228.

66. Pollard JP, Lequesne LP. Method of healing diabetic forefoot ulcers. Br Med J. 1983: 286, 436–437.

67. Bauman JH, Girling JP, Brand PW. Plantar pressures and trophic ulceration. J Bone Joint Surg. 1963: 45B:652–673.

68. Cavanagh PR. Personal Communication, 1989.

69. Wagner FW. The diabetic foot and amputation of the foot. In: Mann RA ed, Du Vries' Surgery of the Foot. 1978: 341–380.

70. Deanfield JE, Dagett PR, Harrison MJ. The role of autonomic neuropathy in diabetic foot ulceration. J Neurol Sci. 1980: 47:203–210.

71. Boulton AJ, Franks CI, Betts RP, Duckworth T, Ward JD. Reduction of abnormal foot pressures in diabetic neuropathy using a new polymer insole material. Diabetes Care. 1984: 711:42–46.

72. Dimonte P, Light H. Pathomechanics, gait deviations and treatment of the rheumatoid foot. Phys Ther. 1982: 62:1148–1156.

73. Radin EL, Paul IL. Importance of bone in sparing articular cartilage from impact. Clin Orthop. 1971B: 78:342–344.

5 Plantar Pressure in the Diabetic Foot

PETER R. CAVANAGH, PH.D.,
AND JAN S. ULBRECHT, M.D.

Attempts to measure the distribution of pressure under the foot or shoe were made at least as early as 1882, but it has only been in the last 25 years that measurements were made in patients with insensitive feet.[1] The contributions of Brand originally focused on prevention of injury in patients with Hansen's disease, and in 1975 the results of pressure distribution studies in a significant number of diabetic patients were published.[2] Systems designed to allow "turnkey" measurement of plantar pressure distribution in a clinical environment have appeared in the last 5 years, but as yet no well-established clinical protocols have been accepted for office or hospital applications. The purpose of this chapter is to review current techniques of plantar pressure measurement and to consider the usefulness of such measurements for the prevention of lesions in the diabetic foot.

RATIONALE FOR PRESSURE MEASUREMENT

Repetitive application of high pressures during the activities of daily life can lead to ulceration on the plantar surface of the insensitive foot.[2-7] No prospective study has shown the association between elevated plantar pressures and plantar ulceration, but cross-sectional studies have shown a clear relationship between the site of ulceration and the presence of elevated pressures in diabetic patients.[2,3] Higher values of plantar pressure have also been found in diabetic patients with ulcers compared to diabetic patients with neuropathy but no ulcers or to age-matched nondiabetic controls.[3]

Circumstantial evidence has shown that elevated plantar pressure is a risk factor for ulceration in the diabetic foot. Elevated plantar pressure, however, even in the presence of sensory neuropathy, has not been proved to cause a plantar ulcer. Peak plantar pressure is one of many cofactors of ulceration including, but not limited to, peripheral sensory neuropathy. This conclusion has developed from seeing patients with loss of sensation, high pressure, and no plantar ulceration.

Among the many putative risk factors for plantar ulceration are sensory, motor, and autonomic neuropathy, foot deformity, vascular disease, soft tissue atrophy or displacement, abnormal gait and foot function, improper footwear, and elevated activity profiles. These have been discussed by many authors[3,4,6,8-10] and by us.[11,13] In the future, it may be reasonable to screen patients routinely with diabetes who have not had foot lesions for a certain combination of the above "necessary" factors, one of which is likely to be elevated plantar pressure. Intervention would then follow to prevent ulceration.

Measurement of pressure distribution can be used to evaluate the validity of a footwear intervention in a patient who has already experienced a plantar ulcer. Even though the exact combination of risk factors that caused the ulcer may be unknown, the patient who has ulcerated exhibits at least the required combination, and is at risk for re-ulceration. Whereas conservative methods for ulcer healing are well established,[14,15] the evaluation of techniques for preventing re-ulceration using "off-the-shelf" or custom footwear are still elementary. The statement "Prescription shoe fitting and shoe correcting are more an art than a science"[16] still seems to be true. Shoe fitting is usually performed by a pedorthist, who often receives a vague prescription as a guide. Follow-up by a physician usually occurs only in an emergency. A common method of evaluating a prescription is trial and error. Some shoe alterations might actually exacerbate a problem that they were theoretically designed to alleviate. Although some rocker bottom shoe designs have been shown to reduce pressures under all measured regions of the foot,[17] others have shown increased heel pressures and a tendency for increased pressure in the lateral metatarsal heads using one rocker design.[18] In-shoe pressure measurement has the potential to revolutionize the way shoe treatments are determined.

Thus, pressure measurement can be useful in the prevention of lesions in patients who have been lesion-free and in the prevention of re-ulceration. It may also lead to a lower rate of lower extremity amputation.[8,19] Given such promise, pressure distribution measurement appears to warrant further study.

TECHNICAL ISSUES

Most orthopedists who treat the foot are familiar with a conventional force plate that measures the three components of the net load acting on the foot in the cardinal planes, but this does not provide any information about the distribution of that load in relation to the anatomic structures.[20,21] It is impossible to tell from a conventional force platform if the patient has concentrations of high plantar pressure. Force and pressure are different quantities, and the terms should not be used interchangeably. Pressure, or, more correctly, stress, is the force per unit area and can be calculated on any plane. The units of pressure are psi (pounds per square inch)

and Pascals (newtons per square meter Pa).* The two most common planes used to measure stress in relation to the foot-floor or foot-shoe interface are the plane of the floor—vertical stress, known as normal stress (or, in lay terms, pressure) and horizontal or shear stress. Shear stress may be more amenable to reduction by footwear intervention than normal stress[22] and may be important as a cause of ulceration.[23] No satisfactory method yet exists for measuring shear stress between the foot and its supporting surface, so the discussion here is confined to normal stress (pressure).

No widely applicable norms are available at present for the clinician to use to determine if a particular patient has abnormally high or low plantar pressures. An important reason for this is that an examination of the same patient on different devices is likely to yield different results. This is not a calibration problem but a function of different element sizes in the measuring devices used. Most devices measure the net force acting on the sensor and the pressure is then estimated from dividing the force by the area of the sensor.

The effect of increasing the linear dimensions of the sensor can be dramatic (Fig. 5-1). Because area varies with the square of length, the same mass of 75 kg distributed over 1 cm^2 could appear to be a pressure of 735 kPa (the correct value), 327, or 184 kPa if the square sensor had side lengths of 1, 1.5, or 2 cm, respectively. Normal values must therefore be collected for each type of device to have any meaning, but this has not been done for most commercially available systems. The above cautions are important when results from optical devices, such as the Pedobarograph, are compared with matrix devices, such as the EMED unit (see Fig. 5-2). Optical devices have a high effective resolution and yield higher values than devices that have larger elements.

---

*The units of pressure that are most familiar in the US and the UK are pounds per square inch (psi), but the SI unit is the pascal (abbreviated Pa) which is defined as 1 newton (N) per square meter (the force under a mass of 1 kg placed on the earth is 9.81 N. Because one pascal is an extremely small pressure, plantar pressures are generally expressed in kilopascals (1,000 Pa = 1 kPa = 14.2 psi) or megapascals (1,000,000 Pa = 1MPa = 142 psi).

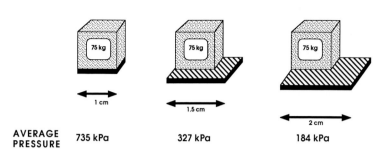

AVERAGE
PRESSURE   735 kPa   327 kPa   184 kPa

FIGURE 5–1 ■ Dependence of average pressure on the size of the measuring element. The same mass of 75 kg distributed over 1 cm² could appear to be a pressure of 750 (the correct value), 334, or 187 kPa if the square sensor had side lengths of 1, 1.5, or 2 cm, respectively.

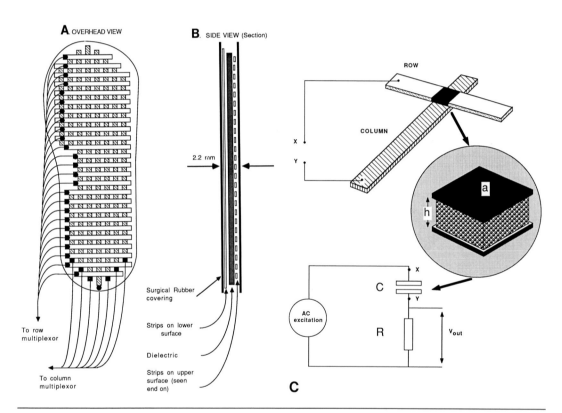

FIGURE 5–2 ■ Schematic of the matrix arrangement used to form individual elements at the intersection of rows and columns in a matrix mat system such as the EMED or FSCAN devices. *A,* Overhead view. *B,* side view (section). The conductive strips on the top and bottom of a spacer are at 90° with respect to each other. They are connected to a multiplexor that can switch each row or column to be the active strip for a brief period. Although the example shown is for an in-shoe device, flat platforms use the same principle. *C,* Schematic of how an individual variable capacitor is formed at the intersection of a row and column when an electrical connection is made between the two. The capacitance (*C*) is proportional to the distance between the plates, which is itself a function of the applied pressure. To estimate the pressure each element in turn is switched into a measurement circuit by multiplexors. In systems in which the sensor acts as a variable resistor, the measuring circuit is basically similar.

When a device is selected such issues as limits, calibration, linearity, hysteresis, and other technical specifications must be acceptable.[11] The technology for pressure measurement is complex and the manufacturer must provide complete, accurate, and readily interpretable information concerning the performance of any system.

MEASURING AND ANALYZING PLANTAR PRESSURE

It is helpful to have a general idea of how devices that measure plantar pressure work and what type of analysis of results is typically performed. Devices that measure plantar pressure are of two types: those that measure pressure at a few discrete locations, and those that measure a distribution of pressure across the entire sole. The interface at which the measurement is made varies with different devices. Some measure pressure between the bare foot and the ground (or shoe and ground), which is sometimes of interest. Others measure interface pressures between the foot and the shoe. Although the latter is functionally relevant, it is difficult to perform. An attractive feature of studying contact between the bare foot and a flat surface—is that it allows the fundamental pattern to be measured and compared with those of other patients and populations, independent of the effects of footwear.

Brand and associates[5] have performed studies with discrete transducers working as variables capacitors. These were placed at areas thought to be at risk under the forefoot and heel.[17] The only commercial device of this type available is the Electrodynogram (EDG).* This device has a waist pack carried by the subject and seven extremely thin sensors that are applied to each foot. Interpretation of the pattern is performed by the computer using an "expert system" approach to evaluation. Although the data processing aspects of the system appear to be suited to the task, attention has been sharply focused on the properties and calibration of the sensors that are on the foot. Brodsky and colleagues[24] have suggested that

the properties of the EDG sensors make the device unreliable and inaccurate, and have discouraged its use.

An objection to measurement using any discrete system is that some a priori assumptions about the pattern of plantar pressure must be made when placing the sensors on the foot. Because a limited number of sensors are used, not all regions can be studied. Even in a foot without deformity this approach is questionable, but sampling in a foot with major structural abnormality can be particularly difficult.

The simplest method available today for plantar pressure distribution measurement is the Harris mat,[4] from an original design by Morton.[25]† The underside of a multilayered, inked rubber mat makes contact with a piece of paper. As the patient walks across the mat a variable density impression is left on the paper, with local density depending on the plantar pressure. Small mats are also available that can be placed inside shoes.[4] Unfortunately, the device only has approximately a four-point scale and saturates at a pressure well within the normal range (about 470 kPa), so that all values above this level result in the same reading.[12] Thus, the Harris mat can provide only a gross indication of plantar pressure distribution.

The three major systems for pressure distribution measurement that are commercially available also differ from each other in their methods of operation and in the nature of their results. The EMED system* belongs to a class of devices characterized as matrix mats, in which the individual sensors are formed electronically at the intersection of rows and columns of conductive material.[26] A rectangular device with 40 rows and 40 columns, each 1 by 48 cm, it appears functionally to be a 1600-element mat with 1 by 1 cm elements separated by a gap of 2 mm. Small flexible units can be made for in-shoe measurements,[18] but at present these are not in routine production. The principle of operation is the same for either a platform or an in-shoe device (Fig. 5-2). An electrical component, usually a capaci-

---

*Langer Biomechanics Group, Inc., 21 East Industry Court, Deer Park, NY 11729.

†Apex Foot Imprint System, Apex Foot Health Industries, 170 Wesley Street, South Hackensack, NJ 07606.
*Novel USA, 511 11th Street, Minneapolis, MN 55415.

tor or a resistor, varies its properties depending on the applied load.

In the EMED system the active element is a variable capacitor, whereas in the FSCAN device[†] the active element is a variable resistor. The FSCAN is sold as a disposable in-shoe sensor with over 1000 active elements. If the electromechanical properties of this device are shown to be reliable and accurate, it could represent a valuable addition to the field.

The final commercially available system for pressure distribution measurement is the Pedobarograph.[*] This system uses a mat with tiny dimples on its surface. The mat is placed, dimples down, on a piece of side-illuminated plate glass. As increasing pressure is applied to the upper flat surface of the mat, the dimples flatten out; this is viewed by a television camera from beneath the plate as a change in light intensity.[27,28] This method is not readily amenable to in-shoe measurement but has the best spatial resolution of any of the available systems.

All these systems require computers that produce displays of varying complexity and visual appeal. They may feature color, three dimensions, animation, regional analysis, impulse measurement, and many other features.[11] Research has not yet progressed to the point at which measurements and methods of analysis critical to identification of the at-risk foot can be stated with certainty. For example, although it seems reasonable that the simple magnitude of pressure is important, it is not yet known whether a lower pressure acting for a longer time and thus resulting in a larger impulse is equally damaging to the tissues of the foot.

Because no accepted standards are available, the following discussion focuses on experience with patients at the Center for Locomotion Studies (at Penn State University). All data presented here, with the exception of the in-shoe data, were collected with a 1000-element piezoelectric pressure distribution mat manufactured at Penn State and analyzed with custom-written software. Although neither this hardware nor software is available commercially, most systems have the capability of generating similar displays.

For illustrative purposes, a pressure distribution pattern is presented of the right foot of a 38-year-old type I diabetic female with pain in the midfoot despite peripheral neuropathy as revealed by vibration and monofilament testing. The starting point for most analyses is a series of photos of pressure distribution at intervals during ground contact (Fig. 5-3). Each diagram is an average of all pressures in one-eighth of the contact phase. These and subsequent plots are viewed as if the observer were looking down on the foot from above, so that the pattern of plantar pressure can be visualized "through" the foot. It is apparent from the sequence that this patient has a functional rocker bottom foot with the base of the fifth metatarsal loaded soon after foot strike. This prominence became the fulcrum of the rocker movement until the area under the second metatarsal head was loaded in the last 250 msec of the contact phase. No pressure is under the toes, and the lateral and medical aspects of the forefoot were minimally involved in the weight-bearing process. A force-time curve is shown in the bottom corner of the display and is similar to the pattern that would be recorded from a conventional force platform. The vertical line on this curve shows the time periods that were averaged to generate the eight individual pressure diagrams.

Figure 5-4 summarizes the largest pressure applied to each area of the foot, regardless of time of occurrence. This display is called a peak pressure plot; it represents a peak memory in which the largest value is retained. The largest pressure on any part of the foot is usually reported with the diagram, and for this patient it was 2.1 MPa. Figure 5-4 and the other diagrams were designed to saturate with the red color at a value of 750 kPa, although the numeric data on the exact pressures are always available. No absolute threshold for damage to the foot has yet been established and the value of 750 kPa represents an arbitrary choice, especially because it is inside the 95% confidence limits for some regions of the foot in a symptom-free population of elderly men using our device (see below, Fig. 5-6). The color coding scheme was chosen to identify patients below critical values, but in need of examination.

Through computer analysis of the digi-

†Tekscan, Inc., 451 D Street, Boston MA 02210.
*Biokinetics, 5413 West Cedar Lane, Bethesda, MD.

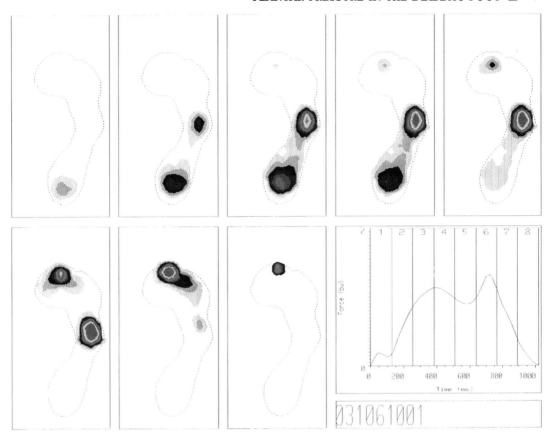

FIGURE 5–3 ■ Pressure sequence showing data from periods during entire contact of right foot of a patient with a functional rocker bottom foot, in whom the base of the fifth metatarsal was loaded soon after foot strike. The second metatarsal head was loaded in the last 250 msec of the contact phase. No pressures were under the toes at any time, and the medial and lateral aspects of the forefoot were minimally involved in the weight-bearing process.

tized footprint, the foot is divided into ten standard regions. Regional peak pressure, regardless of its time of occurrence, is computed for each region and tabulated with standard deviations. For the patient (shown in Fig. 5-4) the regional analysis, shown in Figure 5-5, indicates mean peak pressures of 1.57, 1.02 and 1.64 MPa in the lateral midfoot, first metatarsal head, and second metatarsal head regions, respectively. These values are well above the 95% confidence limits that we have calculated from a symptom-free population. The finding of elevated pressures under the first metatarsal head is an artifact of regional division in this case, because it is clear from Figure 5-4 that this is overflow from the extremely

high pressure under the head of the second metatarsal.

Impulse analysis revealed reversal of magnitude in loading on the two focal areas, with the impulse being greater under the midfoot and the peak pressure greater under the metatarsal heads. This might have been predicted from Figure 5-3, because the area under the metatarsal heads was loaded with a higher pressure but for a much shorter time. The elevated midfoot pressures in this patient were apparently the result of an untreated Charcot fracture.

Figures 5-3, 5-4, and 5-5 provide a fairly complete analysis of foot contact with the ground, which can be compared with previous visits of the same patient, and with

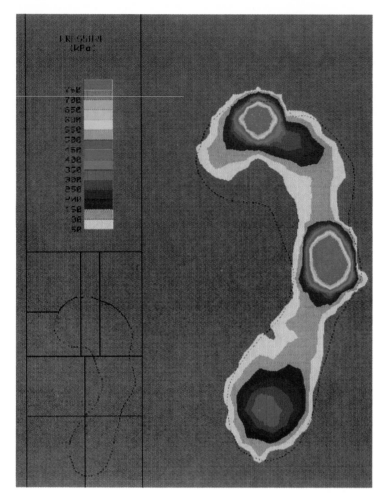

FIGURE 5–4 ■ Peak pressure plot for the right foot contact shown in Figure 5-3. This plot summarizes the highest pressure applied to each region of the foot, regardless of its time of occurrence. This and all subsequent diagrams have been deliberately designed to saturate with the deep red color when a value of 750 kPa is reached, although the numeric data of the exact pressures are always available.

other patients and normal subjects. Such displays are not the only analytic methods that can be used. Peak pressure versus time displays for the whole foot or for individual regions can also be generated, although these can be difficult to interpret, with many overlapping graphs on the same display.[29]

Investigators disagree about the standard activity that should be studied. The choices include standing on both feet or one foot, free walking, or the first step of gait. Duckworth and associates[29] have suggested that walking pressures are more likely to be related to the potential for ulceration than standing pressures. Our preference is to collect all data during the first step onto the measuring platform after the initiation of walking from a standing position. This avoids the problem of targeting for patients

with ataxic gaits or poor eyesight and helps to standardize the measurements within and among patients. Evidence has shown that heel pressures during free gait might be slightly lower than those recorded during first step, but pressures under the anterior regions of the foot appear to be similar between the two methods.[48] Five trials are collected from each foot to estimate the variability of each patient.

LITERATURE REVIEW

Normal Values

The establishment of normal values for a symptom-free population is complicated by the issue of device configuration that was

FIGURE 5–5 ■ Regional analysis of the data shown in Figure 5-4, along with four other trials of the same foot from this patient. The division of the footprint into regions is performed by an automatic algorithm and the peak pressure in each of these ten regions is then located for each of the five trials. The mean, standard deviations, and coefficients of variation are calculated. The location of the peak pressure within each region on each trial is shown by the diamonds on the foot outline; the mean arch index (a measure of foot shape) and the foot placement angle are also shown. See text for further details.

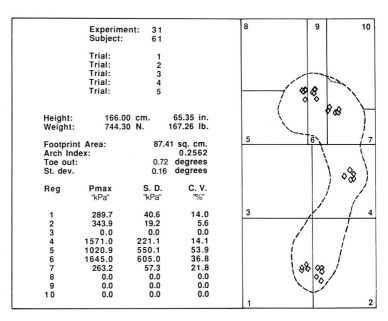

Experiment:	31	
Subject:	61	

Trial:	1
Trial:	2
Trial:	3
Trial:	4
Trial:	5

| Height: | 166.00 cm. | 65.35 in. |
| Weight: | 744.30 N. | 167.26 lb. |

Footprint Area:		87.41 sq. cm.
Arch Index:		0.2562
Toe out:		0.72 degrees
St. dev.		0.16 degrees

Reg	Pmax "kPa"	S. D. "kPa"	C. V. "%"
1	289.7	40.6	14.0
2	343.9	19.2	5.6
3	0.0	0.0	0.0
4	1571.0	221.1	14.1
5	1020.9	550.1	53.9
6	1645.0	605.0	36.8
7	263.2	57.3	21.8
8	0.0	0.0	0.0
9	0.0	0.0	0.0
10	0.0	0.0	0.0

exemplified by Figure 5-1. As mentioned previously, the same patients could record different values on different devices. In addition, preprocessing of data, such as filtering in time or space, can radically affect results. Even if we circumvent these technical problems by using a single device, the normal range is so wide that the usual use of the mean plus and minus two standard deviations places patients at risk for ulceration within the normal range. This emphasizes the tremendous variability in foot structure and function characteristic of the "normal" population. Elevated pressures can be a pre-existing condition in many diabetics, and not necessarily a consequence of diabetes. When the specific diabetes-associated risk factors are added, ulceration can sometimes result.

Figure 5-6 shows this variation in a symptom-free group of elderly nondiabetic men. Each region has its mean; these range from 15 kPa in the medial midfoot to 533 kPa under the second metatarsal head. This broad region-specific range emphasizes the need to consider each region by its own reference value rather than by looking at the peak pressure in the whole foot, regardless of location. Confidence intervals are broad, reaching a maximum value of 976 kPa in

the second metatarsal head region for the upper limit of "normality." Patients with plantar ulcers who exhibit pressures considerably lower than this value, however, have been noted. The shaded area in Figure 5-6 represents values that are over 750 kPa (these appear as deep red in our diagrams). The mean values for peak pressure in the second and lateral metatarsal head regions are both greater than the mean value in the first metatarsal head region. This finding, which confirms earlier work,[30] indicates that the conventional idea of the first metatarsal head as the most highly loaded region of the foot in walking is false.[25] The hallux does, however, experience pressures that are close to the maximum seen in any region of the foot as has been noted by a number of investigators.[31,32] In cases of hallux rigidus, the plantar pressure is likely to be extremely high, with an accompanying high risk of ulceration.

Another approach to establishing normal values is to look at a group of diabetic patients who were otherwise apparently at risk but did not ulcerate. In this way, Boulton and associates,[3,28,29,33,34] who used a Pedobarograph, have identified a value of approximately 1 MPa as their normal limit, regardless of its location on the foot. The

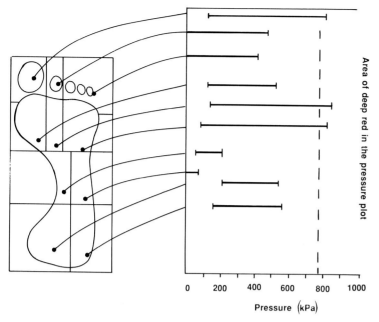

FIGURE 5-6 ■ The 95% confidence limits for the means (in kilopascals) of regional plantar pressures during "first step." Data collected from a sample of 27 symptom-free elderly males. Pressure values at the far right (greater than 750 kPa) are shown as deep red in all contour plots.

discrepancy between this value and those in Figure 5-6 is a combination of the difference in measuring techniques between Boulton and colleagues and those at the Center for Locomotion Studies and a difference in patient populations. Regional norms seem to be a reasonable approach because the midfoot and heel, for example, do not generally experience pressures as high as those in the metatarsal head regions. Values that are dangerous for the midfoot might be tolerable for the metatarsal heads. A single threshold for damage to the foot might exist, however, regardless of location, and this question remains unresolved. If the motivation for ordering a test on a patient is to rule out a particular pathology, it would be concluded at present that pressure distribution measurement cannot provide an answer. However, pressure measurement can provide information on the interaction of the patient's foot with the shoe or ground and information about foot function can be obtained. Such information could not be provided by observation or routine examination. In addition, if values in a lesion-free patient approach or exceed the normative values presented above, then the index of suspicion is heightened and the patient must be considered a candidate for footwear modification.

Another clinical use of pressure distribution measurement is to catalog changes over time that might be too subtle to detect by a routine foot examination. Although it has not yet been conclusively demonstrated, patients with suspected progressive foot deformity[35] or with limited joint mobility syndrome[36,37] can show early increases in plantar pressure distribution before other signs of foot injury are apparent.

Studies of Diabetic Patients

Stokes and co-workers[2] have shown that diabetic patients with plantar ulcers had significantly greater loads than patients without ulcers or control subjects. Because the patients were significantly heavier than the control group, these authors attributed this increase to greater body weight. Experience has shown that peak plantar pressure during standing is not well correlated with body weight. This finding is interpreted to mean that foot deformity is more important than the simple calculation of body weight divided by foot area.[38] Stokes and colleagues[2] also showed significantly decreased load-bearing on the toes, a finding that has been confirmed by subsequent investigators.[33,39] An association was demonstrated between the site of greatest load and the site of ulceration, but in the ten patients with no history of ulceration the most calloused areas were not always those most heavily loaded. This implies that other factors, including shear stress, are also important in the development of callous lesions.

Ctercteko and associates[39] have confirmed the results of Stokes and co-workers.[2] They also determined the site of maximum force and found that all ulcers in the metatarsal region occurred at this site. When compared to controls, both diabetic groups studied showed significantly less pressure under the toes and a medial shift of load-bearing under the forefoot. It was hypothesized that the absence of toe action during gait causes increased pressure to be transferred to the metatarsal heads, and it was suggested that this can predispose to ulceration.[39] They also suggested that foot deformity—whether pre-existing or related to neuropathy—was a common feature, and must be viewed as the reason for localized high pressure.

Boulton and colleagues[3] have collected pressure distribution and other data on 82 diabetics (41 diabetics with neuropathy and 41 diabetics without neuropathy) and 41 nondiabetic controls. The 22 feet that ulcerated, all in the neuropathic group, had peak plantar pressures higher than 1.07 MPa; however, 12 diabetic patients with neuropathy who had pressures above this threshold did not ulcerate. The patients who ulcerated were found to have a significantly longer duration of neuropathy and were significantly heavier than the other patients in the study, and none of them experienced sweating in the feet. In addition to pressure measurement, a vibratory perception threshold greater than 35 in the great toe proved to be the measurement most associated with ulceration. Of the 28 neuropathic patients who had not ulcerated, however, ten also exceeded this value.

In a subsequent study, Boulton and associates[34] modified the foot-floor interface in 35 diabetic patients with clinical evidence of peripheral neuropathy, 11 of whom had a history of plantar ulceration. After a 5-mm thick sheet of viscoelastic polymer was placed over the surface of the Pedobarograph the patients again walked barefoot across the device. Mean reductions of 1 MPa and 382 kPa were achieved for those in the ulcer and nonulcer groups, respectively. Although these measurements were of the pressures between the floor and the polymer sheet, and not between the foot and the polymer sheet, it is likely that considerable reductions in pressure at the latter interface were also achieved by the polymer sheet.

Boulton et al.[33] found high peak pressures in a study of patients with no clinical signs of neuropathy but abnormal nerve conduction velocities and vibration perception. This implies that early structural or functional changes may occur before clinically apparent signs, and these may cause elevated plantar pressure. They also developed a "toe loading ratio" that was significantly reduced compared to that of controls in the diabetic patients with high metatarsal head pressures, but not significantly different in patients with normal forefoot pressures.[33]

Cavanagh and colleagues[40] have completed a 2-year prospective study of pressure distribution in 60 diabetic men and a control group of age-matched nondiabetic controls. Peak pressures underneath the forefoot in the diabetic group increased over the 2-year period, whereas pressures in the control group slightly decreased. The difference between the group responses over time was statistically significant. Again, these findings might be an expression of the progressive foot deformity that has been hypothesized to accompany motor neuropathy.[41,42] Pressure distribution in patients with Charcot neuropathy of the midfoot has also been studied.[43] The mean midfoot peak plantar pressure in 7 feet with midfoot collapse was 748 kPa (±596 kPa, more than 10 standard deviations from the regional mean presented in Fig. 5-6). Although the distribution in grossly deformed feet was predictable, some feet with minor disruption apparent on roentgenograms also had high plantar pressures (see Case Studies).

Studies of Footwear

Although no studies have been published in which the results of footwear intervention in diabetic patients were reported, some researchers have studied symptom-free subjects walking in footwear that is traditionally prescribed for insensitive feet. From in-shoe measurements with discrete transducers, Coleman[17] reported significant reduction of pressure underneath the second and fourth metatarsal heads using various rocker bottom shoe designs. Using a similar experimental arrangement, Sims and Birke[44] found a progressive decrease in metatarsal head pressure as the apex of a rocker was moved posteriorly. Schaff and Cavanagh[18,49] used a 72-element in-shoe capacitance transducer array similar to that shown in Figure 5-2A, and found that a particular rocker bottom shoe reduced pressure by over 30% at the medial forefoot during treadmill walking as compared to a conventional, extra-depth shoe (Fig. 5-7). Peak pressures over the lateral margin of the forefoot were increased, however, indicating that the same design of rocker could not be considered adequate for all types of deformity.

CASE STUDIES

The following case studies from the Diabetic Foot Clinic at Penn State University illustrate the role of pressure distribution measurement in the overall evaluation of diabetic patients. Pressure distribution data are collected from both feet as part of a comprehensive examination of the patients who visit the foot clinic, regardless of their foot complaint. A review of the pressure distribution data is helpful to further our understanding of the mechanics of a particular foot during gait, and to enable us to implicate or eliminate elevated plantar pressure as a possible cause of foot injury.

Case 1

Figure 5-8 shows peak pressure plots collected from a 53-year-old, type I diabetic female with a history of at least six ulcers on the plantar aspect of the right great toe over 8 years. She had patchy loss of sensation, with markedly elevated vibration perception thresholds under both great toes bilaterally. Hallux extension was limited to 42° bilaterally. Pressure distributions (Fig. 5-8) indicated functional cavus feet with pressures lower than 50 kPa in the entire midfoot. Regional peak pressure values from five trials on each foot indicated that all regional values were below the means presented in Figure 5-6, except for the hallux bilaterally. The uncertainty over thresholds

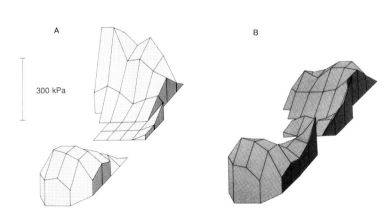

A

300 kPa

B

FIGURE 5–7 ■ Three-dimensional peak pressure diagrams for a single subject during walking in a normal shoe (*A*) and a rocker bottom shoe (*B*). The resolution of the device did not permit a standard contour display; instead, the pressure is shown vertically at the site of each transducer. The scale bar shown is 300 kPa. Note the reduction in pressure achieved by the rocker shoe over the medial and central regions of the forefoot. Pressure is, however, slightly increased in the heel and in the lateral midfoot regions. Data from Schaff and Cavanagh.[18]

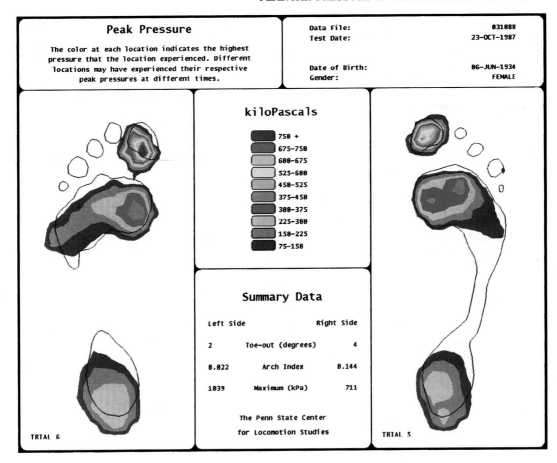

FIGURE 5–8 ■ Peak pressure plots from a 53-year-old, type I diabetic female who reported a history of at least six ulcers on the plantar aspect of the right great toe over an 8-year period. Hallux extension was limited to 42° bilaterally and mean pressures under the hallux from five trials were 150 kPa above the mean shown in Figure 5–6 bilaterally (the values shown in the figure are for a single trial). See text for further details.

for injury and this patient's history of chronic ulceration indicated that this finding was probably significant. The patient was prescribed roomy running shoes that had been made into a rocker configuration, and these were successful in preventing reulceration through a 20-month follow-up.

Case 2

Figure 5-9 illustrates peak pressure plots from a 69-year-old, type II diabetic male farmer referred for pain in his right foot. He had marked clawing of the toes and an equinovarus deformity on the right side secondary to an old crush injury, without a

history of plantar ulceration. Dense callous lesions were present over all metatarsal heads, except the second on the right side. Protective sensation was intact on the left side (as measured by monofilaments), but diminished on the right side. This might have been a spurious finding, given the density of the callous. Vibration perception was, however, diminished bilaterally. The normally appearing distribution of pressure on the left side contrasted with the reduced heel pressures, absence of toe pressures, and exceptionally high pressures (averaging 1.7 MPa) under the lateral metatarsal heads on the right side. Given the questionable status of sensation on the right side, footwear modification was prescribed to reduce fore-

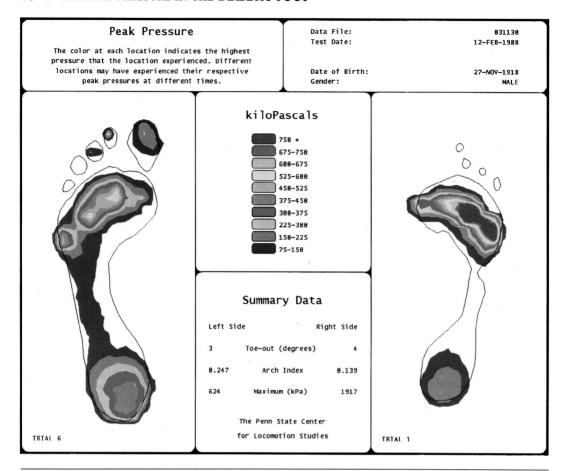

Peak Pressure

The color at each location indicates the highest pressure that the location experienced. Different locations may have experienced their respective peak pressures at different times.

Data File: 031130
Test Date: 12-FEB-1988

Date of Birth: 27-NOV-1918
Gender: MALE

kiloPascals

750 +
675-750
600-675
525-600
450-525
375-450
300-375
225-300
150-225
75-150

Summary Data

Left Side		Right Side
3	Toe-out (degrees)	4
0.247	Arch Index	0.139
624	Maximum (kPa)	1917

The Penn State Center
for Locomotion Studies

TRIAL 6

TRIAL 1

FIGURE 5–9 ■ Peak pressure plots from a 69-year-old, type II diabetic male with marked clawing of the toes and an equinovarus deformity on the right side. Dense callous lesions were present over all metatarsal heads, except the second on the right side. Reduced heel pressures, absence of toe pressures, and exceptionally high pressures averaging 1.7 MPa under the third and fourth metatarsal heads were noted on the right side. See text for further details.

foot pressures and to prevent possible future injury to the plantar surface.

Case 3

The distributions shown in Figure 5-10 were collected as part of the evaluation of a 60-year-old, type II diabetic male with a history of alcoholism. Deformities in the right foot had developed without medical attention. Incision and drainage of a grossly swollen right foot were performed during hospitalization for associated problems. This was followed by a chronic, nonhealing ulcer on which the patient had continued to walk

for 12 months. A cast had failed to effect healing, as had custom-molded shoes. Roentgenography revealed gross disruption of the right midfoot with a rocker bottom deformity and an apparent plantar prominence of the displaced cuboid. The patient had peripheral polyneuropathy, with readings at all sites being off-scale for both vibration and monofilaments. The pressure distribution for the right foot showed the expected pattern, with pressures higher than 1 MPa in the midfoot and no weight-bearing of significance in any other region. The measurement of the apparently uninvolved left foot, however, indicated a collapse of the medial column, with pressures of 1.4

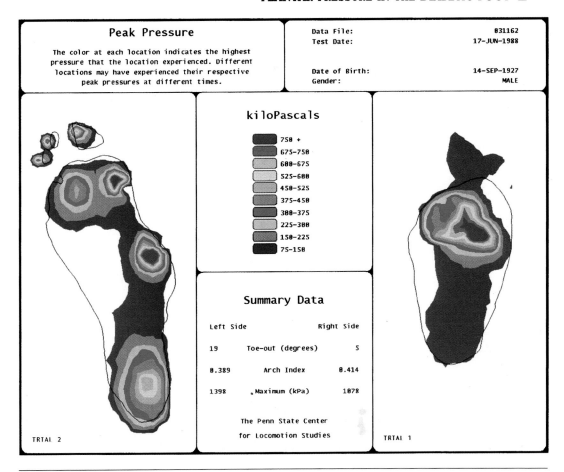

FIGURE 5–10 ■ Peak pressure plots from a patient with a chronic nonhealing ulcer under a rocker bottom deformity in the right midfoot. The pressure distribution for the right foot showed the expected pattern with pressures greater than 1 MPa in the midfoot, but the apparently uninvolved left foot exhibited a collapse of the medial column with pressures of 1.4 MPa.

MPa in the medial midfoot region in addition to pressures of 1 MPa in the forefoot. The immediate recommendation was bed rest and surgery to remove the plantar prominence on the right foot. The examination also focused concern on the apparent changes that were underway in the structure of the left foot, and that were not previously noted.

Case 4

A 54-year-old female had a 23-year history of type II diabetes (Fig. 5-11). She first visited the clinic after an episode of swelling in the right great toe. She exhibited a loss of protective sensation in the forefoot bi-laterally and practiced poor foot care, professing that she "hated to look at her feet." She denied a previous history of plantar ulcers. Hallux extension was adequate bilaterally and no significant forefoot deformity was detected. The peak pressure plots reveal both an unusual distribution and regions of elevated pressure. Both the base and head of the fifth metatarsal were loaded bilaterally with values of more than 850 kPa on the left and higher than 1 MPa on the right. Footwear recommendations were made to relieve these pressures, and an enhanced regimen of foot care was suggested.

One year after the initial visit the patient again complained of swelling in the right foot and, during a routine visit to investigate this

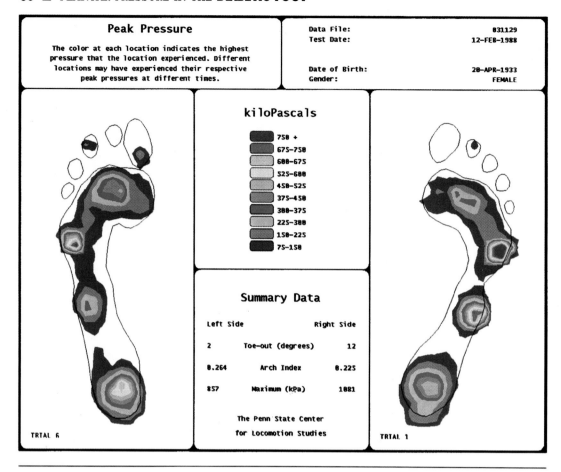

FIGURE 5–11 ■ Peak pressure plots from a 54-year-old female with a 23-year history of type II diabetes. The base and head of the fifth metatarsal were loaded bilaterally with values of more than 850 kPa on the left side and more than 1 MPa on the right. The patient eventually developed a lesion on the plantar aspect of the right great toe, but repetitive trauma was ruled out based on the pressure distribution pattern. The injury was eventually traced to the wearing of open-toed sandals in the previous week, and presumed close encounter with a foreign object between the toe and the shoe. The possibility of progressive bony changes in the midfoot was also being followed carefully.

problem, a lesion was found on the plantar aspect of the great toe, which was unknown to the patient. Pressure data on the initial visit had suggested that the hallux was not involved in the foot-ground interaction, and ulceration from conventional repetitive trauma seemed unlikely. A repeat study revealed no major changes in plantar pressure distribution. The injury was eventually traced to the patient wearing open-toed sandals the previous week, and presumably encountering a foreign object between the toe and the sandal. The areas of high pressure in other regions of the foot continue to be of con-

cern, because the patient has shown a tendency to ulcerate. The possibility of progressive bony change is also being followed. The notable issue here is that pressure distribution measurement ruled out injury through repetitive trauma of the hallux, and the course of treatment and recommendations were made accordingly.

CONCLUSION

We have attempted to present a broad view of plantar pressure distribution measurement and to discuss the role it can have in the evaluation and management of the diabetic patient. This technique is clearly in its infancy, and one can only guess whether it will be shown to be an essential part of the assessment of the diabetic patient. Many techniques and approaches are used in medicine for which the rationale is based entirely on clinical experience. The current enthusiasm for the use of magnetic resonance imaging includes applications for which the result is insightful, but not clearly diagnostic. Although the relevance of plantar pressure distribution measurement to diabetic injury cannot be considered proven, the evidence from cross-sectional studies linking ulceration to elevated pressure is strong.

Because it is generally agreed that most plantar ulcers are the result of repetitive mechanical trauma, it is logical that a method to quantify such trauma would be helpful in the prevention of lesions. The key to predicting which patients will ulcerate, however, is hidden in the combination of the interacting risk factors to which the diabetic patient is subjected.

Even with high plantar pressures, ulceration is unlikely in the presence of intact sensation. What we do not know is why ulceration is not inevitable with high pressures in the absence of sensation. Well-controlled prospective studies might provide answers, and current information seems to favor including pressure distribution measurement in any study of this type. Even though, as we have acknowledged, no well-established norms or even a standard protocol for measurement is presently available, some compelling reasons exist for collecting pressure distribution data routinely on diabetic patients. The informality obtained can only add to the overall clinical picture. Patients usually injure their feet during gait, but most conventional examinations of diabetic feet are static and non-weight-bearing. Thus, pressure measurement provides a window through which the critical interaction of structures and function can be viewed.

References

1. Bauman J, Girling E, Brand PW. Plantar pressures and trophic ulceration. Bone Joint Surg. 1963; 45B:652–673.
2. Stokes IAF, Faris IB, Hutton WC. The neuropathic ulcer and loads on the foot in diabetic patients. Acta Orthop Scand. 1975; 46:839–847.
3. Boulton AJM, Hardisty CA, Betts RP, et al. Dynamic foot pressure and other studies as diagnostic and management aids in diabetic neuropathy. Diabetes Care, 1983; 6:26–32.
4. Brand PW. The diabetic foot. In: Ellenberg M, Rifkin H, eds. Diabetes mellitus. Theory and practice, 3rd ed. vol 2, New Hyde Park, NY: Medical Examination Publishing; 1983; 829–850.
5. Brand PW. Repetitive stress in the development of diabetic foot ulcers. In: Levin ME, O'Neal LW, eds. The diabetic foot, 4th ed. St. Louis: C.V. Mosby; 1988; 83–90.
6. Delbridge L, Ctercteko G, Fowler C, et al. The aetiology of diabetic neuropathic ulceration of the foot. 1985; 72:1–6.
7. Oakley W, Catterall RCF, Martin MM. Aetiology and management of lesions of the feet in diabetes. Br Med J. 1956; (October 27):953–957.
8. Bild DE, Selby JV, Sinnock P, et al. Lower-extremity amputation in people with diabetes. Diabetes Care. 1989; 12:24–31.
9. Edmonds ME. Experience in a multidisciplinary diabetic foot clinic. In: Connor H, Boulton AJM, Ward JD, eds. The foot in diabetes, New York: John Wiley & Sons; 1987; 121–133.
10. Wagner FW. The dysvascular foot: a system for diagnosis and treatment. Foot Ankle. 1981; 2:64–122.
11. Cavanagh PR, Ulbrecht JS. The diabetic foot: a quantitative approach to the assessment of neuropathy, deformity and plantar pressure. In: Jahss M, ed. Disorders of the Foot, 2nd ed. 1990.
12. Silvino N, Evanski PM, Waugh TR. The Harris and Beath footprinting mat: diagnostic validity and clinical use. Clin Orthop Rel Res. 1980; 151:265–269.
13. Weiss KM, Ulbrecht JS, Cavanagh PR, et al. Diabetes mellitus in American Indians: characteristics, origins and preventive health care implications. Med Anthropol. 1989; 11:283–304.
14. Brand PW. Management of the insensitive limb. Phys Ther. 1979; 59:8–12.
15. Coleman WC, Brand PW, Birke JA. The total contact cast: a therapy for plantar ulceration on insensitive feet. J Am Podiatry Assoc. 1984; 74:584–592.
16. Milgram JE, Jacobson MA: Footgear: therapeutic modifications of the sole and heel. Orthop Rev. 1978; VII:57–62.
17. Coleman WC. The relief of pressures using outer shoe sole modifications. In: Mothirami-Patil K, Srinivasa H, eds. Proceedings of the International Conference on Biomechanics and Clinical Kinesiology of the Hand and Foot. Madras, India: Indian Institute of Technology; 1985; 29–31.
18. Schaff PS, Cavanagh PR. Shoes for the insensitive foot: the effect of a "rocker bottom" shoe modification of plantar pressure distribution. Foot Ankle. (In press)
19. Most RS, Sinnock P. The epidemiology of lower extermity amputations in diabetic individuals. Diabetes Care, 1983; 6:87–91.
20. Cavanagh PR, Lafortune MA. Ground reaction forces in distance running. J Biomech. 1980; 13:397–406.
21. Mann RA: Biomechanics. In: Jahss MH, ed. Dis-

orders of the foot, vol 1. Philadelphia: WB Saunders; 1982; WB Saunders; 36–67.

22. Pollard JP, Le Quesne LP, Tappin JW. Forces under the foot. J Biomed Eng. 1983; 5:37–40.

23. Thompson DE. The effects of mechanical stress on soft tissue. In: Levin ME, O'Neal LW, eds. *The diabetic foot,* 4th ed. St. Louis: CV Mosby; 1988; 91–103.

24. Brodsky JW, Kourosh S, Mooney V. Objective evaluation and review of commericial gait analysis systems. Presented at the 19th Annual Meeting of the American Orthopaedic Foot and Ankle Society. Las Vegas; January 1989.

25. Morton DJ. The human foot. New York: Columbia University Press; 1935.

26. Nicol K, Henning EM. Measurement of pressure distribution by means of a flexible large surface mat. In: Asmussen E & Jorgenson K, eds., *Biomechanics VI-A,* Baltimore: University Park Press; 1978; 374–380.

27. Betts RP, Duckworth T, Burke J. Static and dynamic foot-pressure measurements in clinical orthopaedics. Med Biol Eng Comput. 1980; 18:674–684.

28. Duckworth T, Betts RP, Franks I, et al. The measurement of pressures under the foot. Foot Ankle, 1982; 3:130–141.

29. Duckworth T, Boulton AJM, Betts RP, et al. Plantar pressure measurements and the prevention of ulceration in the diabetic foot. J Bone Joint Surg. 1985; 67B:79–85.

30. Collis WJM, Jayson MIV. Measurement of pedal pressures. An illustration of a method. Ann Rheum Dis. 1972; 31:215.

31. Barrett JP, Mooney V. Neuropathic and diabetic pressure lesions. Orthop Clin North Am. 1973; 4:43–47.

32. Birke JA, Cornwall MA, Jackson M. Relationship between hallux limitus and ulceration of the great toe. J Orthop Sports Physical Ther. 1988; 10:172–176.

33. Boulton AJM, Betts RP, Franks CI, et al. Abnormalities of foot pressure in early diabetic neuropathy. Diabetic Med. 1987; 4:225–228.

34. Boulton AJM, Franks CI, Betts RP, et al. Reduction of abnormal foot pressure in diabetic neuropathy using a new polymer insole material. Diabetes Care, 1984; 7:42–46.

35. Harris JR, Brand PW. Patterns of disintegrtion of the tarsus in the anaesthetic foot. J Bone Joint Surg. 1966; 48B:4–16.

36. Brink SJ: Limited joint mobility as a risk factor for diabetes complications. Clin Diabetes, 1987; 5:123–127.

37. Grgic A, Rosenbloom AL, Weber FT, et al. Joint contracture—common manifestation of childhood diabetes mellitus. J Pediatr. 1976; 88 (4 Pt. 1):584–588.

38. Cavanagh PR, Rodgers MM, Iiboshi A. Pressure distribution under symptom-free feet during barefoot standing. Foot Ankle 1987; 262–276.

39. Ctercteko GC, Dhanendran MK, Hutton WC, et al. Vertical forces acting on the feet of diabetic patients with neuropathic ulcerationn. Br J Surg. 1981; 68:608–614.

40. Cavanagh PR, Sims DS, Sanders LJ. Longitudinal changes in the plantar pressure distribution in diabetic veterans. [In preparatiion].

41. Habershaw G, Donovan JC. Biomechanical considerations of the diabetic foot. In: Kozak GP, Hoar CS, Rowbotham JL, et al, (eds.) *Management of diabetic foot problems,* Philadelphia; WB Saunders; 1984; 32–44.

42. Lippman HI, Perotto A, Farrar R. The neuropathic foot of the diabetic. Bull NY Acad. Med. 1976; 52:1159–1178.

43. Ulbrecht JS, Cavangh PR. Plantar pressure distribution in diabetic patients with Charcot neuroarthropathy of the midfoot. Diabetes, 1989; 38(Suppl 2):137A.

44. Sims DS, Birke JA. Effect of rocker sole placement of plantar pressures. In: Proceedings of 20th Annual Meeting of the USPHS Professional Association. Atlanta: 1985; 53.

45. Sims DS, Cavanagh PR, Ulbrecht JS. Risk factors in the diabetic foot. Phy Ther. 1988; 68:1887–1902.

46. Boulton AJM. The importance of abnormal foot pressures and gait in the causation of foot ulcers. In: Connor H, Boulton AJM, Ward JD, eds. *The foot in diabetes,* New York: John Wiley & Sons; 1987; 11–21.

47. Lord M. Foot pressure measurement: a review of methodology. J Biomed Eng. 1981; 3:91–99.

48. Rodgers MM. Plantar pressure distribution measurement during barefoot walking: normal values and predictive equations [Dissertation], University Park, PA: Penn State University; 1985.

49. Schaff PS, Cavanagh PR. The rocker bottom shoe: pressure relief for the insensitive diabetic foot [abstract]. Diabetes 38(Suppl 2):80A, 1989.

6 Vascular Disease of the Diabetic Foot

RICHARD E. WELLING, M.D.,
E. DOUGLAS BALDRIDGE, M.D.,
AND R. TERRELL FREY, M.D.

Peripheral vascular disease (PVD) has a significant impact on the morbidity and mortality of the diabetic patient. Because diabetic patients frequently have associated peripheral neuropathy and attendant foot deformities, many are candidates for reconstructive orthopedic surgery of the foot. To prevent possible complications after reconstructive surgery in an ischemic foot, it is essential for the orthopedist to be able to assess the presence and severity of PVD preoperatively. The purpose of this chapter is to familiarize the surgeon with the incidence, signs, and symptoms of peripheral vascular insufficiency in diabetic patients. This chapter also includes a review of invasive and noninvasive diagnostic techniques and a preliminary discussion of preventative foot care and reconstructive vascular surgery that should precede reconstructive surgery in the diabetic foot.

Although this chapter deals mainly with PVD attendant to the diabetic patient, the associated neuropathy and infection are often inseparable. It is important to identify the most significant component that results in the patient's presentation to the physician and to determine to what extent, if any, the other components contribute.

Peripheral vascular insufficiency in the diabetic foot is the result of macroangiopathy affecting the large, medium, and small blood vessels of the lower extremity. Although microangiopathy is clearly a part of PVD in the diabetic patient, particularly in the retina and the kidney, it is not thought to have a significant clinical impact on PVD in the diabetic patient.

INCIDENCE OF PVD IN DIABETIC PATIENTS

Many studies have documented the increased risk of PVD in diabetic patients.[1-3] In a study of one group of patients who had been diabetic for less than 1 year, 22% had vascular calcifications in the lower extremities, as demonstrated by plain radiographs, 13% lacked one or more peripheral pulses, and 5% experienced claudication.[4]

In 1979, Kannel and McGee reported that PVD, as evidenced by intermittent claudication, was 3.8 times more frequent in diabetic men and 6.5 times more frequent in diabetic women in comparison with those in nondiabetic control groups:[5] Diabetes seems to be a catalyst for atherosclerosis. It has its greatest impact in patients with other risk factors, such as hyperlipidemia, hypertension, smoking, and obesity.[6-13]

The duration of diabetes and the degree of hyperglycemia correlate well with the extent of disease present below the popliteal artery, but do not correlate with the amount of disease present in the aorto-iliac and femoral arteries.[14] One review of 1073 diabetic patients found that 8% had PVD documented by one or more absent pulses at the time diabetes was diagnosed.[15] In those patients who were initially unaffected, 2% per year developed clinically apparent occlusive arterial disease during follow-up. It was estimated that 15% of diabetic patients would manifest PVD, as demonstrated by one or more absent pulses, within 10 years of the initial diagnosis of diabetes mellitus, and 45% would manifest PVD within 20 years of the initial diagnosis.

Diabetic patients also have decreased survival in comparison with those in age-matched control groups. In a study by Tibell, only 20% of diabetic patients hospitalized for PVD between 1949 and 1965 were alive 10 years later.[16] It is clear that diabetic patients have a higher incidence of PVD, an increased amputation rate, and an increased mortality in comparison to their nondiabetic counterparts.

SIGNS AND SYMPTOMS OF PVD

Occlusive PVD in the aorta and the iliac arteries can be present in both diabetic and nondiabetic patients. In the nondiabetic patient, obstructive processes in the arteries distal to the inguinal ligament are frequently not clinically significant. However, in the diabetic patient, these same arterial segments often show evidence of clinically significant occlusive disease as well.[1,3,17] Obstructive disease of the femoral arteries in the nondiabetic patient is frequently unilateral and involves only one arterial seg-

ment. In the diabetic patient, peripheral vascular obstructive disease is multisegmental and is frequently associated with occlusive disease below the popliteal trifurcation (Fig. 6-1).[2,17]

As a result of the occlusive process, the peripheral vascular picture is altered in diabetic patients. Evaluation of these pulses is important to localize the site of arterial occlusion. Aorto-iliac occlusive disease in diabetic and nondiabetic patients is similar as indicated by the absence or diminution of a femoral pulse. Superficial femoral artery occlusion is suspected by the absence of popliteal pulses. Frequently, diabetic patients have palpable popliteal pulses but absent pulses distally. This is a manifestation of a feature of diabetic PVD: occlusive disease in the tibial peroneal trunk and the trifurcation vessels, i.e., anterior tibial artery, posterior tibial artery, and peroneal artery. The extent of occlusive vascular disease is similar in diabetic and nondiabetic patients, but complete occlusion of the peroneal artery is more common in the diabetic patient.[18] The latter observation has not been true in our experience (Fig. 6-2); but this discrepancy

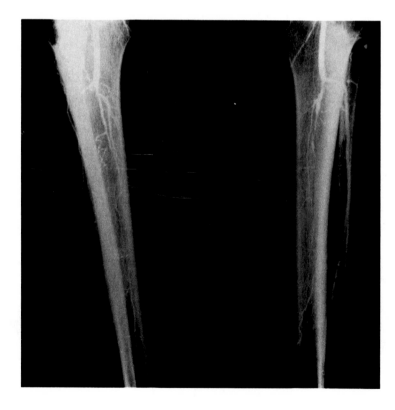

FIGURE 6–1 ■ Occlusive arterial disease below the popliteal trifurcation.

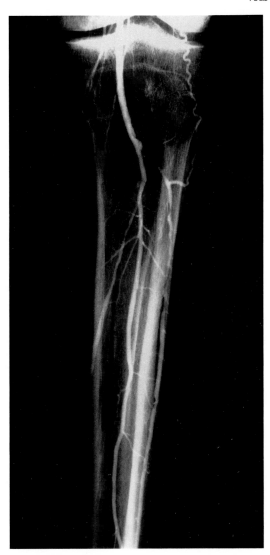

FIGURE 6-2 ■ Patent peroneal artery in a diabetic patient.

might be attributable to the improvements in vascular radiology since 1967. Diabetic patients are less likely to have occlusive arterial disease in the vessels of the foot than nondiabetics.[18] Therefore, angiographic identification of the distal foot circulation, including the pedal arch and its branches, is important in planning reconstructive vascular surgery.

Intermittent claudication, the hallmark of peripheral vascular insufficiency, is similar in diabetic and nondiabetic patients. This must be differentiated from neurogenic claudication, which results from degenerative diseases of the spine. With intermittent claudication, the specific muscle groups involved correlate well with the level of arterial blockage; that is, intermittent claudication of the buttock and thighs indicates aorto-iliac disease, whereas intermittent claudication of the calf indicates femoropopliteal disease.[19] Despite its distressing nature, intermittent claudication is often a stable symptom that the patient experiences for many years. In this state it infrequently leads to limb loss. If, however, it becomes progressive—that is, develops within a shorter distance—it portends a worse prognosis, and a more aggressive therapeutic course is recommended.

Pain in the foot at rest often signifies impending limb loss in the diabetic patient with PVD but without polyneuropathy. Rest pain, however, might be absent or modified in the diabetic patient who has attendant peripheral neuropathy. As a result, impending limb loss in the diabetic patient might first be manifested by ulceration or gangrenous changes in an area of the heel or toes (Fig. 6-3).

When evaluating a patient with ulceration or gangrenous changes of the foot, it is important to look for infection in the surrounding tissue. Because of decreased blood supply, the classic signs of infection might not be present in the ischemic foot. If infection is present it must be treated aggressively, both operatively and nonoperatively, prior to any diagnostic procedures or reconstructive peripheral vascular surgery.

PREOPERATIVE ASSESSMENT

The presence of intermittent claudication or tissue necrosis in the foot associated with diminished femoral or popliteal pulses should alert the orthopedic surgeon to the possibility of significant PVD and the need for evaluation by a vascular surgeon. If the vascular surgeon confirms findings of progressive claudication or an ischemic foot lesion with absent femoral or popliteal pulses, further studies are necessary. These include noninvasive and angiographic assessment of the arterial circulation to the involved lower extremity. On the other hand, many diabetic patients with such history and physi-

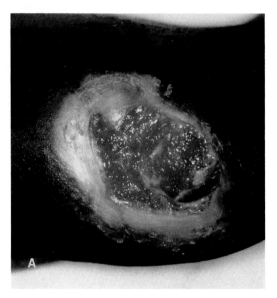
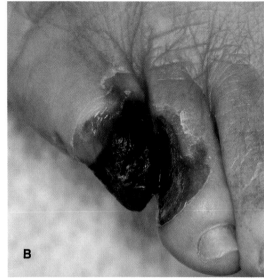

FIGURE 6–3 ■ *A*, Ulceration of the toes. *B*, Gangrene of the toes.

cal findings have a strong popliteal pulse but absent pedal pulses, and such patients are less likely to benefit from arterial reconstruction. The latter finding is frequently associated with arterial occlusion at the tibial-peroneal trunk and the trifurcation vessels. With more distal reconstruction by an in situ autogenous vein bypass, many of these ischemic extremities can be revascularized. During the preoperative assessment it is also important to assess the patient for coronary artery and cerebrovascular insufficiency, because these lesions are often associated with peripheral vascular insufficiency in diabetics and frequently cause perioperative morbidity and mortality.[19,20]

Noninvasive Tests

Noninvasive tests can detect vascular disease in asymptomatic patients and can provide objective confirmation of the results of physical examination in symptomatic patients. They augment the results of angiography by documenting the functional or physiologic significance of anatomic lesions, and therefore assist the surgeon in planning surgery. Such tests are also used serially for intraoperative monitoring and postoperative follow-up. Noninvasive test-

ing is mandatory in the evaluation of any diabetic patient with symptomatic vascular disease.[21]

Current noninvasive tests include determination of segmental pressures by Doppler, pulse volume recording, photoplethysmography, transcutaneous oximetry, laser Doppler velocimetry, duplex ultrasonography, skin temperature measurement, and nuclear magnetic resonance.

SEGMENTAL PRESSURES BY DOPPLER

A Doppler ultrasonic velocimeter consists of two piezoelectric crystals encased in a small probe which is applied to the skin with acoustic coupling gel (Fig. 6-4). An electric signal causes ultrasonic waves to be emitted from one crystal. The waves travel through the tissue and are deflected back to the second crystal, the receiver. When these ultrasound waves encounter a moving particle, such as a blood cell, their frequency is altered, and the change in frequency is transformed into audible sound waves by an amplifier. The Doppler frequency spectrum can be recorded onto videotape or paper. The emission frequency of the Doppler device, usually expressed in megahertz, determines the depth of tissue penetration of the sound beam. To determine segmental pressures a

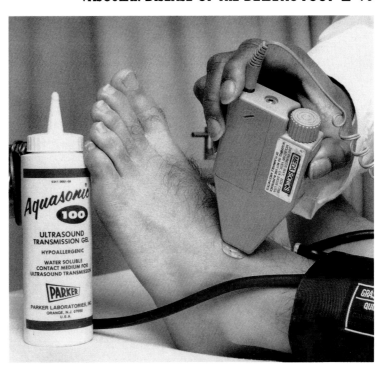

FIGURE 6–4 ■ Doppler device coupled to skin surface by acoustic gel.

5-MHz hand-held Doppler is usually sufficient, allowing tissue penetration to a depth of 6 to 7 cm from the skin surface.[22]

Segmental pressures can be used in diagnosing vascular disease objectively and localizing stenoses to specific arterial segments. By placing inflatable cuffs at appropriate positions, proximally on the thigh, above the knee, below the knee, above the ankle, and on the toes, the physician can determine the blood pressure in each segment of the extremity (Fig. 6-5). A signal is obtained by auscultating with the Doppler over an artery distal to the blood pressure cuff. The pressure cuff is then inflated above systolic pressure, flow is occluded, and a signal is no longer heard. The pressure cuff is slowly deflated and flow resumes when the systolic perfusion pressure exceeds the pressure in the cuff. This corresponds to the segmental pressure. The ankle-brachial index (ABI), one of the most commonly used indices, is the ratio of ankle systolic blood pressure to brachial systolic blood pressure. The use of this index allows comparison of severity of disease, either among different individuals or serially in the same patient. A normal ABI is approximately 1.0 (Fig. 6-

6).[23] An ABI less than 0.5 indicates severe occlusive disease[24] and corresponds to an ankle systolic pressure of less than 55 mm Hg, assuming the brachial pressure is 110 to 120 mm Hg. An index of 0.6 to 0.9 is consistent with claudication in nondiabetic patients. An index of 0.5 or less indicates severe ischemia and usually implies severe stenosis or occlusion at more than one segment of the lower extremity arterial tree.[25,26]

Doppler ultrasound information can also be processed to produce an analog waveform. The normal peripheral arterial waveform is triphasic (Fig. 6-7). Initially, there is a large, steep, positive (upward) deflection during systole. During early diastole, a small, negative, downward wave occurs. This corresponds to the reflection wave caused by the elastic recoil of normal arteries. The second, small, upward wave during the remainder of diastole represents the forward flow of blood propelled by the energy stored in the blood-distended elastic arteries. In diseased arteries, the normal elastic recoil and distensibility of the vessels are lost. The velocity waveform becomes monophasic and progressively dampened. As flow nears zero, the waveform becomes progressively flatter

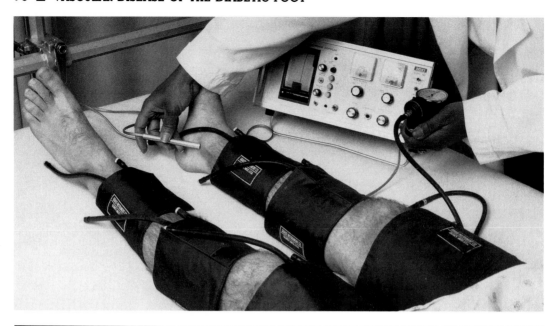

FIGURE 6–5 ■ Segmental pressures by Doppler.

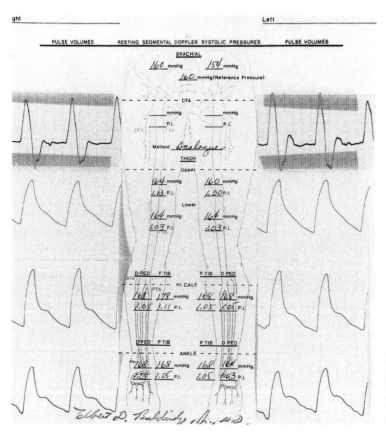

FIGURE 6–6 ■ Normal segmental pressures and pulse volume recordings of the bilateral lower extremities.

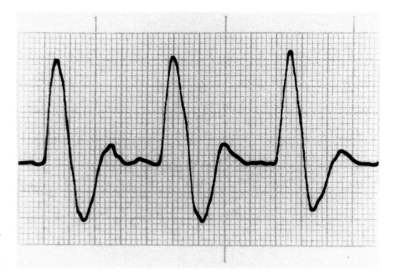

FIGURE 6-7 ■ Normal triphasic Doppler waveform.

and approaches a straight line.

The minimum volume flow rate (ml/min) detected by Doppler depends on the angle of insonation, velocity of flow, diameter of the vessel, frequency of the ultrasound source, and other factors that affect the sensitivity of the instrument. Formerly, reports of Doppler-detected flow rates indicated a lower limit of about 6 ml/min; some new duplex equipment can measure velocities of 0.3 cm/sec, corresponding to lower volumetric flow rates.* It is important to note that the Doppler detects changes in frequency or velocity, and does not measure actual volume flow.

Several caveats apply to segmental pressure determination in diabetic patients. This technique is less useful in diabetics than in nondiabetics. Accurate measurement of segmental pressure depends on the ability of the corresponding blood pressure cuff to occlude flow through vessels beneath the cuff. Vessel rigidity, frequently caused by medial calcification, can falsely elevate systolic blood pressure measurements.[27–29] Diabetic patients tend to have a higher prevalence of small vessel involvement and calcified vessels.[30] Therefore, the ABI is often falsely elevated in diabetic patients (Fig. 6-8).[28] Digital arterial pressure can be measured using small digital cuffs, and these measurements are generally accurate because the small vessels are not usually calcified.[19,31]

By measuring segmental pressures using multiple cuffs at various points along the lower extremity—proximal thigh, distal thigh, proximal calf, ankle, and digits—stenoses and occlusions can be roughly localized.[32,33] Our experience has shown that a decrease of 10 mm Hg between any two levels indicates a hemodynamically significant stenosis between those two cuffs. A gradient of 30 mm Hg indicates severe stenosis or total occlusion. Thus, a decrease between the proximal and distal thigh indicates proximal or midsuperficial femoral artery disease. A difference between the distal thigh and proximal calf indicates disease of the distal superficial femoral artery, popliteal, or proximal trifurcation vessels (Fig. 6-9). A gradient between the proximal calf and ankle pressures indicates tibial artery disease, and so on.

Segmental pressures enhance anatomic information gained from an arteriogram. For example, a moderate stenosis by angiogram might be functionally significant, as demonstrated by a pressure gradient in the Doppler study. Furthermore, lesions that appear significant by angiogram might not result in a pressure decrease, and are not functionally significant. Lesions that are not physiologically significant at rest (basal flow rate) can be functionally important in conditions of stress, such as exercise, reactive hyperemia, and other induced vasodilatory states.

A decreased proximal thigh pressure is often interpreted as inflow (aorto-iliac) dis-

*Quantum Medical Systems, Inc., Issaquah, WA.

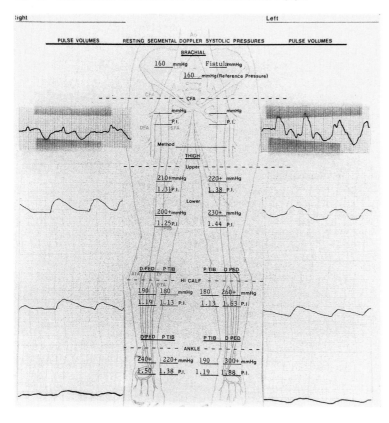

FIGURE 6–8 ■ Falsely elevated segmental pressures with markedly abnormal pulse volume recordings in a diabetic patient with rest pain.

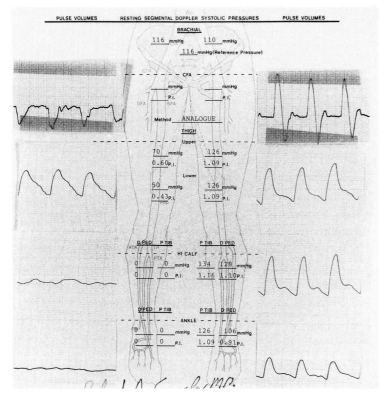

FIGURE 6–9 ■ Localization of disease study of the left lower extremity is normal. The study of the right lower extremity suggests inflow disease and segmental stenosis of the superficial femoral artery, with occlusion of the distal superficial femoral artery or popliteal artery.

ease. Occasionally, this decrease is observed when the cuff is placed over the proximal portion of the profunda and superficial femoral arteries rather than over the common femoral artery. Thus, a decreased proximal thigh pressure might, in fact, indicate either aorto-iliac disease or combined disease of the superficial femoral and profunda femoris artery origins.[34]

PULSE VOLUME RECORDING

Pulse volume recording is a technique in which air-filled cuffs are placed on the extremity. A small but measurable volume change is noted in the extremity with each arterial pulsation. This small change can be processed to produce a wave known as the pulse volume recording. Normal pulse contour shows a steep upstroke, a relative sharp peak, and a rapid downstroke with a dicrotic notch. Increasingly severe disease results in loss of the notch, flattening of the downstroke, rounding of the peak, and a slower upstroke. This produces progressive flattening of the wave profile to the point that no pulsatile flow is observed (Fig. 6-10).

Although its interpretation is more subjective and less quantitative than segmental pressures by Doppler, the pulse volume recording has one distinct advantage: it is useful in patients with noncompressible calcified vessels, in whom segmental pressures

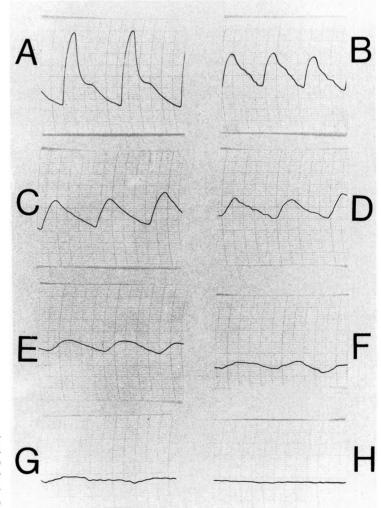

FIGURE 6–10 ■ Serial changes in pulse volume recording with increasing severity of arterial disease. *A* to *H*, Normal to severe.

by Doppler are falsely elevated and unreliable (Fig. 6-8).[3,28,35] Digital cuffs also permit evaluation of small vessel disease. Pulse volume recordings are an important adjunct to segmental pressures in diabetic patients.[28]

PHOTOPLETHYSMOGRAPHY

In photoplethysmography (PPG), infrared light rays are emitted, reflected from blood vessels, and measured by a phototransistor. The reflected light is directly proportional to the blood flow in the microcirculation. The device records pulsation of the cutaneous circulation and can be used to determine blood pressure in a limb or digit (Fig. 6-11). It is particularly helpful in determining pressure in the distal phalanges.

Certain technical limitations must be observed with PPG (Fig. 6-12). First, elevation of the digit or extremity results in more rapid venous emptying and an apparent increase in the pulse obtained by PPG. Similarly, dependency results in flattening of the PPG tracing. Second, undue pressure on the skin surface when applying the PPG cell to the skin surface alters the tracing. Slight pressure augments the pulse, but further pressure on the probe obliterates the pulse. Finally, any factor that causes vasoconstriction, including a cold environment and increased sympathetic tone, tends to flatten the PPG tracing. Conversely, vasodilation, e.g., sympathetic block, exaggerates the pulsatility. Despite its limitations, PPG is useful in the diabetic patient to assess pulsatility in the distal extremity, especially in the digits.

TRANSCUTANEOUS OXIMETRY

Transcutaneous oximetry has been heralded as the most accurate method of evaluating ischemia in both diabetic and nondiabetic patients.[36] First used in 1978 to evaluate PVD,[37] the oxygen monitor consists of a cathode, anode, electrolyte, and oxygen-permeable membrane. The probe contains a heating element that maintains a constant skin temperature. As with PPG, factors that result in vasoconstriction can cause a decrease in the transcutaneous oxygen saturation. Furthermore, factors such as limb position and fraction of inspired oxygen can affect measurements. One particularly useful application of transcutaneous oximetry is the prediction of level of amputation healing. A transcutaneous PO_2 of 35 to 40 mm Hg indicates adequate local blood supply for healing after amputation.[38-42] Most ulcers or amputations heal if the transcutaneous PO_2 is >10 mm Hg.[36]

LASER DOPPLER VELOCIMETRY

Laser Doppler velocimetry was first introduced in the assessment of PVD in 1984.[43] The helium-neon laser Doppler velocimeter employs a laser light source with a wavelength of 632.8 nm. Using the Doppler principle, it records skin blood flow velocity and represents it as a pulse wave. Laser Doppler velocimetry has been reported to be less sensitive than transcutaneous oximetry but slightly more specific in the diagnosis of vascular disease.[36] Use of temperature-controlled probe can increase the sensitivity of the laser Dopper velocimeter. Laser Doppler velocimetry, like transcutaneous oximetry and PPG, reflects perfusion of the skin. A cold environment, increased sympathetic stimulation, and other factors can result in shunting of blood away from the skin. These forms of peripheral circulatory assessment, such as PPG, transcutaneous oximetry, and laser Doppler, are more accurate than ankle pressure measurements in predicting the

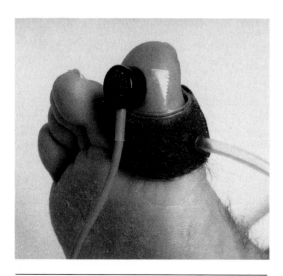

FIGURE 6-11 ■ Photoplethysmography. The probe is applied to the digit with double-stick clear tape.

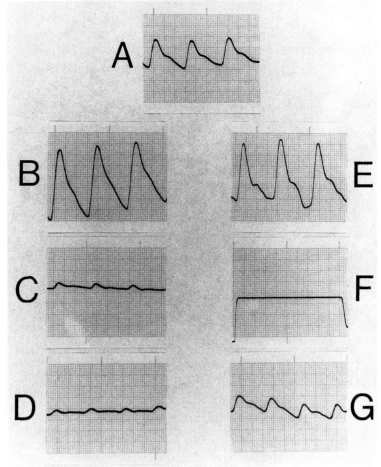

FIGURE 6–12 ■ Factors affecting photoplethysmography. *A,* Normal supine position. *B,* Extremity elevated. *C,* Extremity dependent. *D,* Increased sympathetic tone secondary to Valsalva maneuver. *E,* Slight increase in contact pressure. *F,* Further increase in contact pressure. *G,* Reflexive vasoconstriction induced by cooling adjacent digits.

healing of ulcerations and the outcome of forefoot amputations.[36]

DUPLEX ULTRASONOGRAPHY

In B-mode scanning, ultrasonic waves are deflected at tissue interfaces and reflected back to the receiver. These sound waves are processed to form a visible image. In duplex scanning, a pulse-wave Doppler is coupled to the B-mode image. The pulse-wave Doppler uses a process called range-gating to sample frequency shifts selectively in various areas of the visual image. A cursor on the image screen represents the area of sampling by the Doppler. Thus, various vessels such as the arterial tree of the lower extremity can be visualized and selectively interrogated with the Doppler for elevation of frequencies. In areas of stenosis the blood

velocity is faster, resulting in an increased Doppler frequency shift. Furthermore, in areas of total occlusion, there is loss of visible pulsation and no Doppler signal. The B-mode image also allows visualization of the vessel walls, plaque, and lumen. A good image can permit estimation of the diameter or area of the stenosis. Plaque characteristics such as calcification, irregularity, ulceration, and plaque hemorrhage can often be detected. Occasionally, an intraluminal thrombus can be seen.

New technology has resulted in higher frequency Duplex probes with improved images and better Doppler capability. Computer enhancement has led to more rapid analysis of Doppler information, which can be transformed into a color-coded image; this relatively new technique is commonly known as color Doppler. It is still based on

Doppler frequency shifts, but appears to be superior to standard duplex scanning because it allows thorough interrogation of vessels in a more timely manner.

Duplex scanning can be helpful in diabetic patients with PVD. It provides both anatomic (B-mode image) and physiologic (Doppler) information. No other noninvasive test provides such anatomic information. It is also a useful noninvasive method for preoperative assessment of the saphenous and other superficial veins for adequacy as bypass conduits.[44] This is especially important in diabetic patients, who frequently require distal, i.e., infrapopliteal, bypass. Small veins, varicose veins, and phlebitic veins can be identified by duplex scan, leading the surgeon to search for other veins or choose a prosthetic conduit. Anomalous saphenous systems can also be identified easily. The vein can also be "mapped" to assist in placing the incision directly over the vein, thus avoiding skin flaps, which are prone to infection. Duplex scanning or B-mode imaging can be used intraoperatively to assess the technical results of anastomoses. Finally, conduits can be periodically followed postoperatively to identify problems that could lead to graft failure, such as graft stenosis, anastomotic stenosis, valve remnants, and aneurysms. Noninvasive identification of the failing graft can help to dictate angiographic or operative intervention prior to graft occlusion.

SKIN TEMPERATURE MEASUREMENT

Skin temperature measurement is mentioned only as an adjunctive study that can predict the results of sympathectomy. Rarely, sympathectomy is indicated in diabetic patients who have rest pain or superficial ulceration in the presence of nonreconstructible obliterative disease. Sympathectomy should not be performed unless sympathetic or peripheral nerve block has produced a demonstrable increase in skin temperature of the affected digits.

MAGNETIC RESONANCE IMAGING

Magnetic resonance imaging (MRI) is a noninvasive technique that allows measurement of actual limb flow, and is the only noninvasive test that measures volume flow directly. All other noninvasive tests assess flow indirectly by measuring some other parameter, such as pressure, temperature, or pulsatility. Little information about the technique is available, but early reports suggest that it soon will be a reliable method.[45]

STRESS TESTING

Any discussion of noninvasive tests for assessing PVD in the diabetic patient is not complete without mentioning stress testing. Current noninvasive test results might appear normal in some patients at rest, despite the presence of obliterative arterial disease.[46] These patients usually present with intermittent claudication. Disease severe enough to cause severe claudication, rest pain, or tissue loss inevitably is abnormal at rest. Patients with normal studies at rest should undergo stress testing before the diagnosis of PVD is excluded. Stress testing usually consists either of treadmill exercise or reactive hyperemia.

Treadmill Test. In the treadmill test the patient walks on a treadmill at a standard speed and grade for a specified time. This often reproduces the typical pain of claudication. On completion of the exercise, segmental pressures at the ankle are recorded. If a patient walks to the point of claudication, a decrease in the ankle pressure is always demonstrated. If "claudication" results without a decrease in ankle pressure, another source of the pain should be sought, such as neuropathy or neurogenic claudication. The decrease in ankle pressure and the time required to return to the resting baseline pressure are directly proportional to the severity of occlusive disease.[25] Thus, a patient with a decrease in the ABI to 0.6 that requires 10 minutes to recover to the resting ABI has more extensive arterial disease than a patient whose ABI drops to 0.8 and recovers in 5 minutes, assuming they were exercised under the same treadmill conditions.

Reactive Hyperemia. Stress testing can also be performed by reactive hyperemia. A blood pressure cuff placed on the thigh is inflated and maintained at greater than systolic blood pressure for a given period of time, usually about 5 minutes. This causes tissue hypoxia, with a resultant decrease in peripheral vascular resistance distal to the cuff. When the cuff is released and the limb is reperfused, reactive hyperemia ensues. If stenosis is present the tissue demand for blood flow is not met, and a decrease in pressure can be recorded distal to the area of stenosis. The decrease in ankle pressure is proportional to the degree of stenosis, and the recovery time to baseline is more prolonged with worsening degrees of arterial insufficiency.[47]

Reactive hyperemia is particularly useful in patients who have cardiac or pulmonary insufficiency that precludes treadmill exercise. It also is helpful in assessing the remaining extremity of an amputee, who might be unable to perform a treadmill exercise. It should not be performed in limbs with a patent bypass graft because prolonged occlusion can result in graft thrombosis.

Thus, stress testing can be used to document the presence of arterial disease in patients who have normal resting studies, exclude arterial disease in patients who have pain resulting from a condition other than arterial disease, and quantitate the degree of arterial insufficiency.

Radiographic Tests

ARTERIOGRAPHY

Arteriography is the most complete and accurate method of visualizing the vascular anatomy. It is an invasive procedure, however, and therefore involves some risk for the patient. The risk of serious complication ranges from 1 to 1.5% and death occurs in 0.03 to 0.06% of patients.[48] In addition, arteriography is expensive and not universally available. Thus, noninvasive testing is preferable for the initial diagnosis.

Arteriography should be limited to patients who are candidates for angioplasty or surgical revascularization. Such patients are likely to have one of the following characteristics:[19,49]

1. An ankle ischemic index of ≤0.40
2. Rest pain or night pain not attributable to neuropathy
3. Intractable leg ulcers
4. Gangrene or pregangrenous changes
5. Severe PVD demonstrated by noninvasive tests

Patient preparation. Prior to the arteriogram, the angiographer must evaluate the patient. Risk factors such as bleeding diathesis, hypertension, renal impairment, and anticoagulant therapy must be recognized and corrected prior to the examination. This evaluation process has become more difficult since the advent of outpatient angiography. The angiographer, often a radiologist, rarely meets the patient prior to the day of examination. Careful cooperation and effective communication must be established between the referring physician and angiographer to ensure that such risk factors are not overlooked.

Patients with diabetes must be evaluated for renal impairment. Contrast medium-induced renal failure is more common in patients with renal impairment caused by diabetes than in patients with renal impairment from other causes.[50,51] Diabetic patients with normal renal function have no greater risk of developing renal failure than nondiabetics with normal renal function.[51,52] The angiographer can minimize the risk of contrast medium-induced renal failure by using low osmolality contrast agents (LOCAs), keeping patients well hydrated, and maintaining a sufficient interval between contrast examinations.

Although the mechanisms of contrast medium-induced renal failure are not clearly understood, it is known that LOCAs have a higher LD_{50} than standard contrast agents. LOCAs are less harmful to the renal vascular endothelium, cause less circulatory disturbance, and appear to be less toxic to tubular cells.[48] LOCAs appear to be appropriate for high-risk patients, although their benefits have not yet been well established by clinical studies.

Appropriate hydration is important in minimizing the risk of contrast medium-induced renal failure. Mason and colleagues found no significant renal failure in patients who were properly hydrated.[53] All diabetic outpatients should be permitted oral fluids up to the time of admission, and patients with impaired renal function should be hydrated with intravenous fluids for several hours prior to testing.

Finally, care should be taken to allow sufficient time between examinations that require the administration of radiographic contrast material, e.g., intravenous pyelography and angiography, computed tomography (CT) and angiography. Moreau found no cases of acute renal failure when an interval of 5 days between contrast examinations was observed.[54] The physician should also allow sufficient time between contrast examinations and surgical procedures that might influence renal function, such as aorto-iliac grafting.

Technique. The technique of femoral arteriography has been well documented elsewhere[55,56] and is not presented here in detail. Because vascular access is not always possible through the femoral artery, the angiographer should also be skilled in translumbar and transaxillary angiography.

In femoral arteriography, the catheter is placed in the infrarenal abdominal aorta under fluoroscopic guidance. A total of 60 to 80 ml of 60 to 76% contrast is usually injected over a period of 6 to 10 seconds. Serial filming is performed with rapid film changes and a moving table top. This allows complete examination from the aortic bifurcation to the feet. Such complete coverage is particularly important for diabetics, who are likely to have multiple bilateral lesions and lesions below the popliteal level. Because bypass grafts to the distal runoff arteries can preserve limb function and offer an alternative to amputation, it is important to delineate the distal runoff arteries into the foot clearly.[56–58]

Digital subtraction angiography (DSA) is a computer-assisted arteriography technique. An image of the area of interest, obtained before injection of radiographic contrast, is electronically subtracted from one obtained after injection of radiographic contrast. This technique, which provides high-contrast resolution, is particularly helpful in diabetic patients as an adjunct to the standard film-screen examination. It allows the angiographer to obtain additional projections, e.g., oblique and lateral, to delineate stenoses or collateral flow better while using smaller doses of less concentrated contrast medium (35 to 43%). If the standard examination shows changes of the abdominal aorta, or if the patient has hyperextension, visualization of the renal arteries is indicated. A DSA aortogram can be obtained using 30 ml (15 ml/sec for 2 seconds) of 41% radiographic contrast. The technique can also be used to obtain oblique

views of the iliac arteries and femoral bifurcations in patients with iliofemoral disease.

DSA is an excellent method for evaluating the circulation to the foot and ankle. A lateral view of the foot and ankle can be obtained with excellent vascular opacification after injection of 20 ml (5 ml/sec for 4 seconds) of 41% radiographic contrast (Fig. 6-13). This is important because the integrity of the foot arch greatly influences the patency rate of a bypass graft.[59–61] Unfortunately, it is impractical to use DSA to evaluate circulation of the entire lower extremity. In addition, the technique cannot obtain images with a moving table top. Its field of view is limited to the size of the image intensifier, usually 23 cm, which is smaller than the film-screen field view (36 × 36 cm).

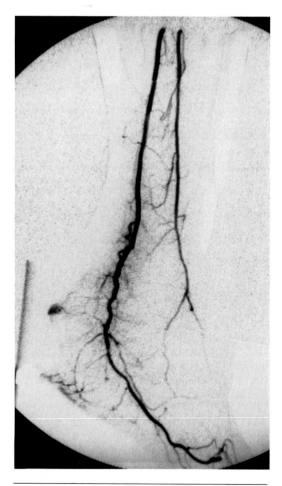

FIGURE 6–13 ■ Lateral digital subtraction angiogram of foot and ankle.

SOFT TISSUE RADIOGRAPHS

Soft tissue radiographs are useful for preoperative evaluation because they can delineate the extent of vessel calcification. Vessels with extensive calcification can be difficult or impossible to anastomose. Some degree of arterial calcification is found in 16 to 25% of patients with adult-onset diabetes.[3,62]

Medial calcifications, which are usually distributed evenly along the length of a vessel, are not typically associated with vascular occlusion (Fig. 6-14).[3,62] Atherosclerosis is seen in soft tissue radiographs as an uneven thickening of the intimal wall, and it is more commonly associated with occlusion and stenosis (Fig. 6-15).

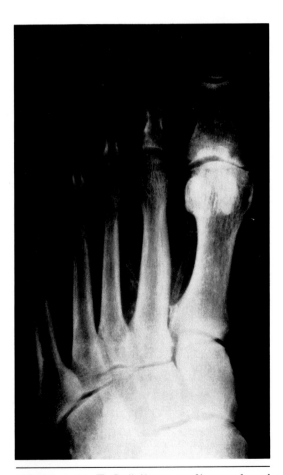

FIGURE 6–14 ■ Soft tissue radiographs of medial calcifications in the arteries of the foot.

XENON-133 WASHOUT

The Xenon-133 washout technique is used to measure blood flow to the muscles. Approximately 50 ml of Xenon-133 dissolved in saline solution is injected into a muscle. The rate at which the radioisotope is cleared from the muscle indicates the capillary blood flow to the area. The technique can be used both at rest and under hyperemic conditions. It has also been used to assess the healing potential of amputation at a given level.[63]

RADIOISOTOPE MICROSPHERE SCANNING

Radioisotope microsphere examination involves the injection of radioisotope-tagged albumin into an artery. This permits evaluation of the blood flow surrounding an area of ulceration. It is also used after lumbar sympathectomy to determine the extent of arteriovenous shunting.

TREATMENT

Although it is not critical for orthopedic surgeons to be intimately familiar with all the technical details of peripheral vascular reconstructive surgery in the diabetic patient, they must be able to diagnose an ischemic foot clinically and must be familiar with the diagnostic and therapeutic options of foot care.

Preventative foot care must be used by the diabetic patient with peripheral vascular insufficiency. Patients should wash their feet daily with mild soap and warm water. Hot water should never be used, and patients should test the temperature of the water before immersing their feet. They should spray their feet with an antifungal spray and apply a moisturizing lotion. Many foot infections in diabetic patients start as cracks in the skin, which allow bacterial penetration and a beginning nidus of infection. Daily application of lotion minimizes this problem and reduces the risk of infection. Diabetic patients must avoid walking barefoot, even on soft surfaces, because the attendant neuropathy permits a minor injury to go unrecognized. They must purchase shoes that fit properly, without undue pressure in any particular area.

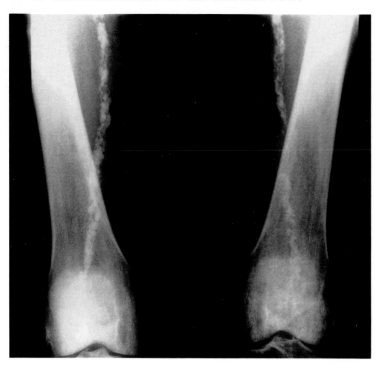

FIGURE 6–15 ■ Soft tissue radiograph of atherosclerotic femoral artery.

The correlation between tobacco use and peripheral vascular disease is important. Proper control of the blood sugar level should be maintained; hyperglycemia can be one of the first indications of a serious foot infection. Patients with intermittent claudication benefit from exercise to increase walking tolerance.[64–67] Management of hypertension and of the cholesterol, lipid, and triglyceride levels also helps to decrease the incidence of peripheral vascular disease.[14,19] Medication to increase the blood supply in the lower extremities has not been proven clinically beneficial in prospective randomized trials,[19,68] nor has nonreconstructive surgery, i.e. sympathectomy, been uniformly successful in increasing the peripheral vascular blood supply in diabetics. Lumbar sympathectomy has been shown to relieve rest pain and reduce the incidence of minor cutaneous skin ulcerations in some studies, but it has no benefit for the patient with intermittent claudication.[1,69–74] Similarly, lumbar sympathectomy has little application in diabetics of 10 or more years' duration, many of whom have had a sympathectomy.[75]

Direct reconstructive vascular surgery is the only therapeutic procedure that has been shown to be beneficial in diabetic patients with PVD, but proper patient selection is essential. Only patients with progressive and disabling claudication or impending limb loss, as manifested by rest pain or gangrenous or pregangrenous changes in the foot, should be considered candidates for vascular reconstruction. Diabetic patients with occlusive peripheral vascular disease in the aorto-iliac and superficial femoral arteries should be treated in the same manner as their nondiabetic counterparts. The long-term success rate of peripheral vascular reconstruction in the aorto-iliac and femoro-popliteal segments is similar in diabetic and nondiabetic patients.[75,76] The profunda femoris artery is an important outflow vessel in aorto-femoral bypass surgery. Frequently, in the diabetic, the occlusive disease process is not limited only to the origin of the artery, but extends to the primary and secondary branches (Fig. 6-16). This must be taken into consideration in planning and executing the distal anastomosis.

Generally, an autogenous saphenous vein graft is the best conduit for reconstruction below the inguinal ligament.[75,77] If a distal anastomosis is possible in an above-the-knee position, however, a synthetic graft is ac-

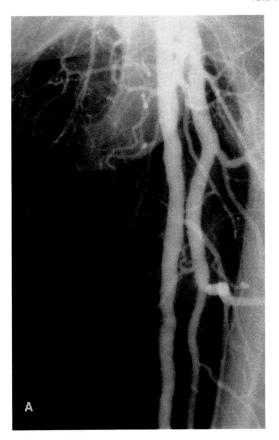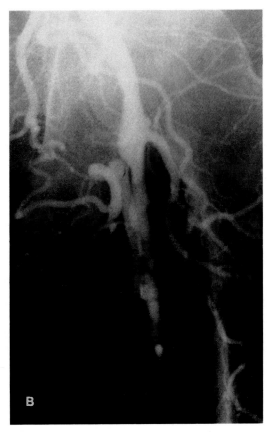

FIGURE 6–16 ■ **A,** Normal profunda femoris artery. **B,** Profunda femoris artery in diabetic patient with peripheral vascular disease.

ceptable and has been shown to have the same long-term patency rate as an autogenous vein graft.[77,78]

Use of the in situ autogenous vein graft as the conduit for vascular reconstruction (Fig. 6-17) has allowed the distal anastomosis to be performed at a more peripheral site, with good long-term graft patency. Because diabetic patients often have peripheral vascular disease in the tibial-peroneal trunk and pedal arch vessels, use of the in situ bypass has allowed more direct arterial reconstruction. Diabetic patients often have adequate arterial inflow into the distal femoral or popliteal artery; using these vessels for the proximal anastomosis, while taking the distal anastomosis to the terminal tibial artery branches or foot vessels, is associated with long-term patency and healing of ulcerated or gangrenous areas on the foot. Frequently, after initial success of a graft and

healing of the skin lesion or toe and forefoot amputation site, re-occlusion of the graft might not result in re-ulceration or breakdown of the amputation site.

With use of the in situ technique, more previously unacceptable autogenous saphenous veins can function as long-term patent conduits, because less endothelial cell injury during preparation of the conduit and a better anastomotic size match result. Preoperative ultrasonographic assessment of the autogenous vein allows the surgeon to make the skin incision directly over the saphenous vein and avoids the risk of skin necrosis. The technique also allows assessment of the size of the autogenous vein, the valves, and the presence of any postphlebitic segments within the vein (Fig. 6-18). Completion of intraoperative ultrasonographic assessment of the anastomosis and conduits can detect defects that could result in early failure. With proper

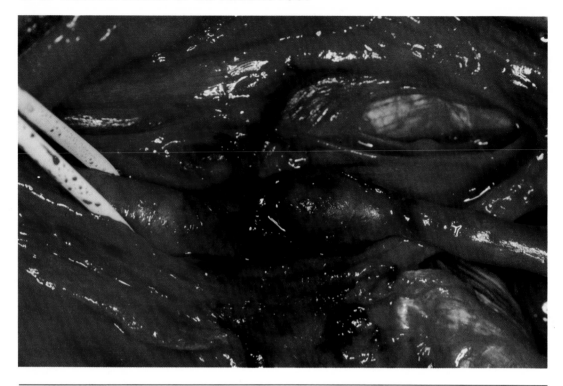

FIGURE 6–17 ■ Anastomosis of in situ antogenous vein graft and distal anterior tibial artery.

corrective action, re-operation or graft failure can be avoided.

The use of angioplasty as an alternative to reconstructive bypass surgery has limited application in diabetic patients. The best results with angioplasty are in those with localized arterial stenoses or occlusions,[79] but this is seldom found in the diabetic patient with peripheral vascular insufficiency. In addition, subintimal dissection can be caused by attempted recanalization, worsen the clinical picture, and result in subsequent urgent reconstructive surgery.

Because of the potential for early graft failure, elective orthopedic surgery at the same time as reconstructive vascular surgery is not recommended. An appropriate period should be allowed after reconstructive vascular surgery before reconstructive orthopedic surgery is undertaken.

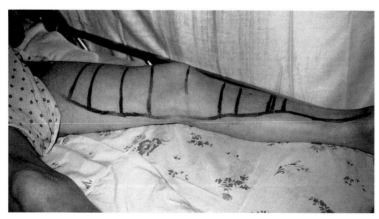

FIGURE 6–18 ■ Mapping of the saphenous vein.

The conduit patency and limb salvage rates after reconstructive vascular surgery are similar for both diabetic and nondiabetic patients. Hurley and colleagues have shown that the cumulative patency rate and limb salvage rate 6 years postoperatively are actually higher in diabetic patients than in nondiabetic patients.[76] Other studies have shown a cumulative patency rate of 94% at 5 years for both diabetics and nondiabetics.[75] It is important to remember, however, that although properly prepared diabetic patients do not have increased morbidity and mortality after major peripheral vascular surgery, they do have a reduced life expectancy as a result of the other manifestations of vascular disease.

Education and proper foot care can avoid many of the accompanying foot complications in the diabetic patient. Before elective orthopedic reconstruction of the foot in diabetics, assessment of the presence and severity of PVD is essential. In properly selected and prepared diabetic patients, the perioperative morbidity and mortality are comparable to those in nondiabetics. Reconstructive vascular surgery, if necessary, should precede other surgery to minimize complications attendant to surgery on an ischemic foot.

References

1. Corson JD, et al. The diabetic foot. Curr Probl Surg. 1986; 23:721–788.
2. Levin ME. The diabetic foot: pathophysiology, evaluation and treatment. In: Levin ME, O'Neal LW, eds. The diabetic foot, 4th ed. St. Louis: CV Mosby; 1988; 1–50.
3. Sicard GA, Walker WB, Anderson CB. Vascular surgery. In: Levin ME, O'Neal LW, eds. The diabetic foot, 4th ed. St. Louis: C.V. Mosby; 1988; 151–181.
4. University Group Diabetes Program. Mortality results. Diabetes. 1970; (Suppl 2) 19:785–830.
5. Kannel WB, McGee DL. Diabetes and cardiovascular disease. The Framingham study. JAMA. 1979; 241:2035–2038.
6. Allison RD, Roth GM. Central and peripheral vascular effects during cigarette smoking. Arch Environ Health. 1969; 19:189–198.
7. Juergens JL, ed. Peripheral vascular disease. Philadelphia: WB Saunders; 1980.
8. Wald N, Howard S, Smith PG, et al. Association between atherosclerotic diseases and carboxyhaemoglobin levels in tobacco smokers. Br Med J. 1973; 1:761–765.
9. Levine PH. An acute effect of cigarette smoking on platelet function. A possible link between smoking and arterial thrombosis. Circulation. 1973; 48:619–623.
10. Beach KW, Strandness DE Jr. Arteriosclerosis obliterans and associated risk factors in insulin-dependent and non-insulin-dependent diabetes. Diabetes. 1980; 29:882–888.
11. Kannel WB, Shurtleff D. The natural history of arteriosclerosis obliterans. Cardiovasc Clin. 1971; 3:37–52.
12. Kreines K, et al. The course of peripheral vascular disease in non-insulin-dependent diabetes. Diabetes Care. 1985; 8:235–243.
13. West KM. Epidemiology of diabetes and its vascular lesions. New York: Elsevier; 1978.
14. Janka HU, Standl E, Mehnert H. Peripheral vascular disease in diabetes mellitus and its relation to cardiovascular risk factors: screening with the Doppler ultrasonic technique. Diabetes Care. 1980; 3:207–213.
15. Melton LJ III, Macken KM, Palumbo PJ, et al. Incidence and prevalence of clinical peripheral vascular disease in a population-based cohort of diabetic patients. Diabetes Care. 1980; 3:650–654.
16. Tibell B. Peripheral arterial insufficiency. Acta Orthop Scand [Suppl]. 1971; 139:51–54.
17. Barner HB. Vasculitis in maturity-onset diabetes mellitus. JAMA. 1976; 235:2495–2501.
18. Conrad MC. Large and small artery occlusion in diabetics and nondiabetics with severe vascular disease. Circulation. 1967; 36:83–91.
19. Levin ME, O'Neal LW. Peripheral vascular disease. In: Ellenberg M, Rifkin H, eds. Diabetes mellitus: theory and practice, 3rd ed. New Hyde Park, NY: Medical Examination Publishing; 1983; 803–828.
20. Fein FS, Scheuer J. Heart disease in diabetes. In: Ellenberg M, Rifkin H, eds. Diabetes mellitus: theory and practice, 3rd ed. New Hyde Park, NY: Medical Examination Publishing; 1983; 851–861.
21. Marinelli MR, et al. Noninvasive testing vs clinical evaluation of arterial disease. A prospective study. JAMA. 1979; 241:2031–2034.
22. Long JW Jr, Stevens R, Lichti E, et al. Reliability of continuous-wave Doppler probes. J Vasc Surg. 1987; 5:558–565.
23. Winsor T. Influence of arterial disease on the systolic blood pressure gradients of the extremity. Am J Med Sci. 1950; 220:117–126.
24. Hurley JJ, Hershey FB, Auer AI, et al. Noninvasive evaluation of peripheral arterial status: The physiologic approach. In: Levin ME, O'Neal LW eds. The diabetic foot, 4th ed. St. Louis: CV Mosby; 1988; 119–130.
25. Sumner DS, Strandness DE Jr. The relationship between calf blood flow and ankle pressure in patients with intermittent claudication. Surgery. 1969; 65:763–771.
26. Carter SA. Clinical measurement of systolic pressures in limbs with arterial occlusive disease. JAMA. 1969; 207:1869–1874.
27. Fronek A, Coel M, Bernstein EF. The importance of combined multisegmental pressure and Doppler flow velocity studies in the diagnosis of peripheral arterial occlusive disease. Surgery. 1978; 84:840–847.
28. Raines JK, et al. Vascular laboratory criteria for

the management of peripheral vascular disease of the lower extremities. Surgery. 1976; 79:21–29.

29. Hobbs JT, Yao ST, Lewis JD, et al. A limitation of the Doppler ultrasound method of measuring ankle systolic pressure. Vasa. 1974; 3:160–162.

30. Guggenheim W, et al. Femoral and popliteal occlusive disease. A report on 143 diabetic patients. Diabetes. 1969; 18:428–433.

31. Gundersen J. Segmental measurements of systolic blood pressure in the extremities including the thumb and great toe. Acta Chir Scand [Suppl]. 1972; 426:1–90.

32. Reidy NC, et al. Anatomic localization of atherosclerotic lesions by hemodynamic tests. Arch Surg. 1981; 116:1041–1044.

33. Barnes RW. Noninvasive diagnostic techniques in peripheral vascular disease. Am Heart J. 1979; 97:241–258.

34. Flanigan DP, et al. Correlation of Doppler-derived high thigh pressure and intra-arterial pressure in the assessment of aorto-iliac occlusive disease. Br J Surg. 1981; 68:423–425.

35. Rutherford RB, Lowenstein DH, Klein MF. Combining segmental systolic pressures and plethysmography to diagnose arterial occlusive disease of the legs. Am J Surg. 1979; 138:211–218.

36. Karanfilian RG, et al. The value of laser Doppler velocimetry and transcutaneous oxygen tension determination in predicting healing of ischemic forefoot ulcerations and amputations in diabetic and nondiabetic patients. J Vasc Surg. 1986; 4:511–517.

37. Tonnesen KH. Transcutaneous oxygen tension in imminent foot gangrene. Acta Anaesthesiol Scand [Suppl]. 1978; 68:107–110.

38. Franzeck UK, et al. Transcutaneous PO_2 measurements in health and peripheral arterial occlusive disease. Surgery. 1982; 91:156–165.

39. Burgess EM, Matsen FA III, Wyss CR, et al. Segmental transcutaneous measurements of PO_2 in patients requiring below-the-knee amputation for peripheral vascular insufficiency. J Bone Joint Surg (Am). 1982; 64A:378–382.

40. Katsamouris A, et al. Transcutaneous oxygen tension in selection of amputation level. Am J Surg. 1984; 147:510–517.

41. Ratliff DA, Clyne CAC, Chant ADB, et al. Prediction of amputation wound healing: the role of transcutaneous PO_2 assessment. Br J Surg. 1984; 71:219–222.

42. Keagy BA, Kotb M, Burnham S, Johnson G Jr. A comparison of four non-invasive methods of preoperative determination of the site of healing in a lower extremity amputation. Presented at the San Diego Symposium on Non-Invasive Diagnostic Techniques in Vascular Disease. San Diego; February 22–26, 1988.

43. Karanfilian RG, et al. The assessment of skin blood flow in peripheral vascular disease by laser Doppler velocimetry. Am Surg. 1984; 50:641–644.

44. Ruoff BA, et al. Real-time duplex ultrasound mapping of the greater saphenous vein before in situ infrainguinal revascularization. J Vasc Surg. 1987; 6:107–113.

45. Salles-Cunh S, Tolan D. Evaluation of a magnetic resonance scanner. Presented at the San Diego Symposium on Non-Invasive Diagnostic Techniques in Vascular Disease. San Diego; February 22–26, 1988.

46. Carter SA. Response of ankle systolic pressure to leg exercise in mild or questionable arterial disease. N Engl J Med. 1972; 287:578–582.

47. Hummel BW, et al. Reactive hyperemia vs. treadmill exercise testing in arterial disease. Arch Surg. 1978; 113:95–98.

48. Ansell G, Wilkins RA. Complications in diagnostic imaging. Chicago: Blackwell/Year Book Medical Publishers; 1987.

49. Salam AA. The role of vascular surgery in the management of arterial insufficiency in diabetes. In: Davidson JK, ed. Clinical diabetes mellitus: a problem-oriented approach. New York: Thieme, 1986; 407–415.

50. Shafi T, Chou SY, Porosh JG, et al. Infusion intravenous pyelography and renal function. Effects in patients with chronic renal insufficiency. Arch Intern Med. 1978; 138:1218–1221.

51. VanZee BE, Hoy WE, Talley TE, et al. Renal injury associated with intravenous pyelography in nondiabetic and diabetic patients. Ann Intern Med. 1978; 89:51–54.

52. Harkonen S, Kjellstrand C. Intravenous pyelography in nonuremic diabetic patients. Nephron. 1979; 24:268–270.

53. Mason RA, Arbert LA, Giron F. Renal dysfunction after arteriography. JAMA. 1985; 253:1001–1004.

54. Moreau JF. Nephrotoxicity of uroangiographic contrast media. In: Ameil M, ed. Contrast media in radiology. New York: Springer-Verlag; 1982; 195–200.

55. Neiman HL, Yao JS. Angiography of vascular disease. New York: Churchill Livingstone; 1985.

56. Bron KM. Femoral arteriography. In: Abrams HL, ed. Abrams' angiography. Boston: Little, Brown and Company; 1983; 1835–1875.

57. Hallin RW. Femoropopliteal versus femorotibial bypass grafting for lower extremity revascularization. Am Surg. 1976; 42:522–526.

58. Reichle FA, Tyson RR. Comparison of long-term results of 364 femoropopliteal or femorotibial bypasses for revascularization of severely ischemic lower extremities. Ann Surg. 1975; 182:449–455.

59. Dardik H, Dardik II, Sprayregen S, et al. Patient selection and improved technical factors in small-vessel bypass procedures of the lower extremity. Surgery. 1975; 77:249–254.

60. Imparato AM, Kim GE, Madayag M, et al. Angiographic criteria for successful tibial arterial reconstructions. Surgery. 1973; 74:830–838.

61. O'Mara CS, et al. Correlation of foot arterial anatomy with early tibial bypass patency. Surgery 1981; 89:743–752.

62. Picus D, Staple TW, Gilula LA, et al. Radiographic imaging and treatment of vascular disease in the diabetic patient. In: Levin ME, O'Neal LW, eds. The diabetic foot. St. Louis: CV Mosby; 1988; 182–202.

63. Moore WS. Determination of amputation level. Arch Surg. 1973; 107:798–802.

64. Lippmann HI. Must loss of limb be a consequence of diabetes mellitus? Diabetes Care. 1979; 2:432–436.

65. [Anonymous]. Management of intermittent clau-

dication [editorial]. Lancet. 1980; 1:404–405.

66. Paffenbarger RS, Hyde RT. Exercise as protection against heart attack [editorial]. N Engl J Med. 1980; 302:1026–1027.

67. Kramsch DM, et al. Cardiovascular effects of exercise in primate atherosclerosis. Circulation. 1979; 59/60:(Suppl 2) II167.

68. Coffman JD. Drug therapy: vasodilator drugs in peripheral vascular disease. N Engl J Med. 1979; 300:713–717.

69. Hoffman DC, Jepson RP. Muscle blood flow and sympathectomy. Surg Gynecol Obstet. 1968; 127:12–16.

70. Smith RB, et al. Effect of lumbar sympathectomy on muscle blood flow in advanced occlusive vascular disease. Am Surg. 1971; 37:247–251.

71. Waibel PP, et al. Increase of arteriovenous shunts after lumbar sympathectomy. J Cardiovasc Surg (Torino). 1975; (Special Issue):638–641.

72. Kreuzer W, Schenk WG Jr. Hemodynamic responses to lumbar sympathectomy. An experimental study of changes in blood flow and limb oxygen consumption in the dog with acute or chronic arterial obstruction. J Cardiovasc Surg (Torino). 1972; 13:532–537.

73. Moore WS, Hall AD. Effects of lumbar sympathectomy on skin capillary blood flow in arterial occlusive disease. J Surg Res. 1973; 14: 151–157.

74. Boulton AJM, Bowker JH. The diabetic foot. In: Olefsky JM, Sherwin RS, eds. Diabetes mellitus: management and complications. New York: Churchill Livingstone; 1985; 255–275.

75. Bradley RF. Cardiovascular disease. In: Marble A, et al. Joslin's diabetes mellitus, 11th ed. Philadelphia: Lea & Febiger; 1971; 417–477.

76. Hurley JJ, et al. Distal arterial reconstruction: patency and limb salvage in diabetics. J Vasc Surg. 1987; 5:796–802.

77. Bergan JJ, et al. Randomization of autogenous vein and polytetrafluoroethylene grafts in femoral distal reconstruction. Surgery. 1982; 92:921–930.

78. Rosenthal D, Levine K, Stanton PE Jr, et al. Femoropopliteal bypass: the preferred site for distal anastomosis. Surgery. 1983; 93:1–4.

79. Fallon JT. Pathology of arterial lesions amenable to percutaneous transluminar angioplasty. Am J Roentgenol. 1980; 135:913–916.

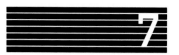

Neurologic Complications of Diabetes in the Lower Extremities

JOHN H. FEIBEL, M.D.

The neurologic manifestations of diabetes mellitus in the foot are among its most important problems. Diabetic neuropathy interacts with hyperglycemia and large vessel arterial and microvascular angiopathy to cause pathologic changes that often result in amputation of the foot or leg. This chapter reviews diabetic neuropathic syndromes in the foot and highlights their presumed pathogenesis, pathology, principles of diagnosis, and treatment. Diabetic neuropathy has also been discussed elsewhere.[1,2]

Diabetic neuropathy is a common complication of diabetes; 10 to 55% of diabetics have objective signs of neuropathy.[2] Differences in prevalence might reflect differences in defining neuropathy and in patient characteristics, such as how long the disease has been present, because the prevalence of neuropathy increases with disease duration. At the time of diagnosis, approximately 8 to 14% of patients have neuropathy. Approximately 50% of patients who have had the disease for 25 years have neuropathy.[3] Other reports indicate a lower prevalence (20 to 25%) at 25 years.[4]

The clinical spectrum of diabetic neuropathy is wide ranging from mild paresthesias in the feet to neuropathic ulceration, joint destruction, and severe pain syndromes. Clinical manifestations also appear to vary significantly. The onset and progression can be abrupt or insidious, the degree of disability varies, and partial recovery can sometimes occur.

Involvement of the peripheral nervous system can result in a single syndrome or in a combination of syndromes, and these can be classified as follows:

1. Symmetric diffuse polyneuropathy
   a. Distal primary sensory neuropathy
   b. Autonomic neuropathy
   c. Proximal motor neuropathy
2. Asymmetric (mononeuropathy and mononeuropathy multiplex) syndromes
   a. Proximal motor neuropathy (diabetic amyotrophy)
   b. Focal and entrapment neuropathies
   c. Cranial neuropathies
3. Combinations of the above

This classification scheme is useful and describes the clinical region affected, but other systems can be used. The predominant function affected can be used as a reference—that is, sensory, motor, or autonomic nervous function is frequently used to classify the neuropathy. Another system uses the predominantly affected preipheral fiber size to differentiate categories—large (more than 2.0 mm) or small, 0.2 to 2.0 mm in diameter. A purely descriptive classification scheme can be used and includes acute painful, ataxic, and acrodystrophic neuropathy categories. A pathogenetic classification can be used to divide neuropathies as distal or proximal and as symmetric or asymmetric because of their distinct differences in pathogenesis.

In this chapter the neuropathies affecting the lower extremity, particularly the foot, are considered. The important symptoms, signs, and differential diagnostic considerations are discussed, as well as the role of diagnostic testing.

CLINICAL SYNDROMES IN DIABETIC NEUROPATHY

Distal Sensorimotor Polyneuropathy

The most common diabetic neuropathy—*distal, predominantly symmetric, polyneuropathy*—begins with sensory symptoms that reflect preferential damage to small sensory fibers. Because small fibers are affected first to this type of neuropathy, it is not surprising that autonomic symptoms and signs are often associated with the somatic sensory findings. In one study,[5] 16 of 27 patients with sensorimotor neuropathy had coexistent autonomic symptoms and signs, and all but one of the patients with autonomic findings had somatic sensory abnormalities.

Typically, symptoms are first present in the toes, the somatic region innervated by the longest axons, which are most vulnerable to metabolic derangements. As the disease progresses symptoms move up the legs. Eventually the hands can be affected, because proportionally less axonal length is required to produce symptoms. This produces the classic clinical picture of stocking-glove distribution. In the most severe cases, even the anterior trunk and vertex of the head can be involved. Because of their shorter axonal length the somatic paraspinal nerves innervating the posterior trunk are spared. This allows the examiner to determine the difference between a true sensory level indicating a myelopathy and diabetic polyneuropathy with truneal involvement (Fig. 7-1). The most common sensory symptoms are paresthesias, such as spontaneous tingling (pins and needles), dysesthesias with an unpleasant, hypersensitive response to touch, shooting pains, and complaints suggesting sensory deficits of numbness and decreased sensitivity to thermal and light touch sensation. Autonomic symptoms, such as dizziness on postural change, which often accompany somatic complaints such as impotence, are frequently an early symptom in males. These sensory symptoms are a result of small fiber nerve involvement, including the sympathetic C fiber, along with autonomic nerve fiber damage.

The neurologic examination in those with early distal sensorimotor neuropathy mir

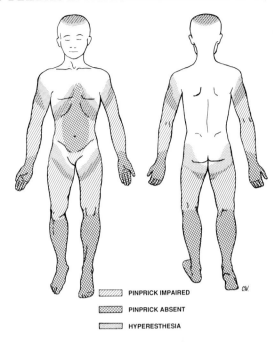

PINPRICK IMPAIRED

PINPRICK ABSENT

HYPERESTHESIA

FIGURE 7-1 ■ Sensory loss in severe diabetic diffuse sensory polyneuropathy. The short nerve roots providing sensation to the back and buttocks are spared. After Sabin TD, et al. Patterns of Clinical Deficits in Peripheral Nerve Disease. In: Waxman SG (ed. Physiology and pathobiology of axons. New York: Raven Press; 1978; 431–438.

rors the predominantly sensory nature of this syndrome. Weakness, if present, is found in the foot muscles, and vibration and proprioception, subserved by larger diameter fibers, are spared. Pain and temperature sensation are reduced distally, whereas tendon reflexes are often spared initially. The diagnostic criteria for diabetic distal polyneuropathy have been reviewed by Dyck and colleagues,[6] who used sural nerve biopsy results as the "gold standard" by which to differentiate diabetics with and without neuropathy. Their findings suggested that polyneuropathy can be diagnosed reliably if two or more of the following investigations are abnormal: neurologic symptoms score, neurologic examination and disability score, nerve conduction testing, and computer-assisted sensory examination. Of 84 neuropathy patients, 95% had abnormal findings on nerve conduction studies, 82% had abnormalities on sensory testing, including touch pressure, vibratory joint position, and pinprick in dorsal great toe, 80% had an abnormal neurologic symptoms score, and another 80% had an abnormal neurologic disability score.[6] Of the 41 patients without neuropathy, 53% had no abnormality on any of these four evaluations. Definite neuropathy can be diagnosed if the following criteria are met: (1) nerve conduction abnormalities are found in two or more nerves (sensory or motor) and (2) ankle reflexes are reduced in those patients less than 70 years of age or absent in those over 70, or vibration perception is reduced in patients under 70 years of age or absent in those over 70. These criteria, although specific and reliable, are not particularly sensitive because (as noted above) many patients with early distal neuropathy can retain tendon reflexes for some time.

Because other diseases present similarly with distal, predominantly sensory, polyneuropathy, it is important to exclude them before diagnosing diabetes as the cause of neuropathy. The history should focus on possible muscle or nerve disease in relatives, including pes cavus and gait problems and on alcohol, drug, or vitamin abuse. A history of other diseases, such as hypothyroidism, B_{12} or other nutritional deficiency, cancer, or exposure to heavy metals or solvents, should be sought.

Small fibers are affected first, but large fiber damage may follow. In a series of 47 diabetics with neuropathy, Guy and associates[7] found that, whereas thermal sensory loss signifying small fiber disease occurred in isolation, vibratory sensory loss signifying large fiber damage did not occur by itself, but did occur simultaneously with thermal loss in many patients. Autonomic and painful neuropathies are associated with small fiber damage, but chronic painless neuropathy with foot ulceration and more severely reduced nerve conductions are associated with large fiber involvement.[8]

One variant of small fiber neuropathy is termed "acute painful neuropathy." This relatively uncommon condition consists of severe burning, distal foot pain, hyperpathia, and hyperesthesia to light touch. The pain can be incapacitating, and the syndrome is often associated with significant weight loss and with impotence in males. Experience in treating alcoholic diabetics reveals that they are particularly vulnerable to this syndrome, which fortunately resolves over several months. Treatment is symptomatic and includes pain control and maintenance of excellent diabetic control. Small fiber damage can also cause so-called treatment-induced neuropathy. In this condition pain and paresthesia occur when insulin treatment is begun, suggesting that improved control of hyperglycemia leads to axonal regeneration and, in the course of axonal sprouting, to sensory symptoms of pain.

NEUROPATHIC FOOT ULCERATION

Chronic, often painless, *foot ulceration* is usually associated with large fiber neuropathy. Large fiber involvement, however, is *not* a prerequisite for the development of diabetic acrodystrophic changes, because patients with small fiber disease can occasionally develop foot ulceration also. Small fiber involvement precedes large fiber involvement, so a combination of the two might be necessary for ulceration to occur. If large fibers are damaged the patient has reduced vibratory and proprioception sensation, and findings typical of posterior spinal cord column involvement are noted. Symptoms of spinal cord involvement include ataxia, initially only with closed eyes, manifested by a positive Romberg sign (swaying or falling on closing the eyes). The patient tends to have a slap-foot gait because of reduced sensory input from the feet, similar to that of tabes dorsalis. Actual joint destruction from diabetic neuropathy is rare, but can occur.[9] If pain and temperature sensory loss (small fiber), impotence, bladder dysfunction (autonomic fiber), and reduced vibratory and proprioceptive sensation with ataxia, absent tendon reflexes, and foot ulceration (large fiber) are all present, the syndrome is known as *diabetic pseudotabes.* Small distal joints (interphalangeal and metatarsophalangeal in the foot and ankle) undergo neuropathic destruction of bone (Fig. 7-2). Osteo-arthropathy in this setting is often preceded by trauma. On the other hand, osteopathy and osteo-arthropathy

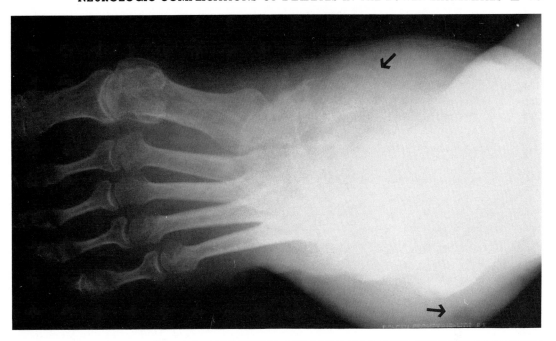

FIGURE 7–2 ■ Radiograph of a foot with diabetic neuropathic (Charcot) midtarsal joints showing destruction with medial displacement of the midfoot (*upper arrow*). Air density in soft tissue (*lower arrow*) resulted from ulcer formation under the weight-bearing portion beneath the lateral malleolus of the ankle.

from neuropathic disease also predispose to pathologic fracture.

The neuropathic ulcer (Fig. 7-3) is a circular, nonhealing lesion situated over the metatarsal heads on the plantar surface of the toes. Ulceration can be precipitated by any trauma, mechanical or thermal, in the susceptible diabetic foot. Impaired sensation prevents the patient from recognizing potential sources of injury and intrinsic muscle weakness and leads to foot deformities that expose the tissue over the metatarsal heads to additional trauma. The foot deformity results from the uncompensated overaction of long toe extensors and flexors caused by weakened foot intrinsics.

Neuropathic foot ulceration occurs experimentally only when both somatic and autonomic neuropathy are present. In the diabetic dog, leg ulceration was produced only after transection of both the lumbar sympathetic and sciatic nerves.[10] Somatic sensory loss, especially that of pain and temperature, increases vulnerability to any type of trauma, and somatic motor weakness is believed to promote ulceration by deforming the foot (claw toes), thus exposing the metatarsal heads to trauma.[11] Peripheral large vessel disease is not a prerequisite for ulceration. Often, neuropathic ulceration is present in patients with excellent foot pulses. Autonomic insufficiency, however, can cause vascular changes that appear to be essential to the production of ulcers. Denervation can also abolish the venivasomotor reflex with a subsequent increase in venous and capillary pressures, especially in the standing position.[12] Increased capillary permeability leads to albumin leakage, with pericapillary edema contributing to increased distal venous pressure and a reduction in arterial flow and venous stasis. Neurogenic foot edema is thereby produced and retards healing of injured tissue. Autonomic neuropathy also leads to sudomotor insufficiency, with reduction of normal sweating. This can dry, fissured skin, especially around calloused areas, which in turn increases susceptibility to infection.

As noted above, *neuropathic foot ulcer-*

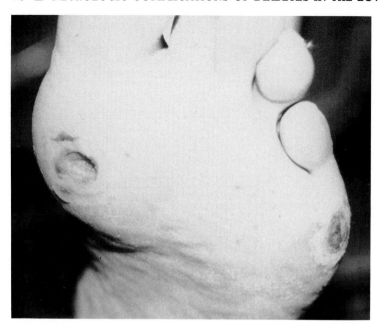

FIGURE 7–3 ■ Neurotrophic ulcer beneath the first and fifth metatarsal heads in a patient with diabetes mellitus.

ation often occurs with intact foot pulses and no evidence of major large vessel disease. In fact, patients with neuropathic ulcers often have increased foot temperature and venous distension.[13] The demonstration of high oxygen concentration in venous blood from the venae comitantes accompanying the dorsalis pedis artery,[7] plus abnormal Doppler arterial patterns from the posterior tibial arteries in ulcer patients,[14] support the presence of arteriovenous shunting caused by sympathetic denervation. Increased arteriovenous shunting leads to capillary ischemia in distal tissues and thus promotes ulceration.[15] Increased blood flow from sympathic denervation has also been demonstrated by isotope bone studies. Increased isotope uptake is present in diabetic neuropathy in the foot. Presumably, sympathetic denervation reduces arterial vasoconstriction and, in bone, leads to osteopenia and pathologic fracture or development of a neuropathic (Charcot) joint.

Neuropathic foot lesions are clearly related to neurogenic dysfunction in the small, unmyelinated, nociceptive C fibers that mediate pain and vasomotor responses. Parkhouse and LeQuesne[16] have demonstrated that foot ulcers and neuroarthropathy in diabetes occur in patients with impaired neurogenic vasodilatation responses to chemi-

cal or mechanical stimulation. Changes in blood flow were measured after chemical production of an axonal reflex flare in five groups of patients: control, long-standing diabetics without foot lesions, patients having miscellaneous lesions with ulceration, those with foot ulceration, and those with neuroarthropathy. The contribution of occlusive vascular disease was eliminated by the presence of intact, direct, non-neurogenically induced local reaction from mechanical stimulation in all groups. Diabetic patients without foot lesions had normal neurogenic responses. Those with a miscellaneous lesion, ulcers, and neuroarthropathy had progressively more impaired or absent chemically induced vasodilatation. *Impaired vasodilatation reduces the inflammatory response to any form of trauma or infection and predisposes to ulceration and arthropathy.* An impaired neurogenic response also correlated with reduced or absent sensation to pinprick. Thus, impairment in nociceptive C fibers results in two separate abnormalities, decreased pain sensation and absent inflammatory response, which correlate with neuropathic foot lesions.

Diabetic autonomic neuropathy frequently accompanies somatic symmetric neuropathy and is important in the pathogenesis of foot ulcers. The gastrointestinal, circulatory, and urogenital systems are involved, along with sudomotor and vasomotor dysfunction. Only a minority of diabetics have major debilitating autonomic insufficiency, such as severe orthostasis. Impotence is common, however, and gastroparesis is not infrequent. Simple noninvasive testing has been recommended for routine clinical monitoring. Participants at a conference on diabetic neuropathy have suggested that routine tests of heart rate response to the Valsalva maneuver, deep breathing, and standing, blood pressure responses to standing, tilting, or sustained hand grip, and tests of sudomotor control, including temperature and chemical-induced (acetylcholine) sweating, be used in diagnosis. Ewing and Clark[17] have quantified these investigations. Heart rate abnormalities occur primarily as result of parasympathetic impairment, whereas blood pressure abnormalities generally reflect parasympathetic impairment.

The role of sympathetic denervation with loss of vascular tone in contributing to ulceration has been shown by the results of studies of the beneficial effect of ephedrine, a sympathomimetic agent, on relieving edema and decreasing blood flow.[18] In addition, the deleterious role of increased blood flow caused by arteriovenous shunting, with subsequent distal ischemia, has been demonstrated by the healing of ulceration after ligation of the dorsalis pedis artery.[19]

TREATMENT OF NEUROPATHIC DIABETIC FOOT PROBLEMS

Gangrene is 50 to 70 times more prevalent in diabetics than in age-adjusted controls. This startling finding is a result of the combination of arterial insufficiency, neuropathic changes, and infection. Treatment of the consequences of distal polyneuropathy is important in preventing amputation and decreasing morbidity. Because a callus predisposes to and accentuates ulceration and infection, it must be carefully removed. Any infection, either cellulitis or abscess, must be debrided, cultured, and treated with the appropriate antibiotic. Because edema and stasis are worsened by the upright position, bed rest during acute treatment of ulceration is often needed. Additionally, care must

be taken to decrease pressure over the affected region; the foot must be insulated as much as possible, which might necessitate making a cast of the foot and molding a shoe around it. For ulcers in weight-bearing areas on the plantar surface, shoes with a rocker sole reduce pressure during walking. These custom-made shoes can decrease the relapse rate from 90 to 19%.[20] Operative procedures designed to decrease mechanical trauma to susceptible areas can limit ulceration. Metatarsal osteotomy or removal of the metatarsal head(s) can be helpful.[21,22] Methods for reducing arterial insufficiency (e.g., proper exercise, cessation of smoking, special diet to decrease cholesterol and lipid levels) and for preventing infection are of paramount importance. A protocol for diabetic foot care is presented in Table 7-1.[23] Use of a multidisciplinary approach in a diabetic foot clinic has achieved a 50% decrease in the number of amputations and a 90% healing rate for ulcers.[24]

Proximal Motor Neuropathies

ASYMMETRIC FORM

The most important asymmetric diabetic syndrome affecting the lower extremity causes severe pain and weakness of the hip and thigh. This entity, previously termed "diabetic amyotrophy,"[25] is now also called asymmetric proximal motor neuropathy.[26] A related disorder, symmetric proximal motor neuropathy, is less common. In one case (see above) the asymmetric form was shown to be a result of microinfarctions in the nerve fascicles of several large nerves, a mononeuritis multiplex.[27] In this case small epineural artery occlusion and severe arteriolar thickening were present.

Clinically, the diabetic patient, usually middle-aged and insulin or noninsulin-dependent, has severe hip and thigh pain associated with acute or subacute developing weakness in the same region. By contrast, almost no sensory deficit is found in typical cases. The pain is worse at night, aching in character, and disappears after several months. The unilateral weakness is followed by atrophy and involves the quadriceps, adductor, and iliopsoas muscles. Weakness is present in the thigh and knee

TABLE 7–1 ■ Foot Care for the Diabetic Patient

DO NOT
Cut corns, calluses, or hangnails.
Trim toenails with fingernail clippers or scissors.
Put talcum or baby powder in shoes.
Rub between toes with rough towel.
Put strong chemicals on feet.
Walk barefoot at any time.

DO
Contact your podiatrist for care of corns, calluses, or ingrown toenails.
Cut toenails straight across with toenail clippers.
Use a good foot powder daily in your shoes.
Bathe feet daily in lukewarm water with mild soap.
Dry carefully between toes.
Use a good foot cream daily before retiring.
Inspect feet daily (bottom, top, and between toes).
Contact your physician if leg becomes red, hard, or swollen.

From Young JR. Foot problems in the diabetic. Cleveland Clin J Med. 1988; 55:458.

and climbing stairs is difficult. Other muscle groups, the glutei and hamstrings, are less often affected. The knee jerk reflex is depressed or absent. If the syndrome is associated with distal polyneuropathy, as is often the case, more widespread reflex depression is present.[28] Weight loss is often associated with the syndrome's onset and weight gain accompanies recovery. Recovery is slow and can take longer than 1 year.

Differential diagnosis of the unilateral neuropathy includes lumbar radioculopathy (L2–L4), inflammation of the lumbar plexus associated with a high sedimentation rate, invasion of a nerve root by carcinomatous cells, and inflammatory myopathy. Other causes of mononeuritis multiplex, such as periarteritis nodosa, might need to be ruled out. Hip disease can cause pain and an apparent weakness. When a structural lesion is suspected myelography or computerized tomography (CT) of the lumbar spine and/or CT of the pelvis to exclude lesions involving the lumbar plexus can be performed. Electrodiagnostic studies are also helpful. Treatment is symptomatic and includes pain control and maintenance of proper nutrition and diabetic control, plus the knowledge that recovery will occur.

SYMMETRIC FORM

The symmetric form of proximal motor neuropathy is slowly progressive and, as in the asymmetric form, is associated with aching pain and weakness in the same mus-

cles. The knee jerk reflex is depressed but sensory loss is minimal. Although the natural history is unknown, Brown and Asbury[29] have suggested that instituting insulin therapy appears to stop disease progress. Recovery is slow and measured over months. Differential diagnosis includes those conditions discussed above for the asymmetric form. The pathogenesis of this condition is also unknown and, like the asymmetric form, may be a result of a bilateral mononeuritis multiplex. Diabetic involvement of the plexus or multiple roots, however, cannot be discounted.

Focal and Entrapment Mononeuropathies

Focal mononeuropathies such as femoral neuropathy are thought to be caused by ischemic processes. Femoral neuropathy is often a component of the asymmetric proximal motor neuropathy syndrome. Focal entrapment and compression neuropathies are twice as common in diabetics.[30] Major compression entrapment neuropathies affecting the foot are peroneal neuropathy at the fibular head and posterior tibial neuropathy with entrapment at the tarsal tunnel. Slow conduction of the peroneal nerve at the fibular head is the most common focal electrophysiologic abnormality in diabetics.[31] Parafootdrop, either unilateral or bilateral, occurs and is usually painless. Sensory loss, if present, is found over the anteriolateral aspect of the leg. No important reflex abnormalities are found. Differentiation from lumbar radiculopathy affecting the L5 root can be difficult; electrodiagnostic testing is helpful. The localized slowing, 15 m/sec slower than distal conduction, is usually superimposed on already slowed conduction and reduced sensory and motor evoked responses caused by the distal polyneuropathy.

Focal entrapment of the posterior tibial nerve at the tarsal tunnel causes dysesthetic pain, sensory loss, and night pain in the foot. Either or both medial and lateral plantar nerve distributions can be involved. Weakness in the intrinsic foot muscles can also be present, but pain and sensory symptoms predominate. No reflex changes are present. Tinel's sign (paresthesia on tapping over the tarsal tunnel behind the medial malleolus) is commonly present. Electrodiagnostic testing demonstrates prolonged distal motor and sensory latencies across the tarsal tunnel, with reduced sensory and motor amplitudes in evoked responses. Denervation in intrinsic foot muscles can also be present. It is essential to note that diabetics usually have some generalized changes on electrodiagnostic testing from distal polyneuropathy, so it is important to compare findings in the symptomatic nerve with those in the lower extremity, motor and sensory, to ensure that focal slowing is present.

PATHOGENESIS OF NERVE INJURY IN DIABETES

The most easily understood presumed cause of diabetic peripheral nerve injury is nerve *infarction* resulting from occlusion of the vasonervosum, the nutrient artery of the nerve. This process appears to cause the asymmetric lesions found in patients with selected mononeuropathies or mononeuritis multiplex. Small vessel infarction has been pathologically proven in isolated cases of cranial[32] and lumbosacral[27] diabetic neuropathy. The patient in the latter case had an 8-month history of diabetes and developed asymmetric weakness, both proximally and distally, in the leg. Micro-infarctions were present in many nerves, including the femoral, obturator, sciatic, and posterior tibial. The nerve roots and spinal cord were not involved. Micro-infarctions are also

thought to account for the mononeuritis multiplex that occurs in patients with vasculopathies such as periarteritis nodosa. This process might also account for asymmetric lesions that occur in nerve roots, such as truncal neuropathy, or in a plexus, such as lumbosacral plexitis. It can cause diabetic amyotrophy, a mononeuritis multiplex, and/or a plexitis involving proximal lumbosacral nerve trunks.

Unlike the angiopathy of small vessels, which can cause nerve damage (as with micro-infarctions in vasonervosum), little evidence has shown that large vessel disease, unless severe, contributes to diabetic neuropathy. So-called "ischemic" neuropathy can occur acutely with catastrophic large vessel occlusion, such as that seen in dissection of the aorta. As discussed previously, neuropathy and large and small vessel disease can interact to worsen diabetes-induced lesions in the feet.

Although distal polyneuropathy is the most common diabetic neuropathy, its pathogenesis is still not completely understood. Biopsies of the distal sensory nerve, such as the sural nerve in those with diabetic distal polyneuropathy, fail to reveal enough small vessel disease and demyelination to be the sole cause of symptoms. Korthals and associates,[33] however, have described thickening of the epineural arterioles in patients with diabetic polyneuropathy. The proliferation of intimal muscle cells significantly increases in the wall of arterioles of the sural nerve, but this does not correlate with the severity of nerve fiber degeneration. Nevertheless, hyperglycemia plus associated metabolic abnormalities might be the cause of intimal proliferation in nutrient vessels, the vaso nervosum, and these alterations can contribute to decreased nerve perfusion and the development of neuropathy.

Because the clinical syndrome begins distally in the feet, it is presumed that axonal damage starts farthest from the cell body, with progressive "dying back" of the axon. *This suggests that a failure of axonal transport of nutrients and trophic factors from distal cell bodies can cause distal polyneuropathy.* The presumed failure of axonal transport might reflect a pathophysiologic mechanism that has not yet been clearly elucidated. Possibly, the longest axons, those to the feet, are involved initially because of their greatest susceptibility to metabolic insult; over time, axonal transport cannot be maintained to more proximal areas, so symptoms gradually spread proximally to the legs and finally to the hands, the so-called stocking-glove distribution. The initial involvement of the axons most distal from their neuron cell bodies does not preclude causes other than failure of axonal transport. Presumably the longest axons would be most vulnerable to any diabetic disease process, including multifocal damage from infarction or other mechanisms.

Possible causes of axonal failure, including hypoxia, myoinositol depletion and abnormal polyol metabolism, have been investigated experimentally. Low and co-workers[34] have postulated that hyperglycemia triggers alterations in the endoneurial fluid content because of rheologic changes— that is, reduced blood flow. Hypoxia in tissues bathing the nerve reduces available energy (ATP), eventually slowing axonal transport and therefore nerve conduction. Others[35] have also found decreased resting energy production in experimental diabetic neuropathy, and this has been associated with a decreased *myo*-inositol level in nerve fibers. *Myo*-inositol, a cyclic hexanol derived from glucose, in an essential constituent of intracellular nerves. This compound is synthesized into a phosphorylated form and then incorporated into various phospholipids that are critical to cell membrane stability. *Myo*-inositol uptake by nerves is competitively inhibited by glucose and is reduced by 20 to 30% in diabetic human nerves.[36] Decreased concentrations of *myo*-inositol are associated with reduced amounts of the important enzyme Na^+/K^+-ATPase and with decreased nerve conduction.[37] One study[38] has found no evidence of *myo*-inositol depletion in diabetic neuropathy, casting doubt on the significance of this compound as a cause of nerve damage.[39]

During hyperglycemia glucose is converted to sorbitol, a sugar alcohol, at high levels through the action of the enzyme aldose reductase. Abnormal sorbitol (a polyol) metabolism may cause neuropathy. In diabetics, increased concentrations of sorbitol are found in nerve tissue[38] and the sorbitol concentration is reduced by chronic treatment with the aldose reductase inhibitor sorbinil. A decrease in sorbitol level is associated with a nearly fourfold increase in regenerated myelinated fibers and with electrophysiologic and clinical improvement in nerve function.[40] These findings, obtained in a randomized study using sorbinil, suggest that a specific preventive treatment might have been found for at least one type of diabetic neuropathy.[38–40] In the sural nerves of patients with symptomatic diabetic neuropathy, the use of magnetic resonance imaging has demonstrated increased hydration. The increased water content was reversed by aldose reductase inhibitors.[41] A double-blind, placebo-controlled, 6-month study using sorbinil, however, failed to document improvement in autonomic or sensory nerve function. Another aldose reductase inhibitor, statil, failed to improve motor or sensory function, but did improve autonomic function as compared with placebo.[42,43]

ROLE OF ELECTRODIAGNOSTIC TESTING

Electrodiagnostic studies are important procedures in the evaluation of diabetics with possible or definite neuromuscular disease. Asymptomatic diabetics can have abnormal results as determined by nerve conduction studies or electromyography (EMG); however, because conduction results depend primarily on the integrity of large myelinated fibers, a normal electrodiagnostic evaluation does not preclude small fiber neuropathy. *Electrodiagnostic studies (EDS) aid in diagnosing diabetic neuropathy and in excluding other conditions, such as entrapment syndromes, polyradiculopathy, motor neuron disease, myopathy, and plexopathy.* They can also help monitor disease progress and the effect of therapy.

In diabetics with early disease and mild symptoms the most vulnerable nerves should be assessed. As noted in the discussion of distal symmetric polyneuropathy, these are distal sensory nerves in the legs, such as the sural nerve. Axonal damage is often the sole abnormality early in the course of the disease. Therefore the sensory or, less likely, the motor evoked response might be diminished compared to normals. Later distal

TABLE 7–2 ■ Protocol for Electrodiagnostic Tests

Motor nerve conduction studies
1. Unilateral studies of ulnar or median nerve, including F waves in upper limb
2. Unilateral studies of peroneal nerve, including F waves in lower limb
3. Measurement of muscle action potential amplitude and latency at each site of stimulation and calculation of segmental conduction velocity.

Sensory nerve conduction studies
1. Unilateral studies of ulnar or median nerve in upper limb
2. Unilateral studies of medial plantar or sural nerve in lower limb
3. Measurement of nerve action potential amplitude and latency at each site of stimulation and calculation of segmental conduction velocity

Studies of additional nerves: might be necessary to characterize abnormalities based on distribution of clinical symptoms or signs

From the Report and Recommendations of the San Antonio Conference on Diabetic Neuropathy. Neurology. 1988; 38:1161–165.

sensory and/or motor latencies (the time from distal stimulation to recording electrode) become prolonged. Finally slowed nerve conduction, which indicates demyelination of large fibers, can then be documented. In unselected diabetics, Mulder and colleagues[44] found that the average conduction in the peroneal nerve was 50 m/sec in normal subjects and 43 m/sec in those in the diabetic group. The amplitude of the motor evoked response was 7.6 mV in normal subjects and 4.0 mV in diabetics. In asymptomatic diabetics conduction values are slower than those of age-adjusted normal subjects and sensory nerves in the legs show more impressive changes; over 50% of asymptomatic patients have significant reduction in sensory nerve (sural) action potential amplitude.[45]

Needle EMG, which indicates neurogenic damage in muscle, can also reveal evidence of denervation (i.e., fibrillation) in asymptomatic patients. The abductor hallucis is the most sensitive muscle in asymptomatic patients; about 25% have EMG changes, indicating denervation. In neuropathy affecting axons the EMG is abnormal, with fibrillations (evidence of denervation) in distal limb muscles. Generally, electrodiagnostic findings reflect the severity of clinical findings. As symptoms and signs worsen, qualitative and quantitative electrodiagnostic changes also worsen progressively.

For screening and for following diabetics with suspected diffuse neuropathy, a sample protocol for EDS is presented in Table 7-2.

Because diabetics routinely have abnormal findings on EDS, the examiner must be cautious in the diagnosis of focal abnormalities (Tables 7-3 and 7-4). Any abnormal finding must be compared with comparable results in the contralateral nerve and in other nerves. Focal slowing and/or conduction block on nerve conduction is considered significant if the motor conduction velocity is more than 15 m/sec slower or if the distal motor or sensory latency is more than 0.5 msec slower than the comparable nerve.[47]

Focal demyelination causing conduction block can be present even if significant slowing is not demonstrable. A 50% reduction in the size (amplitude) of the proximal response compared with the distal motor unit

TABLE 7–3 ■ Classification of Electrodiagnostic Findings in Diabetic Neuropathy

Neuropathic Lesion	EMG Findings	Conduction Velocity	Motor-Sensory Latency	Motor-Sensory Amplitude
Axonal	Fibrillations	> (70%) Normal	Prolonged	Diminished
Demeyelinating (conduction block)	Usually normal	< (70%) Normal	Normal	Usually normal

TABLE 7–4 ■ Normal Electrodiagnostic Values for the Lower Extremities*

Nerve	Distal Motor Latency (msec)	Motor Amplitude (mV)	Distal Sensory Latency (msec)	Sensory Amplitude (mV)	Conduction Velocity (m/sec)
Peroneal	6.1	2.4			40
Posterior tibial	6.2	3.5			40
Sural			4.2	6.0	
F wave					36.0

*Values in any given laboratory vary slightly.

response is diagnostic of conduction block. In practice, amplitude reduction is more commonly found than slowing around the region of conduction block (e.g., the peroneal nerve at the fibular head).[47]

The results of EDS of one or even several diabetic nerves cannot be compared against normal values if a focal neuropathy is suspected. For example, in the diabetic, an apparent focal slowing in the peroneal nerve around the fibular head becomes convincing only when compared with distal values in the nerve, with the contralateral nerve, and with another similar nerve (posterior tibial). The results of EMG complement nerve conduction testing in focal neuropathies by demonstrating asymmetric denervation.

In patients with proximal motor neuropathy, characteristic EDS abnormalities, usually asymmetric, are present. In addition to the usual findings of mild to moderate diabetic distal polyneuropathy, EMG findings indicating severe denervation (e.g., fibrillation in muscles such as the iliopsoas, quadriceps, and adductors innervated by L2–L4) are found. Extensive paraspinal denervation is also found, but its cause is not clearly understood. On the basis of the EDS results, proximal motor neuropathy appears to be a more widespread process than simply mononeuritis multiplex. Lumbosacral polyradiculopathy can also be present.

TREATMENT OF PAINFUL NEUROPATHY

No discussion of treatment is complete without discussing pain alleviation. The pain of diabetic neuropathy, described as lancinating, burning, or aching, can be relentless and is often worse at night, preventing sleep. Diabetic pain syndromes are often associated with depression. Tricyclic antidepressants are effective in the relief of a number of neuropathic pain conditions, including diabetic neuropathy.[48] A randomized, double-blind, crossover study has demonstrated the amitriptyline is superior to placebo in relieving diabetic neuropathic pain in depressed and nondepressed patients. Of 29 patients, 23 reported less pain with amitriptyline as compared to placebo. Patients on high doses had more pain relief. Low doses are given initially, 10 to 25 mg, with a single nightly dose, and slowly increased to 150 mg or more at night, depending on individual tolerance of the side effects and response to the drug. Patients with serum amitriptyline levels below 100 mg might receive benefit from higher drug doses, even more than 150 mg.[49] Other nontricyclic antidepressants, such as the serotonin inhibitor trazodone, can also help control pain.[48] Adding a phenothiazine to a tricyclic antidepressant, as in the combination drug triavil, might potentiate analgesic effects.

Anticonvulsant drugs, particularly carbamazepine (Tegretol) and phenytoin (Dilantin), are helpful in alleviating peripheral nerve-induced pain syndromes such as tic douloureux. In patients with painful diabetic neuropathy, phenytoin was found to be of analgesic benefit in only one of three double-blind studies.[50] Carbamazepine was adjudged more effective than placebo in three of four double-blind comparisons.[51] These drugs are more useful in relieving intermittent lancinating pain than constant burning or aching pain.

The analgesic effects of two nonsteroidal anti-inflammatory drugs, ibuprofen (Motrin, 600 mg, qid), sulindac (Clinoril, 200 mg, bid) were compared with placebo, and it was found that both drugs are significantly better than placebo in relieving diabetic foot pain.[52] Sulindac, which has some aldose reductase inhibiting properties, might be more beneficial than ibuprofen. These drugs must be combined with others to treat severe pain effectively.

Lidocaine infusion (5 mg/kg over 30 minutes) significantly reduced diabetic pain in a placebo-controlled, double-blind study.[53] The effects lasted for 3 to 21 days. A closely related analogue of lidocaine, mexiletine (5 mg/kg), has also been successful in treating painful diabetic neuropathy.[54] The double-blind, placebo-controlled study included 16 patients. The dose given was 150 mg daily for 3 days, 300 mg daily for 3 days, and 10 mg/kg daily thereafter. No serious side effects were noted during either of these treatments.

Continuous subcutaneous insulin infusion (up to 1 year) has been shown to improve metabolic control with lower levels of glycosalated hemoglobin, improve thermal discrimination, and reduce pain.[55] Pain lessened as therapy continued, up to 12 months. Improvement in peripheral nerve function was attributed to reversible changes in small somatic nerve fibers. Continuous subcutaneous insulin infusion has been found to be superior to intensified conventional insulin therapy in improving motor, sensory, and autonomic nerve function.[56] A detailed review of the treatment of peripheral neuropathies, all etiologies, has been published.[48]

Neuropathy affecting the foot is a common and often serious complication of diabetes. Two major syndromes are seen, slowly progressive distal symmetric polyneuropathy and subacute asymmetric proximal motor neuropathy. The former is a result of metabolic damage to distal axons and myelin, whereas the latter results from infarction of the nutrient arteries to the nerve. Neuropathic ulceration occurs in long-standing diabetics secondary to trauma to insensitive tissues, with impaired autonomic responses. Meticulous care to the feet helps to prevent ulcers, infection, and amputa-tion. Preventing and treating infection decreases the risk of neuropathic ulceration. Hopefully, in the future, the use of aldose reductase inhibitors will delay the development of gangrene and neuropathic injuries.

Clinical findings including sensory, motor, and autonomic alterations, supplemented by the results of electrodiagnostic studies—nerve conduction and electromyography—can provide diagnostic clues to the presence and severity of the diabetic neuropathic conditions, some of which are treatable and others, self-limited.

References

1. Brown MJ, Asbury AK. Diabetic neuropathy. Ann Neurol. 1984; 15:1–12.
2. Dyck PJ, Thomas PK, Lambert EH, et al., eds. Diabetic neuropathy. Philadelphia: WB Saunders; 1987.
3. Pirat J. Diabetes mellitus and its degenerative complications. Diabetes Care. 1978, 1:168.
4. Palumbo JP, Elvebach LR, Whisnant JP. Neurologic complications of diabetes mellitus. Adv Neurol. 1978; 19:593.
5. Tackmann W, et al. Autonomic disturbances in relation to sensorimotor peripheral neuropathy in diabetes mellitus. J Neurol. 1981; 224:773.
6. Dyck PJ, Karnes J, O'Brien PC. Diagnosis, staging and classification of diabetic neuropathy and association with other complications. In Dyck JP, Thomas PK, Lambert EH, et al, eds. Philadelphia: WB Saunders; Diabetic neuropathy. 1987; 41.
7. Guy RJC, et al. Evaluation of thermal and vibration sensation in diabetic neuropathy. Diabetologia. 1985; 28:131.
8. Young RJ, et al. Variable relationships between peripheral somatic and autonomic neuropathy in patients with different syndromes of diabetic polyneuropathy. Diabetes. 1986; 35:192.
9. Simhas, Munichoodappa CS, Kozak GP. Neuroarthropathy (Charcot joints) in diabetes mellitus. Medicine (Baltimore). 1972; 51:191.
10. Neilubowocz J, Borkowski M, Baramiewski H. Opening of arteriovenous anastomoses and trophic ulcer formation after peripheral nerve injury. J Cardiovasc Surg. 1975; 48:100.
11. Harrison MJ, Faris IB. The neuropathic factor in the etiology of diabetic foot ulcers. J Neurol Sci. 1975; 28:217.
12. Rayman G, et al. Vascular responses to postural change in the diabetic neuropathic foot. Diabetologia. 1984; 27:324A.
13. Ward JD, et al. Venous distension in the diabetic neuropathic foot. J R Soc Med. 1983; 76:1011.
14. Edmonds ME, Roberts VC, Walkins PJ. Blood flow in the diabetic neuropathic foot. Diabetologia. 1982; 22:9.
15. Kozniewska E, et al. Changes in blood flow and

permeability of vessels to protein preceding the development of cutaneous ulcers in the hind limb of the rabbit. Microvasc Res. 1980; 19:189.

16. Parkhouse N, LeQuesne PM. Impaired neurogenic vascular response in patients with diabetes and neuropathic foot lesions. N Engl J Med. 1988; 318:1306.

17. Ewing DS, Clarke BF. Diabetic autonomic neuropathy. A clinical viewpoint. In Dyck JP, Thomas PK, Lambert EH, et al, eds. Diabetic neuropathy. Philadelphia: WB Saunders, 1987; 66–68.

18. Edmonds ME, Archer AG, Watkins PJ. Ephedrine: a new treatment of neuropathic edema. Lancer. 1983; 1:548.

19. Lefancher C, Bardoux S, Frenaux B. La des arterialisation pediense deus la treatment des troubles trophiques del'acropathic ulcero-multilante. Presse Med. 1975; 4:2325.

20. Edmonds ME, Watkins PJ. Management of the diabetic foot. In Dyck JP, Thomas PK, Lambert EH, et al, eds. Diabetic neuropathy. Philadelphia: WB Saunders; 1987; 212.

21. Frykberg RG: Podiatric problems in diabetes. In Kozak GP, Campbell C, Hoar CS Jr, et al, eds. Management of diabetic foot problems. Philadelphia: WB Saunders; 1984; 5–67.

22. Jacobs RL. Hoffman procedure in the ulcerated diabetic neuropathic foot. Foot Angle 1982; 3:142–149.

23. Young JR: Foot problems in the diabetic patient. Cleve Clin J Med. 1988; 55:458.

24. Edmonds ME, et al. Reduction in the number of major and minor amputations: impact of a new combined foot clinic. Diabetologia. 1984; 27:272A.

25. Garland HT. Diabetic amyotrophy. Br J Clin Pract. 1961; 15:9.

26. Asbury AK. Proximal diabetic neuropathy. Adv Neurol. 1977; 2:179.

27. Ratt MC, Sangalang V, Asbury AK. Ischemic mononeuropathy multiplex associated with diabetes mellitus. N Engl J Med. 1968; 279:17.

28. Subramony SH, Wilbourn AJ. Diabetic proximal neuropathy. Clinical and electromyographic studies. J Neurol Sci. 1982; 53:293.

29. Brown MJ, Asbury AK. Diabetic neuropathy. Ann Neurol. 1984; 15:2–12.

30. Zorilla E, Kozak G. Ophthalmoplegia in diabetes mellitus. Ann Intern Med. 1967; 67:968.

31. Fraser DM, Campbell IW, Ewing DJ, et al. Mononeuropathy in diabetes mellitus. Diabetes. 1979; 28:96.

32. Asbury AK, Johnson PC. Diabetic neuropathy. In Asbury AK, Johnson PC, eds. Pathology of peripheral nerve. Philadelphia: WB Saunders; 1978; 96.

33. Korthals JK, Fieron MA, Dyck PJ. Inferna of epineural arterioles is increased in diabetic polyneuropathy. Neurology. 1988; 38:1582.

34. Low PA, Tuck RR, Takeuchi M. Nerve microenvironment in diabetic neuropathy. In Dyck JP, Thomas PK, Lambert EH, et al, eds. Diabetic neuropathy. Philadelphia: WB Saunders; 1987; 268.

35. Winegard AI, Simmons DA. Energy metabolism in peripheral nerve. In Dyck JP, Thomas PK, Lambert EH, et al, eds. Diabetic neuropathy. Philadelphia: WB Saunders; 1987; 287.

36. Mayhew JA, Gillon KRW, Hawthorne JN. Free and lipid inositol, sorbitol and sugars obtained post-mortem from diabetic and control subjects. Diabetologia. 1983; 24:13.

37. Greene DA, LaHimer SA. Altered *myo*-inositol metabolism in diabetic nerve. In Dyck JP, Thomas PK, Lambert EH, et al, eds. Diabetic neuropathy. Philadelphia: WB Saunders; 1987; 289.

38. Dyck PJ, et al. Nerve glucose, fructose, sorbitol, *myo*-inositol and fiber degeneration and regeneration in diabetic neuropathy. N. Engl J Med. 1988; 319:542.

39. Asbury AK. Understanding diabetic neuropathy. N Engl J Med. 1988; 319:577.

40. Sima AAF, et al. Regeneration and repair of myelinated fibers in sural nerve biopsy specimens from patients with diabetic neuropathy treated with sorbinil. N Engl J Med. 1988; 319:548.

41. Griffey RH, et al. Diabetic neuropathy. Structural analysis of nerve hydration by magnetic resonance spectroscopy. JAMA. 1988; 260-2872.

42. Martyn CN. Six-month treatment with sorbinil in asymptomatic diabetic neuropathy: Failure to improve abnormal nerve function. Diabetes. 1987; 36:987.

43. Sundkuist G, et al. Autonomic and peripheral nerve function in early diabetic neuropathy—possible influence of a novel aldose reductase inhibitor on autonomic function. Acta Med Scand. 1987; 221:445.

44. Mulder DW, et al. The neuropathies associated with diabetes mellitus. Neurology. 1961; 11:275.

45. Daube JR. Electrophysiologic testing in diabetic neuropathy. In Dyck JP, Thomas PK, Lambert EH, et al, eds. Diabetic neuropathy. Philadelphia: WB Saunders; 1987; 171.

46. Katirii MB, Wilbourn AJ. Common peroneal mononeuropathy: a clinical and electrophysiologic study of 116 lesions. Neurology. 1988; 38:1723.

47. Daube JR, Dyck PJ. Neuropathy due to peripheral vascular diseases. In Dyck PJ, Thomas PK, Lambert EH, et al, eds. Peripheral neuropathy, 2nd ed, Philadelphia: WB Saunders; 1984; 1458.

48. Hallett M, Tandon D, Berardelli A. Treatment of peripheral neuropathies. J Neurol Neurosurg Psychiatry. 1985; 48:1193.

49. Max MB, et al. Amitriptyline relieves diabetic neuropathy pain in patients with normal or depressed mood. Neurology. 1987; 37:589.

50. Sandek CD, Werns S, Reidenberg MM. Phenytoin in the treatment of diabetic symmetrical polyneuropathy. Clin Pharmacol Ther. 1977; 22:196.

51. Rull JA, et al. Symptomatic treatment of peripheral diabetic neuropathy with carbamazepine. Double-blind crossover study. Diabetologia. 1969; 5:212.

52. Cohen KL, Harris S. Efficacy and safety of nonsteroidal anti-inflammatory drugs in the therapy of diabetic neuropathy. Arch Intern Med. 1987; 147:1442.

53. Kastrup J, et al. Intravenous lidocaine infusion—a new treatment of chronic painful diabetic neuropathy. Pain. 1987; 28:69.

54. Deigard A, Petersen P, Kastrup J. Mexiletine for treatment of chronic painful diabetic neuropathy. Lancet. 1988; 1:9.

55. Bertelsmann FW, et al. Peripheral nerve function in patients with painful diabetic neuropathy treated with continuous subcutaneous insulin infusion. J Neurol Neurosurg Psychiatry. 1987; 50:1337.

56. Kronert K, et al. Effects of continuous subcutaneous insulin infusion and intensified conventional therapy on peripheral and autonomic nerve dysfunction. J Clin Endocrinol Metab. 1987; 64:1219.

8 Infections in the Diabetic Foot

ISRAEL PENN, M.D.

BASIC CONSIDERATIONS

The magnitude of the problem caused by foot infections in diabetics is revealed by a number of facts: An infected foot is the most common reason for diabetic patients to be admitted to the hospital.[1] Foot infections require more hospital days than any other complications of diabetes. In one study, hospital stay exceeded 1 month in 89% of patients and 3 months in 44%.[2] Approximately $200 million is spent annually in treating foot infections in diabetics.[3] Approximately 50% of all nontraumatic lower extremity amputations performed in the United States are related to diabetes.[4] Three percent of diabetics are amputees.[5]

Once infection becomes established, it tends to be more severe and more refractory to treatment in the diabetic than in the non-diabetic. Diabetic complications, including vascular insufficiency, neuropathy, and hyperglycemia, contribute to the severity and duration of many infections.[6-8] Factors involved include inadequate tissue perfusion, capillary and lymphatic damage, and changes in the bactericidal and chemotactic properties of phagocytes. Foot infections result in a relatively high rate of limb amputation and are associated with a poor long-term prognosis for survival. They occur in patients who have had diabetes for many years and who have developed multiple complications of the disease.[6-8]

Typical Patient Profile

Over the course of 15 to 20 years, many diabetics develop lesions involving a number of organs. Among these are hypertension, myocardial infarction, cerebrovascular accidents, gangrene of a lower limb, peripheral and autonomic neuropathy, retinopathy, cataracts, progressive renal dysfunction, and infections. Once patients have developed a major complication of diabetes, they are likely to have other problems as well. For example, a diabetic with foot problems often has coronary artery disease, retinopathy, and nephropathy.[6-8] A typical patient profile was presented in a study of 55 patients with serious foot infections;[9] it was found that the patients average 54 years in age, are 135% above ideal weight, 71% have type II and 29% have type I diabetes, and they have had diabetes for an average of 18 years. Most are receiving insulin, either alone or in combination with an oral hypoglycemic agent. Control of their diabetes ranges from fair to poor—67% have retinopathy; 78%, nephropathy; 80%, peripheral neuropathy; 91%, decreased pedal pulses; 69%, hypertension; 40%, atherosclerotic heart disease; 58%, a creatinine clearance of less than 90 ml/min; and 44%, proteinuria greater than 150 mg in 24 hours. Another group of diabetics aged 30 to 45 years have had the disease since childhood and have been maintained on dialysis or undergone renal transplantation for end-stage glomerulopathy. The patients' lives are substantially prolonged by control of the uremia, but the ravages of diabetic arterial disease and neuropathy continue to progress, with the result that 10 to 15% of diabetics require lower limb and occasionally even upper limb amputations as well.

Predisposing Causes

Three major factors contribute to the development of foot infections in diabetics: peripheral arterial disease, peripheral neuropathy and, under certain circumstances, an increased susceptibility to infection.[6-8] In some patients neuropathy or vascular insufficiency can be the predominant lesion, but both factors together contribute to the development of foot ulcers in diabetics. This accounts for the greater incidence of foot infections in diabetics compared to patients with other neuropathic disorders, such as paraplegia or syringomyelia. These disorders greatly affect prognosis and treatment. The foot of a patient with early diabetes who has normal circulation and sensation responds to injury and infection like that of a nondiabetic. In the diabetic with neuropathy or vascular insufficiency, or both problems, however, infections that otherwise would be trivial can have disastrous effects, threatening loss of limb or life (Fig. 8-1).

VASCULAR INSUFFICIENCY

Vascular insufficiency is described in Chapter 6. Here I summarize data pertaining to its role in causing foot infections. Approximately 50% of patients have evidence of peripheral arterial disease 10 to 15 years after the onset of diabetes.[10] Atherosclerosis has a higher incidence in diabetics, occurs at an earlier age, is more rapidly progressive, and has a more serious prognosis than in nondiabetics.[6-8,11,12] The distribution of the lesions is different in diabetics than in nondiabetics, in that the more peripheral and smaller vessels tend to be involved. Frequently, occlusions affect the popliteal and tibial arteries and the large vessels of the foot: the dorsalis pedis, the pedal arch, and the metatarsal arteries. In one study significant occlusions were found in 60% of the met-

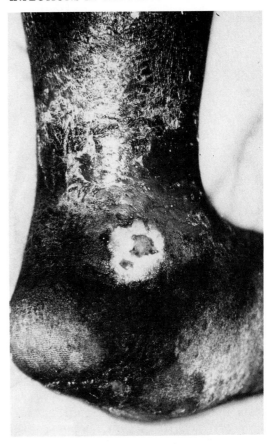

FIGURE 8-1 ■ Diabetic patient with severe neuropathy and vascular insufficiency. Marked osteoarthropathy caused a rocker bottom foot, which resulted in ulceration of the sole. This was successfully treated with skin grafts (not shown). Note the ulceration over the medial malleolus and the poor condition of the skin of the foot. Wet gangrene of the big toe subsequently necessitated a below-the-knee amputation.

atarsal arteries of diabetics compared with 21% of those in nondiabetics.[13] In addition, the digital arteries showed occlusions in 19% of diabetics, compared to 10% of nondiabetics.

Whether all vascular lesions are caused by atherosclerosis or whether the small vessel disease represents a specific diabetic disorder is a subject of controversy. Some investigators have failed to detect any specific small vessel disease peculiar to diabetes.[14]

Small vessel disease is known to occur in the retina (diabetic retinopathy) and in the glomeruli (diabetic nephrosclerosis), however, and similar lesions are believed to occur in small vessels of almost all tissues, including those of the feet and toes.[15] This microangiopathy consists of intimal thickening involving mainly the basement membrane. It is present in 88% of diabetics, as compared to 23% of nondiabetics.[16] Some investigators have suggested that the intimal thickening can occlude the lumen,[17] but others have disputed this conclusion.[13,16] Another hypothesis suggests that the basement membrane thickening interferes with the diffusion of nutrients through the vessel wall and hampers the migration of leukocytes into areas of infection.[16]

A factor that might aggravate arterial insufficiency is edema of the lower limbs caused by congestive heart failure or venous insufficiency.[18] Edema produces increased tissue pressure, with impairment of the collateral circulation. In addition, edema secondary to heart failure is accompanied by decreased cardiac output, which is more harmful in an ischemic limb than in other areas. In 66% of 247 diabetic patients who developed gangrene, a close temporal relationship was found between the development of edema and the appearance of gangrene.[19]

Ischemic ulcers must be differentiated from neuropathic ulcers, because the prognosis and therapy of the two conditions differ.[6-8] Patients with ischemic ulcers often have a history of progressive intermittent claudication. These ulcers are extremely painful and usually occur on the toes. In contrast, neuropathic ulcers are painless and are found on the ball of the foot, over the metatarsal heads, or on the plantar aspect of the hallux.[20]

Because of the more peripheral distribution of arterial lesions and the frequency of multiple occlusions, reconstructive arterial surgery is possible less often in diabetics than in nondiabetics. Nevertheless, in suitable candidates, vascular reconstruction has drastically altered the prognosis for those with diabetic foot problems. Many patients who would formerly have had above-the-knee amputations can now have vascular reconstructions followed by major or minor debridements.[21] These are individuals with

ulceration or gangrene associated with low-grade infection. Bypass grafting, even with autogenous saphenous vein, is contraindicated in the presence of active infection because of the danger of infecting the graft.[18] A primary amputation is preferable under such circumstances. If vascular grafting is feasible it is preferable not to perform debridement at the same time, but several days later. Obtaining a patent bypass graft does not ensure limb salvage. All vascular surgeons have had the frustrating experience of performing a major amputation in the presence of a patent femoropopliteal or femorotibial graft in a diabetic patient, because blood flow failed to improve in the presence of significant distal small vessel disease.

Small vessels adjacent to an area of infection commonly undergo thrombotic occlusion. In the normal foot this process is limited to the margin of the infection. The occlusive process becomes exaggerated in the already diseased vessels of the diabetic foot, however, causing ever-enlarging areas of necrosis. In this way a minor injury or a trivial infection, such as a paronychia, can progress to gangrene. Structures in the foot such as the plantar fascia, tendon sheaths, or ligaments, which would normally retard the spread of infection in the presence of an adequate arterial circulation, tend to succumb to the process of creeping infective angiopathy in the presence of vascular impairment.[21]

The normal foot has a rich collateral circulation. In the diabetic, however, multiple complete and partial occlusions of large, medium-sized, and small arteries, arterioles, and capillaries can convert parts of the foot that are normally perfused by multiple vessels to areas supplied by only a single vessel, analogous to the end-arteries that are normally present in the heart or kidney.[6,7,12] If such an artery becomes occluded by infection, the entire area dependent on it undergoes necrosis. For example, an infection in the inexpansile central plantar space can cause septic arteritis and thrombotic occlusion of the plantar arch and its branches and lead to necrosis, not only of the tissues in the central plantar space but also of those of the second, third, and fourth toes, which receive most of their blood supply from the plantar arch.[12] Because the big and little toes receive some of their blood supply through the medial and lateral plantar spaces, they tend to remain viable.

In long-term diabetics the situation is complicated further by reduction of the maximum vasodilator capacity of the resistance vessels and of the autoregulation of blood flow.[22] The vessels therefore cannot react to the needs of the tissues for increased blood flow to help wall off the infection.

NEUROPATHY

Neuropathy is discussed in detail in Chapter 7. In this section we consider how neuropathy makes the foot vulnerable to infections.

Neuropathy occurs in patients who have been diabetic for 10 to 15 years or more.[6-8] It has variable effects on the motor, sensory, and sympathetic nerve supply of the feet. It can damage the motor nerves of the small intrinsic muscles of the feet, cause diminished sensation or complete absence of pain, and affect the sympathetic nerves, producing dry, nonsweating, vasodilated feet ("autosympathectomy"). The muscular weakness results in deformities such as medial deviation of the lateral three toes, hallux valgus, bunionette of the fifth toe, and hammertoe.[6,7,12,18] Loss of the intrinsic muscles upsets the normal balance between the flexors and extensors, which is necessary for proper weight distribution during walking. The protrusion of the metatarsal heads causes excessive load on the underlying soft tissues during standing or walking. In addition, the amount of weight carried by the toes is reduced and is shifted to the metatarsal area. The result of all these changes is that excessive weight is borne under the metatarsal heads, particularly the first.[5,8,23,24] As a consequence, calluses develop over the bony prominences. In people with normal sensation, such lesions cause pain and force them to reduce weight-bearing. In contrast, diabetics who have diminished or absent sensation in the feet continue with full weight-bearing. As a result the calluses cause pressure necrosis of the underlying plantar skin, leading to neuropathic or mal perforans ulcers, most of which occur under the first, second, and fifth metatarsophalangeal joints (in that order). These ulcers can serve as portals for the spread of infection.

Loss of motor function causes more load to be placed on ligaments and joint capsules; these undergo gradual weakening and destruction, leading to painless, severely osteoarthritic or Charcot joints.[12] Those most frequently affected are the ankle, subtalar, tarsal, and tarsometatarsal joints. The resultant rocker bottom foot, medial tarsal subluxation, digital subluxation, and bone fragments further increase the risks of ulceration, mainly in the midplantar area (Fig. 8-1). The abnormal stresses applied to joint structures can cause an inflammatory reaction that is manifested clinically as swelling and an increase in local temperature, and that might be mistaken for osteomyelitis or pyogenic arthritis.[6,7]

Patients with inadequate sensation in the feet are prone to injure them in various ways. Because of poor eyesight caused by cataracts or retinopathy, they can stub the toes, damage the skin when cutting the nails, or tread on sharp objects. Pressure necrosis can occur when the external pressure exceeds the capillary pressure—for example, on the skin of the heels when insensitive feet lie unprotected against the bed for prolonged periods. Patients can also injure their feet by using hot baths or heating pads, or by applying strong chemical linaments to corns and calluses.

Autonomic neuropathy causes a dry fissured skin that cracks easily, opening up avenues for bacterial infection. Another effect of autosympathectomy is arteriovenous shunting, which can hamper tissue oxygenation. In addition, denervated blood vessels can be hypersensitive to cold, thus increasing skin ischemia further.

SUSCEPTIBILITY TO INFECTION

It is widely believed that diabetics have an increased susceptibility to infection. This is probably not true for the *well-controlled* diabetic, but the poorly controlled patient has impaired immune defenses and is susceptible to infection.[25] The mechanisms are not well understood and various explanations have been presented.[26] Because engulfment and intracellular killing of bacteria are energy-requiring processes, phagocytosis is impaired and bacteria are inadequately killed by the leukocytes of poorly controlled diabetics. Two major factors are involved, hyperglycemia and ketoacidosis. Hyperglycemia causes defective phagocytosis and also facilitates the growth of bacteria that enter the tissues. Ketoacidosis delays the migration of granulocytes to the site of a lesion and depresses the phagocytic and bactericidal functions of these cells. Opinions differ about antibody production in response to bacterial antigens and the opsonic ability of the blood of diabetics. Micro-angiopathy might facilitate the development of infection because of decreased tissue perfusion and lowered oxygen levels. It also impairs the delivery of granulocytes, antibodies, and antibiotics to an area of infection. A host defense that is frequently breached in diabetics is the skin—ulcers caused by ischemia or neuropathy serve as portals for the entry of bacteria.

PORTALS OF INFECTION

Infection in neuropathic or ischemic feet often begins in an apparently trivial break in the skin. The initial lesion frequently starts near the nails, which are often abnormal in ischemic, neuropathic, diabetic feet. Stubbing the toes or wearing new shoes can cause breaks in the skin of patients with long ingrown or incurved nails, or with onychogryphosis. In some patients poor foot hygiene causes excess keratin and debris to collect under the nails and in the nail folds, which can facilitate the growth of bacteria. The accumulation of moist detritus in the webs or the development of epidermophytosis with fissuring of the skin, or both, permits bacteria to enter and results in web space infections. In one study of major foot infections, 60% started in the web space, 30% started in the nail or nail bed, and 10% resulted from direct penetration of the sole.[27] Most cases that required amputation started as web space infections.

What often begins as minor trauma followed by minor infection can progress to a major infection because the circulation is inadequate to control the micro-organisms and because neuropathy permits the spread of infection. Tissue hypoxia resulting from poor blood supply contributes significantly to the incidence of foot infections.[28] In a normal person blood flow is increased at the site of inflammation. The diabetic, how-

ever, responds to infection in areas with inadequate blood supply by developing vascular thrombosis and necrosis in response to the increased tissue demand for oxygen because of reduced delivery. Several factors contribute to this process. Increased tissue turgor from inflammatory edema causes vascular compression, as does liberation of gas by certain bacteria (see below, Microbiologic Types of Infection). Local production of tissue-destroying enzymes, liberated mainly from granulocyte lysosomes, causes local thrombosis and small vessel occlusion. Contributing to this process are endotoxins liberated by the infecting bacteria. This pattern contrasts with gangrene in nondiabetic atherosclerotic patients, which almost invariably is associated with occlusions at or above knee level.

A further problem in diabetics with severe neuropathy is failure to localize infections because affected areas are not at rest, as feet with normal sensation would be, with resultant dissemination of infection along fascial planes. Diabetics often suffer severe infections of the feet, but have little or no discomfort.[6,7]

CLINICAL TYPES OF INFECTION

Infections range in severity from asymptomatic fungal infections of the nails or low-grade paronychias to severe limb-threatening or life-threatening disorders. Patients are often referred after infection has been present for a considerable time. In one study of 55 patients with serious foot infections the process had been present for 23 weeks before referral, and 60% of patients received treatment with oral antibiotics only.[9] Reasons for the delay include the patients' unawareness of pain or discomfort caused by peripheral neuropathy and poor visual acuity and, at times, a lack of awareness by the referring physician of the severity of the disease process. Often the primary care physician is seeing only the tip of the iceberg—a small ulcer and a bead of pus—whereas extensive soft tissue destruction and even osteomyelitis within the foot have already occurred.

Several types of major infection occur in the feet of diabetics.[6,7,12,29] These include the neuropathic ulcer of the plantar surface, necrotizing cellulitis of the dorsum of the foot, and abscess of the deep plantar spaces. In a study of 300 diabetics with major foot infections, deep plantar abscesses comprised 80% of infections, neuropathic ulcers 12%, and dorsal cellulitis 8%.[27] In contrast, in my experience, most infections are neuropathic ulcers.

These ulcers occur in patients with neuropathy, most of whom do not have ischemia (Fig. 8-2). The ulcers arise from breakdown of a pre-existing callus that leaves a rim of hard, thickened skin surrounding the crater. They occur as chronic indolent lesions on the plantar surface, overlying the heads of the first, second, or fifth metatarsal bones. For long periods infection remains limited to the skin and subcutaneous tissues. Quiescent episodes alternate with periods of flare-up of infection, when the adjacent foot becomes swollen and red. Because of the usually good blood supply, a fibrous tissue reaction adjacent to the ulcer obliterates tendon sheaths and tissue spaces. Ultimately, though, the infection destroys the flexor tendon and enters the adjacent joint, causing septic arthritis and osteomyelitis.[12]

The second type of major infection is an abscess in the deep spaces of the sole. The septa of the plantar fascia separate the deep structures of the foot into three compartments.[12,30] The medial compartment is limited laterally by the medial intermuscular septum, which extends from the medial calcaneal tubercle to the head of the first metatarsal. The plantar fascia forms the medial and inferior borders of the compartment. The superior border is the shaft of the first metatarsal. The medial compartment contains the muscles associated with the big toe: the abductor hallucis, hallucis brevis, and flexor hallucis longus. The lateral compartment is bounded medially by the lateral intermuscular septum, which extends from the calcaneus to the head of the fifth metatarsal. Superficially and laterally it is bounded by the plantar fascia. The deep boundary is the fifth metatarsal. The lateral compartment contains the muscles associated with the fifth toe: the abductor digiti quinti, flexor digiti quinti brevis, and adductor to the fifth toes. The central compartment is bounded on either side by the medial and lateral intermuscular septa, superficially by the plantar fascia, and deeply by the metatarsal bones and interosseous fascia. The central compartment contains the flexor digitorum brevis, quadratus plantae, peroneus longus, tibialis posterior, lumbricales, interossei, and adductor hallucis. Experiments with injections of various materials have shown that communications exist among the three compartments, with the dorsum of the foot, and with the deep posterior and peroneal compartments of the leg. Although infection in the sole tends to spread along anatomic pathways it is not necessarily confined by them, because tissue necrosis can

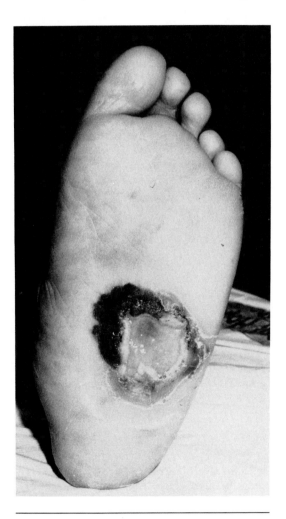

FIGURE 8-2 ■ Patient with diabetic osteoarthropathy and midplantar ulcer that had been treated previously by skin grafting. The central portion of the graft broke down on weight-bearing, leaving a hyperpigmented surviving peripheral area of grafted skin.

permit the spread of infection in other directions.

Deep compartmental infections can cause devastating destruction; 75% of above-the-knee and below-the-knee amputations in diabetics are necessitated by these infections.[30] Usually they involve the central plantar space and, less commonly, the medial or lateral plantar space.[12] Infection in a toe can cause suppurative tenosynovitis of the flexor tendon sheath, which spreads proximally to the plantar space. A web space infection can spread along a lumbrical muscle to reach the central plantar space. Infection from an ulcerated bunion or bunionette can spread to the medial or lateral plantar space, respectively. A patient with neuropathy might tread on a sharp foreign object, which could penetrate a deep plantar space directly and cause infection. The patient may be unaware of any infection until it is well established and he develops constitutional symptoms, notices a foul odor coming from the foot, or has difficulty in getting on his shoe because of swelling of the foot.

In a deep plantar space infection spiking chills, fever, malaise, anorexia, nausea, and other systemic signs of severe infection are frequently present. Hyperglycemia and ketoacidosis often develop. Inflammatory edema causes obliteration of the concavity of the longitudinal arch and disappearance of the skin creases of the sole, followed later by swelling of the dorsum of the foot.[6,7,12] By "milking" the foot from the heel toward the toes, it might be possible to express pus from an ulcer. Crepitus can be elicited if gas is present in the soft tissues of the sole. Gentle probing of an ulcer can reveal a deep sinus tract. Because of neuropathy pain and tenderness are often absent and the patient might continue to walk, thus facilitating the proximal spread of infection. Proximal extension of infection within the space might also be facilitated by the effects of gravity on the bedridden patient, whose foot is kept elevated. Infections initially remain confined to the compartment to which infection has spread from the responsible plantar ulceration. Progressive pressure elevation leads to extension to adjacent compartments along musculotendinous structures that pierce the fascial septa. In the forefoot, where most infections start, central com-

partment disease spreads mainly to the medial compartment along the adductor hallucis and to the lateral compartment by way of the lumbrical and plantar interosseus muscles of the fifth toe. The reverse routes are involved in the spread of infection from the medial or lateral compartments to the central compartment.[31] In untreated patients pus can also spread through the interosseous space onto the dorsum of the foot. In those with advanced disease, infection causes thrombotic occlusion of small and medium-sized vessels and progressive necrosis of the plantar fascia, tendons, bones, and joints. Gangrene of one or more toes can occur. If left untreated, a deep compartmental abscess can spread in various directions.[12,30] Some can point on the sole of the foot and rupture spontaneously through the plantar skin. Infection can also spread proximally up flexor tendon sheaths into the leg, and such extension should be expected if pain is present in the heel or the calf. In late cases, crepitus might be present.[18] Ascending cellulitis and inguinal lymphadenopathy can also be present.

The third variety of major infection consists of a group of necrotizing skin and subcutaneous tissue infections,[29] including necrotizing fasciitis and necrotizing cellulitis. The infection occurs in the loose tissue of the dorsum of the foot. What might initially have been a straightforward cellulitis can progress to varying degrees of necrosis, depending on the presence of vascular insufficiency in the cutaneous and subcutaneous vessels, on the adequacy of the collateral circulation, and on the severity of septic thrombotic arteritis. The dorsum of the foot becomes red and swollen, and can become grossly edematous if the patient continues to walk because of lack of pain. The local picture can be complicated by fever, lassitude, hyperglycemia, and ketoacidosis.

Of patients hospitalized because of diabetic foot problems, 13% have osteomyelitis.[32] In fact, diabetics comprise one-third of all patients with osteomyelitis of the foot.[28] It is usually found in patients between 50 and 70 years of age. Most cases occur as complications of neuropathic ulcers (Figs. 8-3, 8-4, and 8-5), but some follow perforating injuries of the foot. Almost all cases involve the toes or small bones of the feet.[28] Systemic manifestations (e.g., malaise, fe-

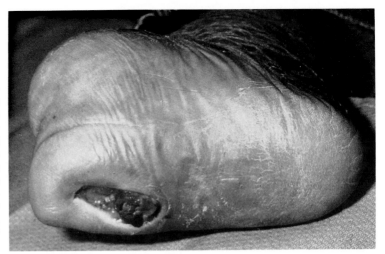

FIGURE 8-3 ■ Diabetic patient with previous transmetatarsal amputation who presented with a neuropathic ulcer of the lateral portion of the sole and osteomyelitis of the underlying bones. The ulcer healed satisfactorily after debridement of all necrotic tissue, including bone.

ver, leukocytosis) are uncommon, but most patients have indolent ulcers with swelling and erythema of the limb. It is sometimes difficult to differentiate osteomyelitis from diabetic neurotrophic arthropathy. The former condition can be associated with leukocytosis and an increased erythrocyte sedimentation rate, as well as with an adjacent neuropathic ulcer, whereas the latter condition can be multifocal and bilateral.[28] Radiographic and radionuclide findings are not always helpful and often the ultimate differentiation is made on clinical grounds by careful sequential observations.

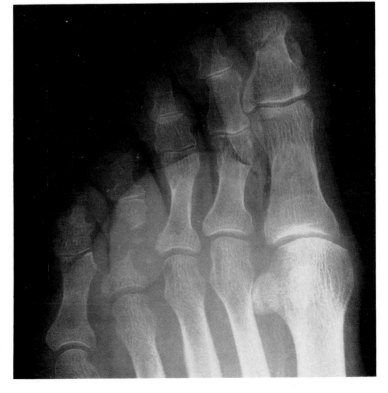

FIGURE 8-4 ■ Radiograph of osteomyelitis with pathologic fracture of the proximal phalanx of fourth toe complicating a neuropathic ulcer of the toe and severe vascular insufficiency. A fourth ray amputation was performed 12 days after a femorotibial bypass graft (in situ saphenous vein), with satisfactory healing. Note the calcified artery in the first interosseous space.

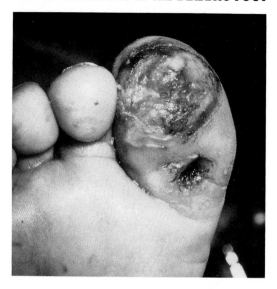

FIGURE 8–5 ■ Patient with long-standing neuropathic ulceration of the ball of the big toe who presented with extensive ulceration and infection of the tip of the toe, and with severe osteomyelitis of the distal phalanx. The blood supply of the foot was adequate and satisfactory healing was obtained after a ray amputation.

DIAGNOSTIC TESTS

A complete history and physical examination are necessary, and not only to determine the extent and severity of the infection, and the presence or absence of neuropathy and vascular insufficiency, but to look for complications of diabetes, such as ketoacidosis or atherosclerotic heart disease.[7] The work-up should include a complete blood count, determination of serum electrolyte, blood glucose and ketone, BUN, serum creatinine, total serum protein, serum albumin, and serum zinc levels, creatinine clearance, urinalysis, 24-hour urine protein excretion, chest radiography, and electrocardiography. Hemoglobin A_{1c} levels and a complete lipid profile can also be determined, if desired. The surgeon should not be lulled into a false sense of security by the absence of leukocytosis, which in one study was present in only 26% of patients.[9]

Aerobic and anaerobic wound cultures should be obtained as soon as possible. Aspiration of fluid from a clinically apparent suppurative focus can be performed preoperatively. At the time of debridement or amputation it is important to obtain cultures from the depths of the wound, because bacteria at these sites can differ significantly from those found in the superficial tissues.[33] Blood cultures should also be obtained at this time.

Radiographs of the foot are necessary to search for foreign bodies, charcot joints (indicative of advanced neuropathy), septic arthritis, or osteomyelitis. In one series, 43% of 55 patients with serious foot infections had radiologic findings suggestive of osteomyelitis.[9] In the presence of gangrene or infection the absence of osteoporosis or other lytic lesions is an unfavorable sign, because good blood flow is necessary to cause such changes.[21] Pathologic fractures through areas of osteomyelitis can be present, most commonly in the distal portions of the first or second proximal phalanges (Fig. 8-4).[34] Radiographs can also reveal evidence of soft tissue infection, including ulceration, edema, or gas collections. In selected cases xeroradiography, which shows the soft tissues as clearly as the bones, can be used to demonstrate early bone erosions or some foreign bodies not visible by routine radiography.[34] Magnification radiography can also be used to detect early osteomyelitis.

When indicated, sinography can demonstrate underlying joint involvement or extension into the deep tissues of the foot.[18] Sinography might underestimate soft tissue involvement, however, because of interference with the spread of contrast medium by inflammatory tissue.[31]

It takes 10 to 14 days for the bony changes of osteomyelitis to become apparent using conventional radiographic techniques. When such radiographs are negative or equivocal, technetium-99m methylenediphosphonate scans can be diagnostic of osseous involvement, but bone scans can be negative in culture-positive bone infection in the presence of impaired blood supply. In addition, they might not differentiate osteomyelitis from cellulitis. If the lesion shows increased radionuclide uptake with time (i.e., late scans at more than 24 hours), however, it is more likely to be osteomyelitis.[28] Gallium-67 citrate scans have been used to identify cases of osteomyelitis that were inconclusively demonstrated by other techniques or to show the proximal extent of soft tissue abnormality,[34] but positive scans can also be obtained with nonsuppurative processes such as neuroarthropathy.[31] Iridium-111 leukocyte scanning has been used to identify early osteomyelitis and to determine the extent of the inflammatory reaction.[34] Although experience with it is limited, promising early results have been obtained. A limitation of radionuclide scanning techniques is that their reliability can be altered by prior antibiotic therapy, because leukocytes might fail to accumulate at a suppurative process.[31]

CT scanning of the foot, although imprecise, can provide useful preoperative diagnostic information. The contralateral foot should also be scanned to serve as a control. CT scans show the bones, joints, and soft tissues, including the three deep compartments of the sole and their contents. Bony abnormalities are well demonstrated. The high resolution of CT scanning in various planes can identify subtle cortical irregularity and loss caused by osteomyelitis that are not visualized by other imaging techniques.[34] Soft tissue densities might represent suppuration, granulation tissue, edema, or fibrosis.[31] CT scanning clearly shows cutaneous ulceration at the site of primary infection, and can detect the extension of superficial foot infections at an earlier stage than existing clinical methods.[31] Associated dorsal soft tissue abnormalities are readily discernible with CT scanning as is the spread of infection to the hindfoot or calf. The use of CT scanning correlates well with the extent of infection as determined by other methods, but cannot predict its proximal limit precisely because of a gradual transition from unequivocally abnormal to normal tissue. Nevertheless, CT scans can be useful in establishing an appropriate level for debridement or amputation.

In patients in whom other imaging methods have not been diagnostic, magnetic resonance imaging (MRI) can be used. It demonstrates bone marrow changes caused by osteomyelitis with greater clarity than other imaging techniques and displays the contrast among soft tissue, medulla, and cortex with greater clarity than other methods.[34] This method is often helpful when other diagnostic studies have failed to delineate the extent of infection.

If any hint of vascular insufficiency is noted, ultrasonographic Doppler blood flow studies and other noninvasive studies should be done on both lower limbs.[6,7] If these demonstrate arterial insufficiency, it might be desirable to use angiography to delineate areas of occlusion and collateral circulation for those in whom vascular reconstruction is possible, in an attempt to save the limb.

MICROBIOLOGIC TYPES OF INFECTION

Infections are caused by a wide variety of organisms and are frequently polymicrobial. In one series, almost 50% of wounds contained three or more micro-organisms, and more than 60% had two or more.[9] The organisms can be gram-positive or gram-negative, aerobic or anaerobic.[6,7,12,29] The most frequent aerobes are gram-negative bacilli (Escherichia coli, Klebsiella, Enterobacter, and Proteus), enterococci, and Staphyloccus aureus. Gram-negative bacilli, especially Bacteroides and Fusobacterium, Clostridia, and anaerobic cocci are the most common anaerobes encountered. Anaerobes outnumber aerobes more than tenfold.[35] Anaerobic infections should be suspected whenever a fetid discharge, crepitus, or subcutaneous gas is present. If bacteremia is present, it is most frequently caused by Bacteroides fragilis or Staphyloccus aureus.[35,36]

The great variety of bacteria in the lesions necessitates the use of broad-spectrum antibiotics. Bactericidal rather than bacteriostatic agents are preferable because of possible defects in leukocyte function.[9] In view of possible poor tissue perfusion and possible leukocyte dysfunction, large doses should be used to achieve high tissue concentrations.[9] If the patient has impaired renal function, however, care must be used in prescribing aminoglycosides because of their potential nephrotoxicity and ototoxicity; if used, their blood levels should be carefully monitored. Antibiotic therapy might have to be prolonged, particularly if bone or joint infection is present, requiring an average of 4 to 6 weeks of treatment compared with an average of 10 to 14 days with infections confined to the soft tissues. Disagreement about which antibiotics to use is widespread. A few of the more widely used agents or antibiotic combinations are mentioned here. If the patient is afebrile, has no recent changes in mental status, and appears relatively nontoxic, a mixture of ticarcillin and clavulanic acid (Timentin) can be given parenterally.[28] Ticarcillin provides coverage against a wide range of aerobes and anaerobes and clavulanic acid inhibits the β-lactamases of Staphylococcus aureus and most strains of Bacteroides fragilis. If the patient is febrile, lethargic, or delirious, and appears toxic, or has extensive cellulitis, an aminoglycoside should be added.

Other traditional antibiotic regimens have included clindamycin (for gram-positive and anaerobic organisms) combined with any aminoglycoside (for gram-negative organisms) and ampicillin (for enterococci).[30] The effects of cefoxitin and ceftizoxime were compared in a randomized, prospective, double-blind trial.[3] Cefoxitin has broad-spectrum activity against gram-positive, gram-negative, and anaerobic organisms, including Bacteroides fragilis. Ceftizoxime is effective against aerobes, facultative bacteria, and many anaerobes, and therapeutic levels can be obtained with less frequent dosing than with cefoxitin. It was shown that both agents are safe and effective, but satisfactory clinical responses are seen more frequently with ceftizoxime.[3]

When osteomyelitis is present, the antimicrobial concentrations that are obtained in bone as percentages of their serum concentrations should be kept in mind: oxacillin, 11 to 14%; ceftizoxime, 19%; cefoxitin, 15 to 21%; gentamycin, 30%; oral rifampin, 19 to 41%; and clindamycin, 29 to 49%.[37] In an occasional patient with low-grade chronic osteomyelitis in the base of an ulcer, the infection can be suppressed by long-term (up to 12 months) antibiotic therapy, and thus a major operation on the foot can be avoided. Such an approach requires meticulous patient follow-up.

METABOLIC COMPLICATIONS OF INFECTION

A severe infection in a diabetic induces a series of catabolic disturbances,[25] including a negative nitrogen balance, increased gluconeogenesis, hyperglycemia, mobilization of fatty acids, and acidosis. The net result

is an increase in insulin "resistance" and a consequent increase in insulin requirements for maintenance of control. Thus, a vicious cycle is established: poorly controlled diabetes, with accompanying hyperglycemia and ketoacidosis, impairs host defense mechanisms, which in turn facilitates progression of the infectious process.[25]

Infections of various organs, including those of the foot, are the most common precipitating cause of diabetic ketoacidosis. In different series they accounted for 28 to 77% of such cases.[7,38,39] Infections are a major cause of mortality and morbidity in diabetics. In a study of patients with ketoacidosis the overall mortality was 6%, but 43% of the deaths were caused by infection.[39]

PREVENTION OF INFECTION

Advances in the self-monitoring of the blood glucose level and in the self-administration of insulin have provided better control of the metabolic abnormalities of diabetes, and perhaps can reduce the vascular, neurologic, and infectious complications associated with poorly controlled diabetes.[40,41] Long-term follow-up of such patients with conventionally treated controls might provide the answer to this important question. In addition, it might be possible to reduce the risk factors associated with vascular disease by controlling obesity, hyperglycemia, hypercholesterolemia, hypertriglyceridemia, and hypertension and by avoiding cigarette smoking and sedentary habits.[42,43] Preventive measures include a diet containing reduced amounts of saturated fats, cholesterol, and total calories and a high fiber content. Drugs that lower the serum cholesterol or lipid level are also being used. At present pancreatic transplantation is only being used in diabetics with advanced complications. With more experience this operation might be done earlier, before the onset of serious problems and, hopefully, by providing a source of insulin that responds to the body's varying needs, might enable complete control of diabetes and arrest the progression of vascular disease, neuropathy, and nephropathy.[7]

Patients must be seen at regular intervals by their physicians, who during a complete evaluation, should pay particular attention to the condition of the cardiovascular, neurologic, renal, and ophthalmic systems and to the lower extremities.[6,7] Patients must be taught to recognize signs of infection, such as fever, malaise, redness, swelling, or discharge, and should report promptly to their physicians if these changes occur or if they develop a significant break in the skin that fails to heal. The lower limbs should be evaluated in particular. The feet should be examined for nail abnormalities, fungal infections, corns, calluses, and bony exostoses. Correction of these abnormalities can help prevent the development of more serious complications. In selected patients prophylactic surgery, including bone resection, osteotomy, and soft tissue release, can be undertaken to correct forefoot and midfoot deformities, including ingrown toenails, hammertoes, soft corns, bunions, and nonweight-bearing exostoses. A study of prophylactic operations in 32 patients indicated a 31% incidence of complications, including soft tissue infections, osteomyelitis, and localized amputations.[44] To reduce these problems to a minimum, the authors recommended stringent guidelines involving adequate blood supply, minimal neurologic deficit, proper nutritional status, nature of the deformity, bacteriologic evaluation of any ulcers, and evaluation of any other diabetic problems that affect the general condition of the patients.

A great effort must be made to educate patients, particularly those who already have neuropathy, about the care of their feet. Some patients are remarkably unconcerned about their problems, have little insight, and are guilty of self-neglect.[45] Proper foot care is essential.[5,7,29] This includes daily examination of the feet by patients or by their spouses if their vision is poor. The feet should be kept clean and dry and tight-fitting shoes or socks should not be worn. Patients should avoid using mended socks or socks with seams and should change their socks daily. If their feet are cold at night they should wear bed socks, but should not use hot water bottles or heating pads. They should avoid trauma to the feet, including application of strong chemicals in the form of "corn removers." Patients should not walk barefooted, especially on hot surfaces such as sandy beaches and around swimming pools. Shoes should be inspected daily for foreign objects, nail points, and torn linings. Toenails, corns, and other minor foot problems should be given proper care, usually by a podiatrist. Epidermophytosis should be treated promptly. Patients or spouses should be given a set of written instructions outlining the various preventive measures. Patients must be taught to seek medical care promptly, even for a trivial lesion such as an ulcerated callus or an infected ingrown toenail because, if left unattended, it might progress to a potentially life-threatening complication requiring a major amputation.

TREATMENT OF INFECTION

The diabetic with a septic foot needs emergency treatment.[7] Large doses of broad-spectrum antibiotics should be given until culture and sensitivity tests have been completed, when changes in antibiotic therapy can be made, if indicated. Because infection can cause loss of control of the diabetes, it might be necessary to treat the patient temporarily with regular insulin and to monitor the blood glucose level frequently until the infection is under control. If septic shock or severe ketoacidosis is present, a Swan-Ganz catheter should be placed to help monitor blood volume replenishment. Usually 6 to 12 hours of treatment are necessary to prepare the patient for operation. During this time ketoacidosis and hyperglycemia are controlled, extracellular fluid volume is replenished, and adequate blood levels of antibiotics are secured.[18] During hospitalization great care must be taken to protect the feet and other susceptible areas from developing decubitus ulcers.[6,7]

Surgery is indicated in all patients except those with superficial ulcers, which can be managed conservatively, or a superficial cellulitis (without necrosis) that responds to bed rest and antibiotics. The need for prompt surgical drainage, debridement, or amputation, when such procedures are indicated, must be stressed.[6,7] Unfortunately, needless delays on the part of the patient or primary care physician often occur, which result in spreading infection, vascular thrombosis, and proximal extension of the destructive process, threatening the patient's limb and even life.

Surgical treatment can range from minor

debridement of a paronychia and removal of an ingrown toenail to major amputation of a foot that has been destroyed by infection.[21] Aggressive local treatment is possible only if an adequate blood supply is present. A patient with severe sepsis and extensive popliteotibial occlusive disease should have a guillotine amputation just above the ankle.[18]

Drainage and Debridement

If the foot has an adequate blood supply, extensive drainage and debridement of all infected and necrotic tissues should be performed without regard to subsequent reconstruction. This can include removal of several digits and metatarsals. The amount of devitalized tissue is invariably more extensive than that suggested by the initial clinical examination of the foot. Often patients are treated by making small stab incisions to drain deep plantar abscesses; these are totally inadequate.

Whenever performing debridement or drainage procedures in diabetic feet, adjacent tissues must be handled gently because of associated neuropathy or impaired blood supply. The goal is to avoid amputation or to perform it at the lowest possible safe level.[21] Rough handling of the tissues can defeat this objective by causing necrosis of the wound margins. Local anesthesia should be avoided because the volume of fluid injected might aggravate ischemia. Skin hooks should be used in preference to forceps. Absorbable ligatures should be used in the wound, which should be left open but not be tightly packed. The use of constricting dressings or bandages should be avoided.

In treating a neuropathic ulcer, its depth should be assessed clinically and radiographically to ascertain whether tendon, bone, or joints are affected.[6,7] If the ulcer involves only the skin and subcutaneous tissues it will heal if the patient avoids weight-bearing and local care is given to it. A sinus tract must be laid wide open and all necrotic tissue, including infected bone, should be removed (Fig. 8-3). Because the circulation in a neuropathic foot is often good, small ulcers can heal spontaneously; if the defect is large, however, skin grafting might be required. Weight-bearing must be avoided by bed rest or the use of crutches. Patient compliance is often a problem because poor vision and the absence of pain create a false sense of complacency.

Once the lesion has healed, a weight-transferring prosthesis must be fitted to the shoe to prevent recurrent problems. If a neuropathic ulcer involves an underlying joint, a ray amputation removing the toe and the head of the related metatarsal is often the procedure of choice.[6,7] If more than one ulcer is present in the distal foot, a transmetatarsal amputation yields the best results. This not only removes the ulcers but, in those in whom neuropathy is confined to the forefoot, places insensitive skin on a nonweight-bearing part of the foot.

Necrotizing skin and soft tissue infections should be treated with antibiotics and by prompt surgical drainage and debridement.[6,7] Amputation might be necessary if extensive necrosis has occurred.

An abscess of the medial or lateral plantar space can be drained dorsal to the print line of the sole to avoid a scar on the weight-bearing surface.[21] The incision can be extended proximally as far as necessary toward the lower margin of the medial malleolus and up posterior to it, if required. The incision can also be extended forward to include amputation of the big toe (if this is needed), and can be used to excise as much of the first ray as necessary. An associated neuropathic ulcer underlying the first metatarsal head should also be excised and left open to granulate.

A similar incision on the lateral side of the foot is used to drain lateral plantar space abscesses, and can be extended as far proximally as required. It can be combined with amputation of the little toe or as much of the fifth ray as necessary.

An abscess of the central plantar space is opened through a plantar incision, starting at the affected metatarsal head and extending as far proximally as the extent of infection. If necessary, the incision can be extended to the area of the medial malleolus and up behind it into the leg. A plantar incision represents the most direct approach to the central plantar space. The subsequent development of potentially painful scars is not a concern, because the great majority of patients have insensate feet (as a result of neuropathy). If an abscess has extended through into the dorsum of the foot, a dorsal counterincision is made to provide through-and-through drainage. If one or more toes are beyond salvage they should be excised. If a metatarsophalangeal joint or metatarsal bone is involved, a ray resection of all diseased bone can be performed. All necrotic and devitalized tissue should be removed, and, at the end of the procedure, all wound surfaces should be bleeding. The primary aim is to control sepsis.[6,7,21] A formal amputation at a higher level might be necessary at a later date if so much destruction of the soft tissues has occurred that the foot cannot be used for walking. If infection has extended proximally along tendon sheaths the incision must be continued proximally into the leg as far as necessary.

In a patient with limb-threatening ischemia complicated by wet gangrene, ulceration with cellulitis, osteomyelitis, or soft tissue closed space infection, an aggressive approach to vascular reconstruction is advocated by some surgeons.[46] In a series of 69 such limbs (in a group of patients of whom 74% were diabetic), 28% required prebypass drainage, debridement, or amputation, 55% had concurrent debridement or amputation, and 63% had postbypass debridement.[46] Prebypass procedures were performed in patients whose foot infections were complicated by systemic sepsis, whereas concomitant bypass procedures and debridement or amputation were performed in those patients in need of definitive wound management who urgently required blood flow restoration to prevent rapidly progressing necrosis, infection, or both. Patients with pedal sepsis had a lower 30-day limb salvage rate and higher morbidity and mortality rates than control patients without sepsis (34 limbs), but the long-term salvage rates of both groups by life table analyses were not statistically different, remaining at the 70% level 3 years postoperatively.

Amputation

In patients with septic feet amputation might be required on an emergent basis to remove a necrotic toe or part or all of the foot, or it might be an elective procedure, when distal sepsis is under control, and amputation is done to dispose of nonfunctional tissue, promote healing, and facilitate rehabilitation. In the former instance the wound is usually left open, and in the latter formal closure of the amputation site can safely be done. The primary objective of treatment is to save as much of the foot as possible to permit the patient to continue walking. If possible, the definitive operation should be the first one. This might not be possible when severe sepsis is present, however, and the initial procedure needs to be wide drainage and debridement or a guillotine amputation. The lower the amputation level, the better, because healed amputations in the foot permit walking without prostheses. Large parts of the foot can be excised, with eventual healing and successful ambulation.[47] Fortunately, a minor amputation is frequently possible because of the distal location of vascular occlusion in many diabetics or because of the presence of a neuropathic ulcer without vascular compromise. In one series the initial treatment was a minor amputation in 40% of diabetics as compared with 4% of nondiabetics.[48] Prolonged hospitalization to obtain the most distal amputation is justified, because overall mortality is related to the length of the contralateral extremity. On the other hand it is important to recognize those patients in whom a distal amputation is contraindicated at an early stage, and thus avoid prolonged hospitalization during which successive amputations progressing up the foot and leg are performed.

A tourniquet must not be used when performing any amputation, because it could damage an already tenuous blood supply. Tissues must be handled gently and complete hemostasis obtained. Drains should be avoided, if possible, because they can serve as portals for infection. The skin flaps should be approximated without tension with fine monofilament sutures.

The most common amputation is of an individual toe, with removal of part or all of the toe.[47] If the latter is necessary, amputation through the distal part of the metatarsal bone is preferred to disarticulation through the metatarsophalangeal joint, because exposed avascular cartilage delays healing.[21]

If infection involves not only the toe but also the metatarsophalangeal joint or metatarsal bone, a ray amputation can be performed if the foot has good circulation.[6,7] Sometimes it might be necessary to excise more than one ray. Although a satisfactory result can be obtained after excision of two lateral rays, it is possible with only one central ray.[30] Depending on control of infection, it might be possible to close the wound primarily around a closed suction drain. Otherwise the wound is packed open and closed later, when infection is under control, by delayed suture or with Steri-strips, or the wound can be allowed to granulate in. When ulceration involves two or more toes a transmetatarsal amputation can be the procedure of choice. A satisfactory blood supply in the distal foot is essential to ensure healing after all these operations. A Syme's amputation is rarely done.[6,7] It is used mainly in patients who do not have enough healthy skin to permit a transmetatarsal amputation or in whom a transmetatarsal amputation has failed. It is indicated in patients with visual disturbances or in those who would do poorly with crutches or prostheses.[21] A palpable posterior tibial pulse is essential to ensure healing of the stump.

Amputation below the knee (BKA) or above the knee (AKA) might be necessary when extensive tissue destruction has occurred. It is possible to save the knee in more than 80% of diabetics,[4,7] provided that a BKA is not contraindicated by the level of infection or ischemia or by a flexion contracture of the knee. Primary closure of the stump is safe if no evidence of spread of infection above the ankle is seen.[18]

The rate of primary wound healing is similar in diabetics and nondiabetics,[47] but the incidence varies in different series. Healing occurs in 33 to 71% of toe amputations, 50 to 70% of transmetatarsal procedures, 28 to 80% of Syme's amputations, 68 to 83% of BKAs, and 82 to 100% of AKAs. Failure of healing occurs as a result of inadequate arterial blood supply, excessive surgical trauma, uncontrollable invasive infection, or combinations of these problems.

POSTOPERATIVE CARE

After drainage of a major foot infection the wound must be reassessed on a daily basis. If pus is found on the dressings an inadequately drained pocket, which must be opened widely, should be suspected.[6,7]

The wound granulates in and closes spontaneously if the blood supply is satisfactory and the defect is small. Meshed split-thickness skin grafts can be applied to large defects to shorten the duration of the healing process. Occasionally a viable toe is sacrificed to provide a full-thickness pedicle flap to close a fairly large distal defect.[18] When two or more toes have been lost, a transmetatarsal amputation is often the best treatment.

In some patients the wound fails to heal, despite satisfactory drainage of infection, because of an inadequate blood supply. Such patients should be evaluated for vascular reconstruction. Thus, bypass grafting procedures in limbs that are infected distally might have to be performed, bearing in mind the risk of involvement of the operative wound. The danger should be minimized with the use of autogenous material, whenever possible, the use of monofilament sutures, and appropriate antibiotic coverage.[49] If the patient is not a satisfactory candidate for arterial reconstruction, and daily examinations reveal extension of necrosis in the skin edge or in exposed muscles, an amputation at a level with an adequate blood supply is necessary.

Zinc deficiency (present in 62% of patients in one series)[9] interferes with wound healing and can impair the immune response to infection. It should be corrected with the administration of oral or intravenous zinc sulfate supplements.

PROGNOSIS

The immediate outlook for limb and life depends on the extent of soft tissue and bone destruction and on the general condition of the patient. For example, central plantar compartment abscesses have a less favorable prognosis regarding limb salvage than lateral or medial compartmental abscesses.[30]

Formerly, amputations in diabetics involved a mortality rate of 20 to 40%, and most were AKAs. More recent reports have shown decreased mortality rates and a definite trend toward the use of more distal amputations. The improvement results from a more aggressive approach to lower extremity revascularization, improved perioperative management, and the concentration of patients in a single surgical service.[47] One study showed that death after lower limb amputation in diabetics occurs mostly in terminally ill, bedridden patients and that the rate can be kept down to about 5%, a similar figure to that obtained in nondiabetics.[47]

Although satisfactory immediate control of foot infections is frequently obtained, one study showed that relapses of infection are common during long-term follow-up.[3] Only one-third of patients had long-term satisfactory outcomes without relapse within 12 months. Foot problems are frequently bilateral, and at least 30% of all diabetic amputees lose the contralateral limb within 3 years.[50]

The importance of complications at other sites (causing ischemia of the heart, brain, and kidney) is underscored by a significantly decreased life expectancy, irrespective of the age at which diabetes developed.[6,7,51] In fact, diabetes with its complications is the third most common cause of death in the United States.[20] After amputation of a leg, two-thirds of patients die within 5 years.[12]

Foot infections are the most common indication for hospital admission of diabetic patients. Once infection becomes established, it tends to be more severe and more refractory to treatment than infection in the nondiabetic. The typical patient with foot infection has other signs of long-standing diabetes, including retinopathy, nephropathy, and atherosclerotic heart disease, all of which influence the patient's long-term prognosis. Lower extremity ischemia and/or neuropathy, by breaking down the skin barrier, are major predisposing causes to infection. Once infection becomes established a vicious circle can develop, with loss of metabolic control of diabetes, increasing hyperglycemia and ketoacidosis, and impairment of the host's immune defenses against infection. Infections can range in severity from asymptomatic dermatophytosis to severe sepsis that threatens loss of limb or life. Three major types of severe infection include neuropathic ulcers of the sole, abscesses in the deep compartments of the sole, and necrotizing cellulitis of the dorsum of the foot. The patient work-up requires evaluation of the patient as a whole, including a search for other complications of diabetes (particularly those involving the cardiovas-

cular system), evaluation of systemic signs of sepsis, and meticulous examination of the foot, paying special attention to its blood supply and neurologic state. Ancillary tests of the foot can include plain radiography, sinography, radionuclide, CT and MRI scanning, noninvasive vascular studies, angiography, and cultures of purulent material.

Until we learn how to prevent the progression of diabetes, particularly its effects on the cardiovascular and nervous systems, the long-term prognosis of diabetics with foot problems remains guarded. At least 30% of diabetic amputees lose the contralateral limb in 3 years and two-thirds of amputees are dead within 5 years.

Most infections are polymicrobial, involving various aerobes and anaerobes. Appropriate antibiotic therapy is combined with surgical incision, drainage, debridement, or amputation, depending on circumstances. Most feet can be saved if the infection is treated early enough. Sometimes such feet can have an unattractive appearance if parts have been removed but, if they permit ambulation, are preferable to any prostheses. Effort needs to be expended to educate patients, their spouses, and even their physicians about foot care to help prevent the types of injuries, often minor, that can lead to foot infections and about recognizing early signs of infection so that these can be vigorously treated before much tissue destruction has occurred.

References

Owing to space limitations, relatively few references from a vast literature can be cited. Many other references are found in the following publications listed below.

1. Pratt TC. Gangrene and infection in the diabetic. Med Clin North Am. 1965; 49:987–1004.
2. Larsson U, Anderson GBJ. Partial amputation of the foot for diabetic or arteriosclerotic gangrene: results and factors of prognostic value. J Bone Joint Surg. 1978; 60B:126–130.
3. Hughes, CE, et al. Treatment and long-term follow-up of foot infections in patients with diabetes or ischemia: a randomized, prospective, double-blind comparison of cefoxitin and ceftizoxime. Clin Ther. 1987; 10(Suppl A):36–49.
4. Ecker ML, Jacobs BS. Lower extremity amputation in diabetic patients. Diabetes. 1970; 19:189–195.
5. Bouton AJM. Detecting the patient at risk for di-

abetic foot ulcers. Practical Cardiol. 1983; 9:135–145.

6. Penn I. The impact of diabetes mellitus on extremity ischemia. In: Kempczinski RF, ed. The ischemic leg. Chicago: Year Book Medical Publishers; 1985; 56–69.

7. Penn I. Diabetes mellitus and the surgeon. Curr Probl Surg. 1987; 24:535–603.

8. Levin ME, O'Neal LW. The diabetic foot, 4th ed. St. Louis: CV Mosby; 1988.

9. Leichter SB, et al. Clinical characteristics of diabetic patients with serious pedal infections. Metabolism. 1988; 37:22–24.

10. Brandman O, Redisch W. Incidence of peripheral vascular changes in diabetes mellitus. Diabetes. 1953; 2:194–198.

11. Haimovici H. Peripheral arterial disease in diabetes mellitus. In: Ellenberg M, Rifkin H, eds. Diabetes mellitus: theory and practice. New York: McGraw-Hill; 1970; 890–911.

12. O'Neal LW. Surgical pathology of the foot and clinicopathologic correlations. In: Levine ME, O'Neal LW, eds. The diabetic foot, 4th ed. St. Louis: CV Mosby; 1988; 203–236.

13. Ferrier TM. Comparative study of arterial disease in amputated lower limbs from diabetics and nondiabetics (with special reference to feet arteries). Med J Aust. 1967; 1:5–11.

14. Strandness DE Jr, Priest RE, Gibbons GE. Combined clinical and pathologic study of diabetic and nondiabetic peripheral arterial disease. Diabetes. 1964; 13:366–372.

15. Williamson JR, Vogler NJ, Kilo C. Regional variations in the width of the basement membrane of muscle capillaries in man and giraffe. Am J Pathol. 1971; 63:359–370.

16. Banson BB, Lacy PE. Diabetic microangiography in human toes, with emphasis on the ultrastructural change in dermal capillaries. Am J Pathol. 1964; 45:41–58.

17. Goldenberg S, Alex M, Joshi RA, et al. Non-atheromatous peripheral vascular disease of the lower extremity in diabetes mellitus. Diabetes. 1959; 8:261–273.

18. Towne JB. Management of foot lesions in the diabetic patient. In: Rutherford RR, ed. Vascular surgery, 2nd ed. Philadelphia: WB Saunders; 1984; 661–669.

19. Lithner F, Tornblom N. Gangrene localized to the lower limbs in diabetics. Acta Med Scand. 1980; 208:315–320.

20. Stemmer EA. Vascular complications of diabetes mellitus. In: Moore WS, ed. Vascular surgery: a comprehensive review. New York: Grune and Stratton; 1983; 415–429.

21. O'Neal LW. Debridement and amputation. In: Levin ME, O'Neal LW, eds. The diabetic foot, 4th ed. St. Louis: CV Mosby; 1988; 237–248.

22. Kastrup J, Lassen NA, and Parving HH. Diabetic microangiopathy: a factor enhancing the functional significance of peripheral occlusive arteriosclerotic disease. Clin Physiol. 1984; 4:367–369.

23. Ctercteko GC, Dhanendran M, Hutton WC, et al. Vertical forces acting on the feet of diabetic patients with neuropathic ulceration. Br J Surg. 1981; 68:608–614.

24. Lippman HI, Farrar R. Prevention of amputation in diabetics. Angiography. 1979; 30:649–658.

25. Johnson JE III. Infection and diabetes. In: Ellenberg M, Rifkin H, eds. Diabetes mellitus: theory and practice. New York: McGraw-Hill; 1970; 734–745.

26. Casey JI. Host defense and infections in diabetes mellitus. In: Ellenberg M, Rifkin H, eds. Diabetes mellitus: theory and practice, 3rd ed. New York: McGraw-Hill; 1970, 667–678.

27. Bose K. A surgical approach for the infected diabetic foot. Int Orthop. 1979; 3:177–181.

28. Little JR, Kobayashi GS. Infection of the diabetic foot. In: Levine ME, O'Neal LW, eds. The diabetic foot, 4th ed. St. Louis: CV Mosby; 1988; 104–118.

29. LeFrock JL, Molavi A. Foot infections in diabetic patients: In: Andriole VT, ed. Mediguide to infectious diseases, vol 3. West Haven, CT: Miles Pharmaceuticals; 1983; 3:1–5.

30. Goldman FD. Deep space infections in the diabetic patient. J Am Podiatr Med Assoc. 1987; 77:431–443.

31. Sartoris DJ, et al. Plantar compartmental infection in the diabetic foot: the role of computed tomography. Invest Radiol. 1985; 20:772.

32. Kozak GP, Rowbotham JL. Diabetic foot disease: a major problem. In: Kozak GP, Campbell D, Hoar CS, et al, eds. Management of diabetic foot problems. Philadelphia: WB Saunders; 1984; 1–8.

33. Sharp CS, et al. Microbiology of superficial and deep tissues in infected diabetic gangrene. Surg Gynecol Obstet. 1979; 149:217–219.

34. Hardy DC, Staple TW, Picus D, et al. Imaging of the diabetic foot. In: Levine ME, O'Neal LW, eds., The diabetic foot, 4th ed. St. Louis: CV Mosby; 1988; 131–150.

35. Sapico FL, et al. Quantitative aerobic and anaerobic bacteriology of infected diabetic feet. J Clin Microbiol. 1980; 12:413–420.

36. Sapico FL, et al. The infected foot of the diabetic patient: quantitative microbiology and analysis of clinical features. Rev Infect Dis 1984; 6(Suppl 1):S171–S176.

37. Gerding DN, et al. Extravascular antimicrobial distribution in man. In: Lorian V, ed. Antibiotics in laboratory medicine, 2nd ed. Baltimore: Williams & Wilkins; 1986; 938–994.

38. Nabarro JDN. Diabetic acidosis: clinical aspects. In: Leibel BS, Wrenshall GA, eds. On the nature and treatment of diabetes. New York; Excerpta Medica; 1965; 545–562.

39. Soler NG, Bennett MA, Fitzgerald MG, et al. Intensive care in the management of diabetic ketoacidosis. Lancet. 1973; 1:951–954.

40. Skyler JS. Self-monitoring of blood glucose. Med Clin North Am. 1982; 66:1227–1250.

41. Unger RH. Benefits and risks of meticulous control of diabetes. Med Clin North Am. 1982; 66:1317–1324.

42. Dunn FL. Hyperlipidemia and diabetes. Med Clin North Am. 1982; 66:1347–1360.

43. Christlieb AR. Treating hypertension in the patient with diabetes mellitus. Med Clin North Am. 1982; 66:1373–1388.

44. Gudas CJ. Prophylactic surgery in the diabetic foot. Clin Podiatr Med Surg. 1987; 4:445–458.

45. Delbridge L, Appleberg M, Reeve TS. Factors as-

sociated with the development of foot lesions in the diabetic. Surgery. 1983; 93:78–82.

46. Rubin JR, Pitluck HC, Graham LM. Do operative results justify tibial artery reconstruction in the presence of pedal sepsis? Am J Surg. 1988; 156:144–147.

47. Porter JM, Baur GM, Taylor LM Jr. Lower extremity amputations for ischemia. Arch Surg. 1981; 116:89–92.

48. Steer HW, Cuckle HS, Franklin PM, et al. The influence of diabetes mellitus upon peripheral vascular disease. Surg Gynecol Obstet. 1983; 157:64–72.

49. Jacobs RL, Karmody AM, Wirth C, et al. The team approach in salvage of the diabetic foot. In: Nyhus LM, ed. Surgery annual, vol. 9. New York: Appleton-Century-Crofts; 1977; 231–264.

50. Goldner MG. The fate of the second leg in the diabetic amputee. Diabetes. 1960; 9:100–103.

51. Goodkin G. Mortality factors in diabetes: a 20-year mortality study. J Occup Med. 1975; 17:716–721.

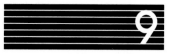

Cutaneous Manifestations of Diabetes Mellitus

ARTHUR C. HUNTLEY, M.D.

Diabetes mellitus is a common disorder in the United States—it has been estimated that 11 million persons have this condition. With such a high prevalence, a physician can expect a high proportion of patients to have diabetes. Most primary care physicians and dermatologists who care for patients with diabetes might not treat disease-related problems daily. Those specialists, including foot and ankle surgeons who deal mainly with foot disease, might have diabetic patients as a sizeable portion of their practice.

The skin involvement of diabetes is noteworthy because of the many and varied complications of the disease. It has previously been estimated that the proportion of those with skin manifestations of diabetes was about 30%.[1] In fact, the actual figure probably approaches 100%, especially if the metabolic effects on the microcirculation and changes in skin collagen are included.

It is useful to recognize the skin findings of diabetes because they are often the presenting manifestations of the disease. Other skin findings can indicate serious, even life-threatening, problems. In addition, relatively minor skin manifestations involving the feet can potentiate major complications. Recognition is the key to treatment and prevention.

Some cutaneous findings can also reflect the degree of long-term control in this disease. The metabolic condition of hyperglycemia affects most tissues of the body, including the skin. The resulting manifestations can at some point be used as an indicator of metabolic control.

This chapter reviews the cutaneous manifestations of diabetes mellitus, and emphasizes those features that are common in the diabetic foot. These conditions are discussed in related groups according to assumed pathophysiology. Because the pathophysiology is not always known, however, some findings are discussed separately. Many diabetic manifestations are purported to be the product of hyperglycemia, so the first section reviews normal skin and discusses some of the biochemical effects of hyperglycemia.

NORMAL SKIN

The skin is a specialized organ that forms the surface of the body. As the largest organ of the body it has many and varied functions, including thermoregulation, protection from physical, chemical, and biologic insult, maintenance of internal hydration, metabolism of vitamin D, sensory interface, and excretion. It is plastic and elastic, allowing joint movement to be unhindered. Several components of this organ are specialized to serve these functions.

Keratinocytes

The epidermis, the outer layer of the skin, consists mostly of a basal layer of undifferentiated cells that are continuously generating cells that migrate toward the surface and differentiate. These cells develop keratin, lose their nuclei, become a protective horny layer, and are then shed. Epidermal cells, or keratinocytes (so called because their primary product of differentiation is keratin), are attached to one another by bridges known as desmosomes. They also attach to the basement membrane by similar bridges, hemidesmosomes. Within the upper layers of the epidermis the keratinocytes also produce lipid-containing packets, membrane-coating granules, which are subsequently excreted and play a role in the barrier function of the skin.

Melanocytes

Interspersed in the basal layer of cells, about one cell in ten, are dendritic, pigment-producing melanocytes. These pigment cells manufacture small packets of melanin, melanosomes, which are then transferred to neighboring keratinocytes by way of the dendritic processes. The keratinocyte positions the melanosomes above the nucleus, forming an umbrella that protects the genetic material of the cell from some incidental electromagnetic radiation, including much of the ultraviolet light (UVL).

Racial differences in skin color are the result of melanosome size, and packaging, and the number of melanosomes. Persons with light skin have smaller melanosomes, which are packaged together by the keratinocyte, whereas persons with darker skin have larger melanosomes, which tend to be dispersed singly. Tanning consists of UVL stimulation of melanocytes, which results in an increased production and transfer of melanosomes to keratinocytes. Because the pigment occurs in keratinocytes, which have a continuous rate of turnover, skin that is dark because of tanning loses its color when the stimulus to the melanocytes is no longer present and the darker keratinocytes are shed.

Increased pigmentation of the skin can also follow inflammation. This is the result of pigment incontinence by the disturbed melanocytes rather than of transfer of melanosomes to the keratinocytes. The pigment is "dropped" into the underlying dermis. This is clinically visible as focal areas of darker skin at the sites of previous inflammation. Unlike a tan, which tends to resolve relatively quickly once the stimulus has been withdrawn, postinflammatory hyperpigmentation is reversed by macrophage removal of pigment, a process that takes months to years to complete.

Langerhans' Cells

Also within the epidermis are another set of dendritic cells, the Langerhans' cells. These are related to circulating macrophages and process and present antigen to lymphocytes. Langerhans' cells probably play a major role in immune surveillance in the epidermis. They are also involved in the sensitization and elicitation phases of allergic contact dermatitis. Langerhans' cells can be temporarily suppressed by the application of topical corticosteroids or by exposure to high doses of UVL (i.e., sunburn).

Dermis

The dermis is a thick fibrous layer that provides nutrient and structural support for the overlying epidermis. The major cell of this layer is the fibroblast, whose products include collagen, elastin, and glycosaminoglycans. Most of the dry weight of the skin consists of collagen, a helical protein that accounts for most of the structural integrity of this organ. Interspersed within the dermis is elastin, the protein responsible for returning the skin to its original shape following deformation. The third major product, glycosaminoglycans, are hydrated molecules that serve to cushion the skin from point trauma. The dermis is divided into an upper papillary dermis and a lower reticular dermis. The term "papillary" refers to the upward protrusions of the dermis into the epidermis. The papillary dermis extends down to the superficial vascular plexus and is characterized by wispy collagen, capillary loops ascending into the dermal papillae, and occasional mast cells. These latter cells produce and release mediators of inflammation. Most of the dermis is situated in the area below the superficial vascular plexus down to the subcutaneous fat, and is called the reticular dermis. This layer is characterized by thick bundles of collagen, a deep vascular plexus, and occasional neural bundles.

Adnexal Structures

The adnexal structures of the skin consist of sweat glands, sebaceous glands, hair, and nails. The eccrine sweat glands are present over most of the body surface. They are innervated by the sympathetic nervous system and primarily serve the function of thermoregulation. Taken as a whole, their output volume can exceed that of the kidneys. Apocrine sweat glands exist primarily in the axillae and groin and their secretion is metabolized by skin flora, resulting in a malodorous product. Sebaceous glands develop at puberty and are found mainly on the head and upper chest regions. The function of these glands is not completely understood. Hair is an adnexal structure found on most of the body surface except for the palms and soles. Much of the body hair is fine (vellus) and can be best appreciated with a hand lens. Nails serve to protect the ends of the digits. These specialized keratinous structures are produced by the nail matrix, which is situated underneath the proximal nail fold.

Vasculature

The dermal vasculature consists of deep and superficial networks of vessels and a superficial arcade of capillary loops that nurture the epidermis. The superficial plexus lies at the junction of the papillary and reticular dermis. The predominant portion of the cutaneous microcirculation consists of the capillary venous loops, which serve the dermal papillae.

BIOCHEMICAL CONSIDERATIONS

Rahbar, in 1968, observed that patients with diabetes mellitus have oddly behaving hemoglobin.[2] It was subsequently demonstrated that this is a result of nonenzymatic condensation of glucose with hemoglobin to form stable covalent products. Not only does glucose bind to hemoglobin, but this nonenzymatic glucosylation also occurs with other proteins. In addition, proteins can be complexed by other carbohydrates, such as galactose, ribose, mannose, fructose, and fucose.[3] Because this attachment seems to result in some functional derangement, it is interesting that, among the sugars, glucose actually seems to have less avidity for this union and might therefore be more compatible with biologic systems.[4]

Glucose in solution exists as a stable pyranose ring structure in equilibrium with the open chain aldehyde form. The reaction of monosaccharides with proteins involves the covalent linkage of the double-bonded oxygen of the aldehyde function with an NH_2 group, either on the α-amino group of the N-terminal amino acid or on the ϵ-amino group of lysine. This condensation step, resulting in the formation of a Schiff base or aldimine, is a reversible reaction. Following the formation of the Schiff base, however, is an internal reconfiguration of the molecule, the so-called Amadori rearrangement, which results in the formation of a ketoamine that tends not to revert back to the Schiff base. The rate of reaction of various carbohydrates with protein correlates with the extent to which the sugar exists in the open ring (aldehyde) form. Relative to other monosaccharides glucose exists in a more stable ring structure and has less avidity for this condensation with protein.

Following the condensation and reconfiguration, the Amadori products undergo a series of further reactions with amino groups on other proteins to form glucose-derived intermolecular crosslinks.[5] One of these advanced glycosylation products is a yellow compound, 2-(2-furoyl)-4(5)-(2-furanyl)-1H-imidazole, and has been identified.[6] The identification of this product and the characterization of its spectrophotometric properties might allow some quantitation of the tissue glycosylation reaction.

The process of nonenzymatic glycosylation occurs to a minor extent at normal blood sugar concentrations. This gradual glycosylation of proteins might be responsible for some of the changes associated with the aging process. In patients with elevated blood sugar levels, this process is accelerated. Most proteins studied seem to be involved in this reaction. The result of glycosylation on protein can be a change in its physical and chemical properties. Glycosylation of the red cell membrane is apparently responsible for the stiffness of diabetic erythrocytes.[7] Glycosylation of collagen results in biochemical changes such as increased stiffness and resistance to enzymatic degradation, mechanical changes of collagen that are also characteristic of aging.

Although other biochemical changes occur in diabetes mellitus, the focus is currently on the relationship of protein glycosylation to many of the disease complications. Changes in the tertiary structure and solubility of proteins could result in many of the clinical phenomena observed in diabetes, especially increased dermal thickness and micro-angiopathy.

SKIN INVOLVEMENT IN DIABETES

The following sections group similar complications together because of presumed similarities in their pathogenesis. For example, all microvascular complications are combined because they are assumed to have common underlying factors. In some instances, however, this might not be a valid assumption. For example, in the next section, it is clear that hyperglycemia is the predisposing factor for cutaneous infections caused by Candida but not for those caused by Pseudomonas. Another problem associated with grouping complications into broad categories is the need for a miscellaneous category because, for several manifestations, the pathogenesis is unclear. Nevertheless, this grouping is still useful for understanding many differing but etiologically related manifestations of diabetes.

Cutaneous Infections

Before antibiotics (and insulin) were available, the prevalence of some dermatologic infections such as furunculosis, carbunculosis, and erysipelas was much higher in diabetics than in nondiabetics.[8] In the diabetic population of today these types of infections do not seem to account for much morbidity. Current estimates do not substantiate a generalized increase in the frequency of infections in diabetics.[9,10] Several infections do occur characteristically in persons with diabetes mellitus, however, and some of these infections can threaten life and limb (Fig. 9-1).

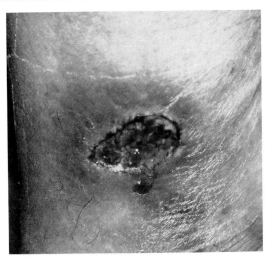

FIGURE 9–1 ■ Ecthyma of the posterior aspect of the lower leg in a 73-year-old, non-insulin-dependent diabetic woman. This wound, resulting from a minor injury, enlarged and became ulcerated with surrounding deep erythema. Cultures grew mixed flora, including Pseudomonas, and the lesion resolved with antibiotic therapy.

CANDIDIASIS

Yeast infections caused by Candida are common in established diabetic patients. Stomal and vaginal candidiasis is almost universal among long-term diabetic patients.[11,12] Yeast infections might even be the presenting manifestation of the disease. Candidal infection of the foot also occurs. When such an infection enters into the differential diagnosis, it is helpful to determine if other body sites are affected (Fig. 9-2).

Successful treatment usually involves normalizing the blood sugar level and treating the vagina and vulva with topical medication. Because these patients generally have a reservoir of Candida in the colon, oral nystatin is also frequently administered.

Candidal paronychia involves the hands and feet. It begins at the lateral nail folds as erythema, swelling, and separation of the fold from the lateral margin of the nail. Further infection can result in involvement of the proximal nail fold and in separation of the cuticle from the nail. Moisture trapped in the resultant space favors further growth of the yeast and repeated episodes of inflam-

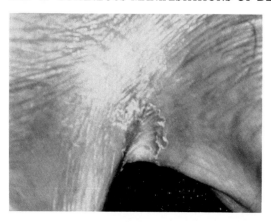

FIGURE 9-2 ■ *Candida albicans* infection of the web space of the hand. The web spaces of both hands and feet can trap moisture, which promotes the growth of yeast. Support for growth of this organism presumably results from maceration of the epidermis caused by the apposition of the skin in a moist environment.

mation. At times there is a purulent discharge from the involved nail fold, a clinical finding suggesting bacterial paronychia. The diagnosis of yeast infection can usually be established by performing a KOH preparation on extruded serous material from this space. Treatment involves controlling the blood sugar level, keeping the digits dry, and using a topical antifungal agent, such as nystatin cream. Antifungal solutions might offer some advantage over creams in regard to reaching the infection.

Candidal infection of the foot commonly presents in one of two ways. The most common manifestation is infection of the fourth to fifth web space of the toes. This area has a tendency to retain moisture as a result of occlusion from apposing surfaces of skin. Presumably, the increased sugar content of the skin encourages establishment of this infection. The clinical appearance is that of a white patch of skin, often with central peeling. It is often mistaken for a dermatophyte infection, but the diagnosis can be confirmed using a KOH preparation. Also included in the differential diagnosis are infection by Pseudomonas aeruginosa, erythrasma, intertrigo, and a soft callus. P. aeruginosa and erythrasma can be diagnosed by characteristic fluorescence on ex-

posure to an ultraviolet (Wood's) lamp. Intertrigo is a diagnosis of exclusion. Because infection of the diabetic foot can lead to serious consequences it is imperative that the correct diagnosis be established and treatment begun.

The second and less common presentation of candidal infection of the foot is involvement in the nail plate. Dystrophic toenails are often assumed to be the result of dermatophyte infection (onychomycosis), for which the current first-line treatment is oral griseofulvin. Nail plate cultures performed to confirm the diagnosis occasionally demonstrate the pathogen to be Candida sp. (usually not C. albicans), for which griseofulvin would be inappropriate therapy. Clinically, nail plate infection with either dermatophyte or Candida sp. presents with distal yellowing or whitening and thickening of the toenail. Living tissue does not appear to be involved. If it is especially risky for the diabetic host to have this nail plate infection, it has not been demonstrated.

PHYCOMYCOSIS

Other micro-organisms thrive in a high-glucose medium. Hyperglycemia can allow nonpathogenic organisms to establish an infection in traumatized skin, even resulting in gangrene and loss of limb. Diabetic patients with leg ulcers or nonhealing surgical wounds, especially those of the lower extremities, might have a complicating phycomycetous infection.[13] Such an infection should be suspected when lower extremity ulcers or post-traumatic lesions are unresponsive to therapy. Diagnosis can be confirmed by culture and by the histologic demonstration of fungal elements invading vascular channels.

Uncontrolled diabetics with ketosis can be predisposed to deep mycotic infections, including mucormycosis.[14] Treatment consists of correction of acid-base imbalance, aggressive debridement of necrotic tissue, and intravenous amphotericin.

PSEUDOMONAS AERUGINOSA INFECTIONS

Although pseudomonas aeruginosa occasionally cause a life-threatening infection of the external ear in persons with diabetes,[15,16] the common and more benign site of involvement is of the foot. Pseudomonas aeruginosa commonly causes infection of the toe web spaces or under the toenails. Often, persons with onychomycosis develop a lifting of the nail plate from the nail bed (onycholysis). The resulting space between plate and bed can become colonized with P. aeruginosa, resulting in a green discoloration of this area.

As mentioned previously, web space infection of the feet is usually assumed to be dermatophytosis, but this assumption might be incorrect. The differential diagnosis includes candidiasis, infection caused by P. aeruginosa, erythrasma, and intertrigo. If examination of a scraping from the affected web space fails to reveal hyphae, a Wood's lamp examination can reveal the coral fluorescence of erythrasma or the green fluorescence of Pseudomonas aeruginosa. Topical treatment usually suffices to eradicate this infection but, in those with more advanced cellulitis, oral Ciprofloxacin is the antibiotic of choice.

DERMATOPHYTOSIS

Dermatophyte infections of the foot (tinea pedis) are probably not more common in diabetics than in nondiabetics,[17] but they are of special concern. Toe web space infections can lead to inflammation and fissuring and thus serve as a portal of entry for bacterial infection in a compromised diabetic foot. The oxygen demand of the subsequent inflammation might exceed the ability of the diabetic microcirculation, leading to gangrene. Therefore, tinea pedis should be aggressively managed in patients with neurovascular compromise.

Infection of the toenails by dermatophytes (onychomycosis) is common among elderly diabetics, as it is in the general population. The infection itself is of little consequence, but the nail dystrophy that results can make proper nail care more difficult for the patient. Current treatment for onychomycosis consists of 8 to 15 months of oral griseofulvin or ketoconazole. In a patient with good circulation to the toes, this antifungal administration period can be shortened by avulsion of the affected nails, but this is often not an available option for diabetics. Currently available topical antifungal agents do not eradicate this infec-

tion, although they are often prescribed as adjunctive therapy.

Dermal Manifestations

DIABETIC THICK SKIN

Persons with diabetes usually have thicker skin than nondiabetics. Three considerations are relevant to this observation. Diabetics generally have a clinically inapparent but measurable increase in skin thickness compared to that of controls; this is unassociated with symptoms and goes unnoticed by patients and most physicians. The diabetic hand syndrome consists of the development of scleroderma-like skin changes involving the fingers and dorsum of the hand. Infrequently, the syndrome of diabetic scleredema, in which the patient develops markedly thickened dermis on the upper back region, can occur.

Adult skin is approximately 1 mm thick. It is thicker on the palms and soles because of an increased stratum corneum and thicker on the back because of a greater volume of dermis. Quantitative estimations of skin thickness have been determined by microscopic measurement, caliper measurement of skin folds, ultrasonography, and radiologic investigation.[18] These measurements demonstrate a variation of skin thickness by body site and by age and sex.[19] The skin increases in thickness from birth until adulthood, and decreases from about the age of 20 years to senility. From adulthood on women tend to have thinner skin than men. The skin on the trunk is generally thicker than that of the extremities. Except for the soles and the volar finger skin, about 95% of skin thickness is of dermal and 5% of epidermal origin.[20] Skin thickness can be influenced by endocrinologic conditions such as acromegaly, with increased skin thickness, and Cushing's syndrome, with decreased skin thickness.

The presence of diabetes mellitus is usually associated with measurably thickened skin. Using pulsed ultrasound it can be demonstrated that diabetics have thicker forearm skin than their age and sex-matched nondiabetic counterparts.[21] Contrary to nondiabetics, skin thickness in diabetics can increase with age, but this might be associated with increased duration of the disease. Most studies have used upper extremity skin in the evaluation of skin thickness, but it might not be valid to conclude that diabetic skin is thickened at other sites. In our laboratory at the University of California, Davis, increased skin thickness on the dorsum of the feet, but not of the back, has been demonstrated, suggesting that increased skin thickness is not necessarily universal in diabetes. It can be said, however, that patients with diabetes mellitus generally have detectably thicker skin on their extremities (Fig. 9-3).

DIABETIC HAND SYNDROME

Special mention is made here of the diabetic hand syndrome because similar manifestations probably occur on the feet. The diabetic hand syndrome consists of thick-ened skin over the dorsum of the digits and limited joint mobility, especially of the interphalangeal joints. The earliest description revealed that insulin-dependent diabetes is occasionally complicated by painful, stiff hands.[22] Rosenbloom and Frais have described three adolescent patients with the syndrome of long-standing diabetes mellitus, restricted joint mobility, thick, tight, waxy skin, growth impairment, and maturational delay.[23] Rosenbloom and colleagues later reported in a study of 309 diabetics (mostly juveniles) that 30% had joint limitation and one-third of these had thick, tight, waxy skin that the examiner could not dent, mostly involving the dorsum of the hands.[24] Their results have been confirmed by others and have also been extended to patients with type II diabetes mellitus.[25]

At least 20 to 30% of diabetic patients have skin thickening. Clinical clues that

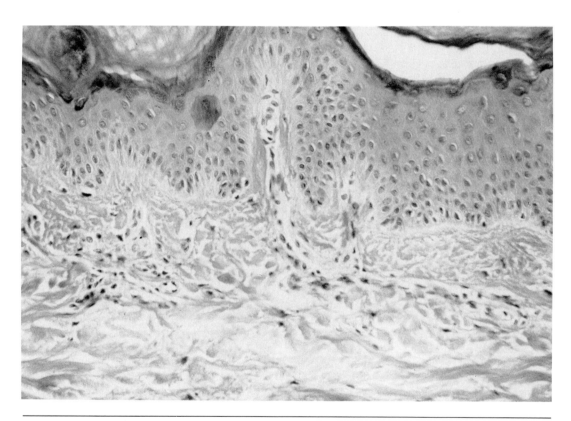

FIGURE 9–3 ■ Thickened extremity skin in diabetes mellitus. The epidermis is slightly hypercellular, but otherwise normal. The collagen in the upper (papillary) dermis is thickened instead of wispy, as is normally found. Well seen on this section is a widely dilated capillary loop ascending from the superficial vascular plexus (at the junction of the papillary and reticular dermis) and entering the dermal papilla.

suggest such a thickening include difficulty in tenting the skin, pebbled or rough skin on the knuckles or peri-ungual region,[26] and decreased skin wrinkling following immersion in water.[27] Occasionally, skin thickening of the hands becomes so exaggerated as to be scleroderma-like.

Largely ignored in the literature is the fact that digital sclerosis often involves the feet as well (Fig. 9-4). Using ultrasound, the skin on the dorsum of the foot has been found to be measurably thickened in most of our diabetic population.

The medical literature suggests that digital sclerosis (thick skin) of the hand and feet is significant because it is a marker for retinal microvascular disease, but a spectrum of thickening of the skin exists that ranges from thickening that is only detectable by ultrasound to the more obvious. For less than

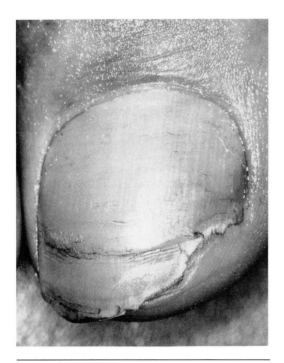

FIGURE 9–4 ■ Thickened skin on the dorsum of the great toe in a patient with insulin-dependent diabetes mellitus. Of the many clues to this thickening, a pebbled or rough appearance is one of the more common indications. Whereas thickening of the skin on the plantar surface would result in a callus, thickening on the dorsum is often seen clinically by the appearance of minute pebbling, as seen here.

digital sclerosis, the significance of thick skin in diabetics is uncertain at present.

As for many other complications of diabetes today, many believe it is a result of nonenzymatic glycosylation. One study of skin biopsies from clinically affected children demonstrated on average a tenfold increase in collagen glycosylation[28] but questions regarding this hypothesis still remain. First, whereas nonenzymatic glycosylation of collagen is supposed to be a slow process, with the build-up of collagen caused by the decreased ability of collagenase to cleave the molecule, clinically thickened skin can be detected in newly diagnosed diabetics. Second, it would be expected that this process is slowly or not at all reversible, and one study found normalization of skin thickness (as measured on multiple sites by ultrasonography) following good control of diabetes.[29] An alternate mechanism has been proposed, that collagen hydration secondary to polyol accumulation is responsible.[30] To date the pathogenesis has not been conclusively demonstrated.

In regard to treatment for the thick skin syndrome, one study has suggested that tight control of the blood sugar level is helpful. Lieberman and associates reported that four diabetic patients with thick skin had a decrease of skin thickness following pump administration of insulin and achievement of tighter diabetes control.[29] In their study skin thickness was measured ultrasonically on six body areas and the sums of pretreatment and post-treatment determinations were compared; however, they did not report thickness measurements for any one area. No treatment is known for diabetic scleredema.

It is apparent, then, that persons with diabetes mellitus have thickened skin on the extremities. Best described for the hands, this phenomenon is also evident in the feet. The pathogenesis of this thickening is not fully known, but the significance might be that of a marker of poorly controlled diabetes with microvascular complications.

LIMITATION OF JOINT MOBILITY

Restriction of joint mobility occurs in about 50% of patients with diabetes.[31] Although this phenomenon has been described mainly for its hand involvement, other joints can also be involved. Perhaps the flexion contractures noted in the toes of some diabetic patients are a result of this process. It seems likely that the hand and foot manifestations would be similar for this disease (Fig. 9-5).

YELLOW SKIN

Patients with diabetes mellitus often have a yellow hue to their skin. It might seem odd to group this with dermal complications of diabetes, because it was traditionally assumed to be caused by carotenemia. Carotenemia produces yellowing of the epidermis and areas of the body with a thickened epidermis, such as the palms and soles, are the easiest sites for demonstrating this in patients with diabetes. The main problem with using carotene to explain the distinctly yellow hue of diabetic skin is that the serum carotene levels of diabetics are not elevated.[32] The carotenemia noted in studies years ago was probably a manifestation of the diet of diabetics of the time.

What is responsible for the yellow color of diabetic skin? Perhaps the yellow glycosylation end products present in proteins with a long turnover time are responsible. One of the advanced glycosylation products that has been identified, 2-(2-furoyl)-4(5)-(2-furanyl)-1H-imidazole,[6] has a distinctly yellow hue (see above, Biochemical Considerations). Proteins that have a long turnover time, such as dermal collagen, undergo glycosylation and become yellow.

Whatever the cause, yellow skin is a common finding in the skin of patients with diabetes. It is probably best appreciated on the palms and soles because of sparse competition with melanocytic pigment in these areas. Currently, no significance is associated with this finding, other than that of a time-proven observation.

Macro-angiopathy

Diabetics have a higher incidence and prevalence of large vessel disease.[33] They are known to develop myocardial infarctions and strokes at a much younger age than their nondiabetic counterparts. Large vessel disease can also be present in the lower extremities. Atherosclerosis of the arteries in the legs is said to result in skin atrophy, hair loss, coldness of the toes, nail dystrophy, pallor on elevation, and mottling on dependence.[34] One reliable sign of large vessel disease is dependent rubor, with delayed return of color following pressure on the skin. A delayed return of color longer than 15 seconds is considered abnormal (Fig. 9-6).

Micro-angiopathy

A major complication of diabetes mellitus is known as micro-angiopathy. This term has traditionally been applied to the small blood vessel changes affecting the retinal and renal vasculature, which are responsible for blindness and kidney failure. Microvascular pathology has also been assumed to play a role in diabetic neuropathy and in the diabetic foot. Histologic changes considered diagnostic of micro-angiopathy, however,

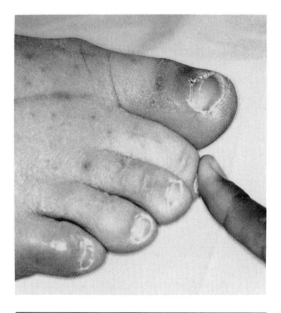

FIGURE 9–5 ■ Limited joint mobility of the toes in a 44-year-old man with long-standing, insulin-dependent diabetes mellitus. The examiner is attempting to flex the toe fully, demonstrating the limitation. This patient also had moderately thickened skin on the dorsum of the toes (note the minute pebbling on the dorsum of the great toe) and multiple red-yellow papules histologically demonstrated to be eruptive xanthomas.

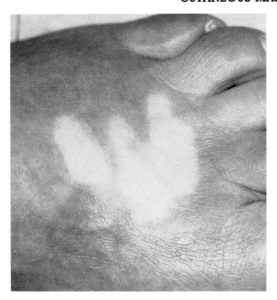

FIGURE 9-6 ■ Delayed return of erythema indicative of large vessel disease. The three marks on the dorsum of the foot of this elderly diabetic patient are impressions left from pressure of the examiner's fingers approximately 20 seconds previously.

have not always been demonstrable in the skin.

The clinical hallmark of micro-angiopathy generally consists of changes observed in the eyegrounds. The sine qua non of diabetic retinopathy is the presence of microaneurysms. In those with more severe involvement hemorrhages, exudates, and even some devascularized areas are also seen.

Histologically, biopsies of diabetic tissue reveal a PAS (periodic acid-Schiff)-positive thickened capillary basement membrane. Electron microscopy of skeletal muscle capillaries reveals reduplication of the basal lamina. Why isn't the skin, such easily accessed tissue, biopsied routinely to assess the status of a patient's micro-angiopathy? The small blood vessels of the skin develop less basal lamina thickening than skeletal muscle, which is also easily accessed using needle biopsy. When investigators used skin and muscle biopsy to assess micro-angiopathy it was not a sensitive enough assay—that is, some patients with severe microcirculatory problems, such as gangrene of the foot, appeared to have normal capillaries. The *structural* changes that occur in the micro-

circulation, though, cannot account for all the problems associated with this condition. From this last observation arose the concept of *functional* micro-angiopathy. Clinical observations support this hypothesis, such as retinal venous dilatation, red face, and periungual telangiectasia, all of which can be early manifestations of the disease and which can improve with control of diabetes.

The phenomenon of functional micro-angiopathy is complex. It has been noted that nonenzymatic glycosylation affects many blood components, including hemoglobin, the red blood cell membrane, fibronectin, fibrinogen, and platelets. Glycosylation of the red blood cell has been shown to inhibit cell pliability and to decrease the ability of this cell to pass through pores smaller than 7 μ. The lumen of some capillaries can be as narrow as 3 μ, and ordinarily red blood cells elongate into a more sausage-like configuration to traverse this loop. A stiffened membrane inhibits or limits this passage.

In addition to stiffened red blood cells, diabetics have an increased plasma concentration of fibrinogen and suffer from capillary leakage, leading to loss of albumin and water and an increased tendency for diabetic platelets to aggregate. The result is increased whole blood or plasma viscosity and sluggish microcirculation.

Patients with diabetes therefore have micro-angiopathy that can be attributed both to structural and functional abnormalities. The following discussion reviews some cutaneous manifestations that might be linked to this micro-angiopathy.

DIABETIC DERMOPATHY

Diabetic dermopathy (Fig. 9-7), or shin spots, is the most common cutaneous finding in diabetes.[35] It is usually noted as atrophic hyperpigmented macules on the shins. These irregularly round or oval, circumscribed, shallow lesions vary in number from few to many. They are usually bilateral but are not symmetrically distributed. They are asymptomatic and often overlooked by patient and physician.

The genesis of these lesions is unclear. Some authors have described a preceding, distinct, red papular eruption that is independent of trauma to the skin.[36] Lithner, however, was able to duplicate these lesions

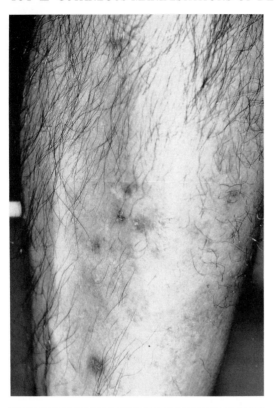

FIGURE 9–7 ■ Diabetic dermopathy. This middle-aged diabetic man has multiple, atrophic, hyperpigmented macules on his shins. These "shin spots" are often present in persons with diabetes but, when there are multiple lesions, as seen here, the patient usually also has diabetic retinopathy.

by local thermal trauma.[37] Many patients who develop these depressed lesions have antecedent trauma or mild pyoderma, such as folliculitis. In many respects these lesions appear to be consistent with post-traumatic atrophy and postinflammatory hyperpigmentation in poorly vascularized skin.

The lesions presented might represent the cutaneous manifestation of structural micro-angiopathy. Histologic characteristics of acute lesions are edema of the epidermis and papillary dermis, extravasated erythrocytes, and a mild lymphohistiocytic infiltrate.[38] Older lesions have thick-walled capillaries in the upper dermis, occasional extravasated erythrocytes, and a positive Perls' stain reaction for iron. One electron microscopic study, however, has demonstrated the presence of a thickened basal lamina in some patients.[39] Based on the available studies, evidence exists both for and against a relationship to structural micro-angiopathy.

How often one expects to encounter diabetic dermopathy, and the significance of its occurrence, depends on its operational definition. Defined as one or more spots, the original report noted their presence in 55% of 293 diabetics (65% of males and 29% of females).[40] Thus, defining diabetic dermopathy as one or more spots results in high sensitivity but low specificity for diabetics.[41] In a study that defined dermopathy as the presence of four or more lesions, however, the lesions were absent in nondiabetics and present in about 14% of diabetics (24% of men and 3% of women).[42] The multilesional definition also found a high correlation with retinovascular disease.

The presence of pretibial pigmented patches is also significant. They are a common finding in diabetes mellitus. When several are present they can be a cutaneous sign of microvascular disease in other tissues. Their presence in patients seen for other conditions should prompt an evaluation for diabetes mellitus. The pathomechanism of this condition, however, is not known.

PIGMENTED PURPURA

Pigmented purpuric dermatosis (Fig. 9-8) is a condition that results from red blood cell extravasation of the superficial vascular plexus involving the skin on the lower extremities. It is characterized by patches of orange to tan pigmentation and "cayenne pepper" spots on the shins, often extending down to involve the ankles and dorsum of the feet. It has been described as a manifestation in older diabetic patients, about 50% of whom had diabetic dermopathy.[43] In most of these patients, cardiac decompensation with edema of the legs was determined to be a precipitating factor for the purpura. Except for the frequent association with diabetic dermopathy, this condition appears clinically consistent with Schamberg's disease.

With little insight into the pathophysiology, this condition appears to be a marker of structural micro-angiopathy.

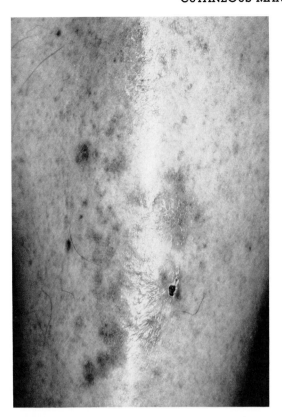

FIGURE 9–8 ■ Pigmented purpura of the lower extremities. One apparent manifestation of microvascular disease of the skin in the diabetic is the occurrence of petechial purpura followed by the deposition of hemosiderin and the yellow-brown appearance of the affected area. Darker spots can be appreciated within some of these lesions; these represent focal extravasation of individual vascular loops within the papillary dermis.

RED SKIN AND RUBEOSIS FACEI

The prototypical site of involvement of functional micro-angiopathy is the face. The intensity of red coloration that can be appreciated in the "complexion" is a function of the degree of engorgement of the superficial venous plexus. Hyperglycemia apparently predisposes to sluggish microcirculation and venous engorgement in the microcirculation. Affected individuals develop a functional microangiopathy that is clinically evident by venous dilatation.[44] The venous dilatation is present in the eye-

ground and on the skin. This erythema has been well described for the face, but is also present in the feet. It can be seen in newly diagnosed diabetics and, more importantly, the venous engorgement can return to normal when the blood sugar level is controlled. In a prospective study of 150 medical hospital admissions comparing facial redness with diabetic parameters, persons with diabetes had markedly red faces.[45]

This sign appears to be an interesting marker of functional micro-angiopathy of the skin, including the foot. One problem in practice, however, is that it is difficult to grade this phenomenon. Fortunately, a more objective means of evaluating cutaneous functional micro-angiopathy is available.

PERIUNGUAL TELANGIECTASIA

The skin can be examined directly to evaluate the microcirculation of the superficial dermis. Any area of skin can be examined but, because the capillary loops at the nail fold are in a horizontal axis (relative to the surface of the skin), this area offers an excellent view of the entire microvascular loop. To see past the stratum corneum it is helpful to apply mineral oil to the skin surface initially and to wait a few minutes until this layer becomes translucent. A low-power microscope (Fig. 9-9) or simply an ophthalmoscope (+40 lens for 10 × magnification) can be used. Generally, the microcirculation of less pigmented individuals is easier to visualize. One study has found venous capillary dilatation in the nail folds of 49% of 75 diabetic patients compared to 10% of 65 controls.[46] It is important to note that connective tissue disease can also result in periungual vessel changes, but that these changes are morphologically different. In diabetes isolated homogeneous engorgement of the venular limbs is seen. In connective tissue disease the patterns seen are megacapillaries or irregularly enlarged loops.[47]

Periungual microcirculatory changes appear to be more important than just another marker of diabetes. Evidence has shown that venous dilatation of the cutaneous microcirculation is an excellent indicator of functional micro-angiopathy and of long-term control of the disease. Furthermore, struc-

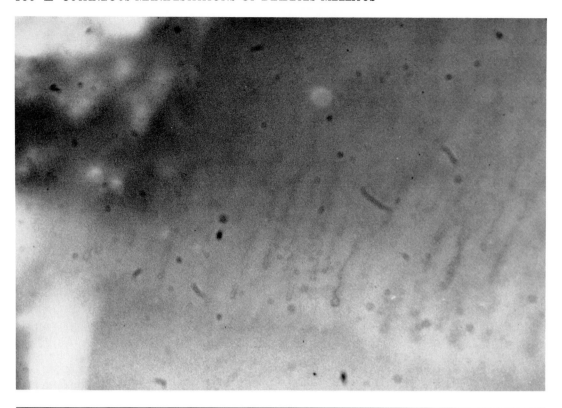

FIGURE 9–9 ■ Periungual telangiectasia as seen through the microscope. Examined here is the fold of skin, which extends over the proximal portion of the nail. A palisade of capillary loops can be seen. Instead of being simple hairpin-shaped many of these capillaries are tortuous and moderately dilated, suggesting long-standing diabetes mellitus with poor control.

tural changes can be noted, usually venous tortuosity, which seem to indicate long-term micro-angiopathy. Thus, a newly diagnosed patient is likely to have simple capillary loops with a dilated venous portion. A long-term diabetic patient who has had poor control for a number of years, but who now has excellent control, can exhibit venous tortuosity without dilatation. More extensive micro-angiopathy can be heralded by small hemorrhages and by dropout of areas of the microcirculation.

ERYSIPELAS-LIKE ERYTHEMA

Another reported phenomenon of microcirculatory compromise in diabetic patients is the development of well-demarcated erythema on the lower leg or dorsum of the foot, which seems to correlate with radio-logic evidence of underlying bone destruction and indicates incipient gangrene.[48,49] The condition was at first mistaken for erysipelas (hence, the name erysipelas-like erythema), but no associated pyrexia, elevated erythrocyte sedimentation rate, or leukocytosis is seen. If these observations are supported, they would seem to be an important sign of localized functional micro-angiopathy.

Other Skin Markers

YELLOW NAILS

As noted by Lithner, persons with diabetes mellitus tend to have yellow nails.[43] He observed this phenomenon in 50% of 36 diabetics and in one of nine controls. Our patients seem to have a similar incidence of yellow nails, except we also see it occasionally in elderly controls and in some patients with onychomycosis. Although all the nails can be yellow, it most often occurs on the distal aspect of the nail of the hallux.

The cause of the yellow color is *not* usually underlying dermatophytosis. Similar to the yellow color observed in diabetic skin, yellowing of the nails probably represents glycosylation end products. Whereas keratin of the epidermis is only present for 1 month before being shed, that of the nail plate can be present for more than 1 year. The protein-glucose reaction continues to evolve in the aging nail, resulting in the yellowest pigment at the distal aspect of the slowest growing nail. The presence of yellow glycosylation end products in the nail plate has not been confirmed to date, but one study of fingernails has demonstrated that diabetics have high levels of fructose-lysine, another marker of nonenzymatic glycosylation.[50]

The yellow nails of diabetics are best seen on the toenails. Most diabetic patients manifest some degree of this yellowing. Minimal involvement consists of distal yellow or yellow-brown discoloration of the hallux nail plate. Marked involvement consists of canary yellow discoloration of all toe-nails and fingernails. It is not a specific finding in diabetes mellitus, because it is also observed with normal aging. Like the yellow hue that is generally appreciated in the skin of persons with diabetes, the significance of this observation is undetermined. The obvious question is whether yellow nails and yellow skin can be used as quantifiable indicators of the degree of nonenzymatic glycosylation for other tissues of the body.

DIABETIC BULLAE

Another curious phenomenon in those with diabetes mellitus is the spontaneous appearance of blisters, diabetic bullae (Fig. 9-10), on the extremities (usually confined to the hands or feet). These lesions are not the result of trauma or infection, and tend to heal without treatment. The most common type is spontaneous and nonscarring.

Current studies indicate that diabetic blisters are a heterogeneous phenomenon. They present as clear, sterile blisters on the tips

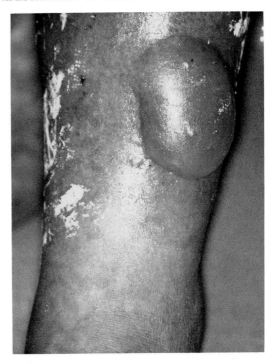

FIGURE 9–10 ■ Diabetic bullae. Patients with long-standing diabetes mellitus occasionally develop spontaneous bullae on distal portions of the extremities. These lesions resolve spontaneously.

of the toes or fingers and, less frequently, on the dorsal and lateral surfaces of the feet, legs, hands, and forearms. Spontaneous healing occurs within 2 to 5 weeks.[51] These patients were reported to have good circulation to the affected extremity, but also tended to have diabetic peripheral neuropathy. In patients in whom histopathology has been performed, an intra-epidermal cleavage without acantholysis is found.[52,53]

Other reports of diabetic bullae differ from the preceding reports in that the bullae were found to heal with scarring and slight atrophy.[54,55] These blisters can also be hemorrhagic. They differ from the common type of diabetic bullae in that the reported cleavage plane is below the dermo-epidermal junction.

The third type has been described in a case report as multiple, tender, nonscarring blisters on sun-exposed and deeply tanned skin on the feet, legs, and arms. Immunofluorescence and porphyrin studies were negative.

Electron microscopy placed the cleavage plane at the lamina lucida.[56]

Despite the differing levels of cleavage plane reported in the literature, these blisters share a common feature: they seem to be unique to diabetes mellitus.

NECROBIOSIS LIPOIDICA DIABETICORUM

Necrobiosis lipoidica diabeticicorum (NLD) is an uncommon manifestation of diabetes mellitus, occurring in about 0.3% of diabetics (Fig. 9-11).[57] This skin manifestation is not always associated with diabetes mellitus; less than two-thirds of patients with necrobiosis lipoidica are diabetic. Necrobiosis lipoidica has been documented to occur prior to the onset of diabetes mellitus.[58] Certainly, any patient who presents with necrobiosis lipoidica should be evaluated for diabetes.

The initial lesions of NLD begin as well-circumscribed erythematous papules. Evolving radially, the sharply defined lesions have hard, depressed, waxy, yellow-brown, atrophic, telangiectatic centers through the underlying dermal vessels, which can be visualized. When the lesion is active the periphery is slightly raised and erythematous. Ulceration has been reported in about one-third of those with leg lesions, mostly in large lesions following minor trauma. The lesions of NLD sometimes resolve spontaneously, but more often do not. They seem to occur and persist independent of the degree of control of the hyperglycemia.

Whereas most lesions of NLD present on the legs, about 15% are found elsewhere, including on the hands, forearms, abdomen, face, and scalp. When necrobiosis lipoidica occurs in areas other than the lower extremities, the patient is less likely to have diabetes mellitus.[59]

Histopathology. Ackerman has given a clear description of the histopathology.[60] Early lesions reveal a neutrophilic necrotizing vasculitis. With progression collagen degeneration and destruction of adnexal structures occur. Lesions evolve through granulomatous and sclerotic stages, with most of the sclerosis occurring in the lower reticular dermis. The upper dermis contains fatty deposits that can be demonstrated by oil red O or Sudan black stain. These deposits give the lesions their yellow color.

Treatment. An effective treatment for this condition has yet to be found. Application of high-potency topical steroids or intralesional injection of steroids into the active margin can arrest the progression. Previous reports of aspirin and dipyridamole producing significant improvement[61-63] were unsubstantiated by the results of double-blind trials.[64] Current studies include some encouraging therapeutic trials using hemorrheologic agents, such as pentoxifylline. Because the pathophysiology of necrobiosis is not understood, however, it is difficult to design rational therapy.

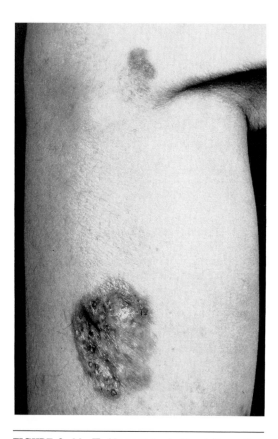

FIGURE 9–11 ■ Necrobiosis lipoidica diabeticorum. Occurring in less than 1% of diabetics are these peculiar erythematous plaques, which develop central atrophy. Although the early histologic events include a vasculitis of the deep dermal blood vessels, the pathogenesis of this condition is not understood.

Diabetic Neuropathy

AUTONOMIC NEUROPATHY

Autonomic neuropathy can have troubling manifestations in the diabetic patient, including postural vertigo, diarrhea, and constipation. These problems are fortunately rare, but other involvement of the autonomic nervous system, especially of the peripheral autonomic nerves, is common. It has been suggested that nonmyelinated nerve fibers, such as those of the autonomic nervous system, might be the first nervous tissue affected in diabetics.[65] Clinical evidence of autonomic neuropathy involving the feet seems to be the rule rather than the exception.

The key physical finding in making the clinical diagnosis is a disturbance of sweating (usually absent sweating) of the feet. Occasionally patients complain of oversweating elsewhere, a compensatory mechanism for loss of the ability to regulate the temperature in the involved area. It has also been reported that autonomic neuropathy (as measured by quantitation of the sweating deficiency) correlates well with the severity of loss to painful sensation.[66] It might safely be assumed that patients who have diabetic sensory neuropathy also have accompanying autonomic involvement.

At least two areas are of clinical significance with peripheral autonomic neuropathy. First, the patient might complain that the feet are abnormally cold, burning, or pruritic. The absence of sweating is also a problem. Perspiration on the feet seems to maintain hydration of the stratum corneum. A thickened stratum corneum, such as callosities without hydration, tends to become brittle and, with pressure, can fissure and form a portal for infection. Thus, symptoms and signs of autonomic peripheral neuropathy in the diabetic patient are an indication for extra attention to foot care.

MOTOR NEUROPATHY

Although diabetic motor neuropathy can involve other areas, the foot is most often affected (Fig. 9-12). The clinical presentation is characterized by a wasting of the interosseous foot muscles, which results in two major mechanical problems. First, the foot tends to splay on weight-bearing, resulting in a wider foot. Second, the toes tend to draw upward and the plantar fat pads move forward, leaving the metatarsal heads riding on the plantar skin without the benefit of padding.

Motor neuropathy can appear suddenly or occur gradually over several years. Acute and reversible motor neuropathy can follow an episode of ketoacidosis,[67] and can also occur as the result of insulin excess. More usual is the insidious progression of motor

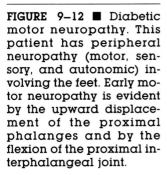

FIGURE 9–12 ■ Diabetic motor neuropathy. This patient has peripheral neuropathy (motor, sensory, and autonomic) involving the feet. Early motor neuropathy is evident by the upward displacement of the proximal phalanges and by the flexion of the proximal interphalangeal joint.

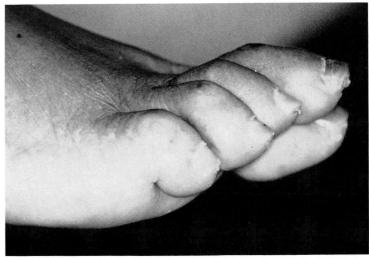

nerve deterioration involving the lower extremity.

The clinical significance of motor neuropathy is noteworthy. Motor polyneuropathy in diabetes mellitus is almost always accompanied by a sensory neuropathy. Changes in the shape of the foot follow the imbalance of its internal musculature and result in ill-fitting shoes. If the changes go unnoticed the patient might continue to wear previously purchased shoes, which could traumatize the foot. Because of the accompanying sensory loss, displacement of the plantar fat pads can result in uncushioned weight-bearing at the metatarsal heads. Callosities and eventually ulceration of the weight-bearing skin or of the skin being rubbed by the now ill-fitting shoes result (neuropathic ulcers). Chronic motor neuropathy of the foot often necessitates the use of specially widened shoes with molded inserts to redistribute weight-bearing to accommodate and protect the compromised foot.

SENSORY NEUROPATHY

Diabetics often develop sensory neuropathy of the feet, especially those with long-standing disease (Fig. 9-13). The clinical presentation usually involves reports of tingling and numbness starting in the toes. The level of neuropathy varies from mild numbness of the distal toes to profound anesthesia and neuropathic ulcers.

Sensory neuropathy is clinically significant. Although tingling and numbness tend to be the complaint, the lack of sensation can allow trauma to go unnoticed and result in a traumatic ulceration. Depending on the status of the microcirculation, these ulcers can present difficult therapeutic problems. Neuropathic patients who walk barefoot can sustain damage during routine ambulation because they have inadequate sensation to withdraw the foot when it encounters noxious stimuli. Occasionally this unsensed trauma during ambulation causes fractures, resulting in the Charcot foot (Fig. 9-14).

Patients with sensory neuropathy need to be instructed to ensure that their shoes contain no foreign objects before they put them on. As simple as it sounds, patients who do not follow this rule occasionally sustain severe damage by wearing shoes that, unknown to them, had objects in them, even children's toys.

The Diabetic Foot

One of the major complications of diabetes mellitus, the diabetic foot, is largely a cutaneous manifestation of the disease. It is actually the total of multisystem involve-

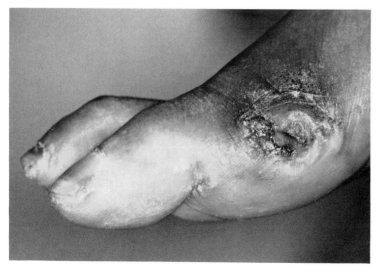

FIGURE 9–13 ◼ Sensory neuropathy. The medial aspect of the foot shown in Figure 9-12 demonstrates a traumatic ulcer of which the patient was unaware. Because of the motor neuropathy, the foot had become wider and friction from her shoe affected the medial aspect of the metatarsal head. Because her feet were numb she did not sense this traumatic ulceration as it occurred. This illustrates the importance of inspecting the feet of diabetic patients, even though they might report that no problems exist.

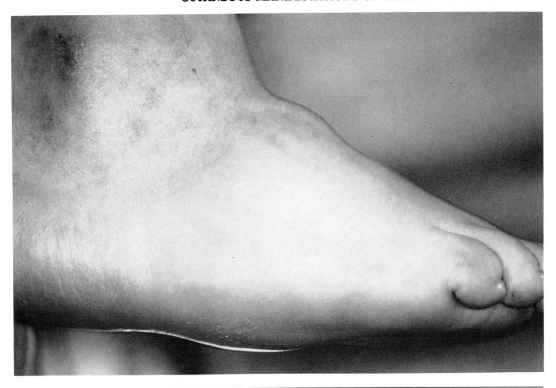

FIGURE 9–14 ■ Charcot foot. This patient, with sensory and motor neuropathy, broke the rule of always wearing protective shoes. She was barefoot when she ran out of the house to scold the neighbor's children. The snapping sound she heard as she ran was apparently fracturing of the small bones in her feet. Note the resulting distortion of the shape of the foot.

ment, including angiopathy, neuropathy, and cutaneous infection.

In the presence of both micro-angiopathy and macro-angiopathy, the cutaneous circulation in the foot can be minimally adequate. When the supply decreases—that is, with congestive heart failure or a decrease in hematocrit—oxygen delivery at the tissue level is inadequate and necrosis (gangrene) ensues. The supply might remain at a minimum level and the tissue demand increase because of a minor infection (such as inflammatory tinea pedis) or because of tissue injury (trauma not avoided because of the sensory neuropathy).

Gangrene can vary in the clinical presentation, depending on the underlying predisposing factors. With atherosclerosis, simple blockage of large arteries or arterioles results in loss of circulation to an area, which then develops "dry gangrene." A decrease in oxygen saturation in an area that already

has borderline circulation results in tissue necrosis even though the circulation continues, so-called "wet gangrene." Obviously, combinations of these two forms are found—patients often present with both microvascular and macrovascular disease.

The most effective treatment for complications of the diabetic foot is prevention. This begins with a careful assessment of the circulation, including intermittent claudication. Physical examination for patency of the large vessels includes feeling the popliteal, posterior tibial, and dorsalis pedis pulses. Although full pulses usually indicate good circulation, it is important to note that medial calcinosis transmits bounding pulses even in the presence of severe circulatory compromise. Restoration of the circulation for many patients with macrovascular disease can be the treatment of choice.

Evaluation of the microcirculation of the skin on the lower extremity can be performed by direct visualization (see above). Venous engorgement of the capillary loops is an indication of functional micro-angiopathy. Tight control of the blood sugar level by such methods as home glucose monitoring can result in improvement in functional micro-angiopathy. There are currently clinical trials to determine if pentoxifylline and other hemorrheologic agents might improve microcirculation in the diabetic.

A careful assessment of neuropathy can determine whether the patient needs to wear special protective footwear. The presence of neuropathy is also an indication for tighter control of the blood sugar level and, in some cases, might be used as a motivating factor. Although some controversy exists, many physicians believe that normalization of the blood sugar level and/or the use of hemorrheologic agents can result in improvement of the neuropathy.

Other important considerations include the presence of toe web space infections and dystrophic nails. Even minor web space infections can result in gangrene in the compromised foot, either because of increased tissue oxygen requirements or because of the resulting gap in the epidermal barrier, which allows the entry of other pathogens. Dystrophic nails can abrade adjacent toes and cause breakdown of the epidermal barrier and infection.

It is necessary for diabetic patients to have their feet examined whenever they undergo follow-up medical evaluations. This part of the examination is often overlooked, especially when the patient is unaware that a problem exists. Not only does this re-examination serve to reinforce proper foot care for the patient, it allows the practitioner to monitor whether the current therapeutic regimen is sufficient. Diabetes has many manifestations that can be observed in the feet, and any changes noted should be used to modify therapy accordingly.

GENERAL THERAPEUTIC CONSIDERATIONS

Diabetes is associated with increased collagen cross-linking, which has been alleged to be responsible for many diabetic complications. One report has suggested that systemically administered aminoguanidine, a hydrazine compound, can prevent the formation of glucose-derived collagen cross-links.[5] Because glycosylated protein develops (among other compounds) an intermolecular cross-link, which has a specific fluorescence, the extent of this reaction can be measured. It was found that aminoguanidine administered to rats inhibits diabetes-induced accumulation of advanced glycosylation products and reduces abnormal cross-linking of arterial wall connective tissue.[5] It remains to be seen whether the results of such animal research can be translated into new therapy for diabetic patients.

Diabetes mellitus is a common condition, often encountered by dermatologists and primary care physicians. Because glucose attaches to long-lived proteins, it can have a profound effect on the tertiary structure of that protein. Chronic hyperglycemia can be responsible for the pathogenesis of many diabetic complications. It has been suggested that increased cross-linking of collagen in diabetic patients is responsible for the fact that their skin is generally thicker than that of nondiabetics. Advanced glycosylation end products are probably responsible for yellowing of skin and nails. The increased viscosity of blood resulting from stiff red blood cell membranes results in engorgement of the postcapillary venules in the papillary dermis, detected as erythema of the face or as periungual erythema. Skin changes might eventually be used as a reflection of the patient's current and former metabolic status.

References

1. Gilgor RS, Lazarus GS. Skin manifestations of diabetes mellitus. In: Rifkin H, Raskin P, ed. Diabetes mellitus, vol. 5. Bowie, RJ Brady; 1981; 313–321.
2. Rahbar S. An abnormal hemoglobin in red cells of diabetics. Clin Chim Acta. 1968; 22:296–298.
3. Kirschenbaum DM. Glycosylation of proteins: its implications in diabetic control and complications. Pediatr Clin North Am. 1984; 31:611–621.
4. Bunn HF, Higgins PJ. Reaction of monosaccharides with proteins: possible evolutionary significance. Science. 1981; 213:222–224.
5. Brownlee M, Vlassara H, Kooney A, et al. Aminoguanidine prevents diabetes-induced arterial wall protein cross-linking. Science. 1986; 232:1629–1632.
6. Pongor S, Ulrich PC, Benesath FA, et al. Aging of proteins and identification of a fluorescent chro-

mophore from the reaction of polypeptides with glucose. Proc Nat Acad Sci USA. 1984; 81:2684–2688.

7. Otsuji S, Kamada T. Biophysical changes in the erythrocyte membrane in diabetes mellitus. Rinsho Byori. 1982; 30:888–897.

8. Greenwood AM. A study of the skin in 500 diabetics. JAMA. 1927; 89:774–776.

9. Edwards JE, Tillman DB, Miller ME, et al. Infection and diabetes mellitus. West J Med. 1979; 130:515–521.

10. Gilgor RS. Cutaneous infections in diabetes mellitus. In: Jelinek JE, ed. The skin and diabetes. Philadelphia: Lea & Febiger; 1986; 111–132.

11. Sonck CE, Somersalo O. The yeast flora of the anogenital region in diabetic girls. Arch Dermatol. 1963; 88:846–852.

12. Knight L, Fletcher J. Growth of Candida albicans in saliva: stimulation by glucose associated with antibiotics, corticosteroids, and diabetes mellitus. J Infect Dis. 1971; 123:371–377.

13. Tomford JW, Whittlesey D, Ellner JJ, et al. Invasive primary cutaneous phycomycosis in diabetic leg ulcers. Arch Surg. 1980; 115:770–771.

14. Batra VK, Gaiha M, Gupta PS. Mucomycosis in a diabetic. Postgrad Med J. 1982: 58; 78r2.

15. Petrozzi JW, Warthan TL. Malignant external otitis. Arch Dermatol. 1974; 110:258–260.

16. Wilson DF, Pulec JL, Linthicum FH. Malignant external otitis. Arch Otolaryngol. 1971; 93:419–422.

17. Alteras I, Saryt E. Prevalence of pathogenic fungi in the toe-webs and toenails of diabetic patients. Mycopathologica. 1979; 67:157–159.

18. Arho P. Skin thickness and collagen content in some endocrine, connective tissue and skin diseases. Acta Dermatol. Venereol. 1972; 52(Suppl 69):1–48.

19. Lee MM. Physical and structural age changes in human skin. Anat Rec. 1957; 129:473–493.

20. Southwood WFW. The thickness of the skin. Plast Reconstr Surg. 1955; 15:423–429.

21. Collier A, Matthews AM, Kellett HA, et al. Change in skin thickness associated with cheiroarthropathy in insulin-dependent diabetes mellitus. Br Med J. 1986; 292:936.

22. Lundbaek K. Stiff hands in long-term diabetes. Acta Med Scand. 1957; 158:447–451.

23. Rosenbloom AL, Frais JL. Diabetes mellitus, short stature and joint stiffness—a new syndrome. Clin Res. 1974; 22:92A.

24. Rosenbloom AL, Silverstein JH, Lezotte DC, et al. Limited joint mobility in childhood diabetes mellitus indicates increased risk for microvascular disease. N Engl J Med. 1981; 305:191–198.

25. Fitzcharles MA, Duby S, Wadell RW, et al. Limitation of joint mobility (cheiroarthropathy) in adult noninsulin-dependent diabetic patients. Ann Rheum Dis. 1984; 43:251–257.

26. Huntley AC. Finger pebbles: a common finding in diabetes mellitus. J Am Acad Dermatol. 1986; 14:612–617.

27. Clark CV, Pentland B, Ewing DJ, et al. Decreased skin wrinkling in diabetes mellitus. Diabetes Care. 1984; 7:224–227.

28. Buckingham BA, Uitto J, Sandborg C, et al. Scleroderma-like syndrome and the non-

enzymatic glucosylation of collagen in children with poorly controlled insulin-dependent diabetes (IDDM). Pediatr Res. 1981; 15(Pt 1):626.

29. Lieberman LS, Rosenbloom AL, Riley WJ, et al. Reduced skin thickness with pump administration of insulin. N Engl J Med. 1980; 303:940–941.

30. Eaton PR. The collagen hydration hypothesis: a new paradigm for the secondary complications of diabetes mellitus. J Chron Dis. 1986; 39:753–766.

31. Pal B, Anderson J, Dick WB, et al. Limitation of joint mobility and shoulder capsulitis in insulin- and non-insulin-dependent diabetes mellitus. Br J Rheumatol. 1985; 25:147–151.

32. Hoerer E, Dreyfuss F, Herzberg M. Carotenemia, skin color and diabetes mellitus. Acta Diabetol Lat. 1975; 12:202–207.

33. West KM. Epidemiology of diabetes and its vascular lesions. New York: Elsevier North-Holland; 1978; 353.

34. Haroon TS. Diabetes and skin—a review. Scott Med J. 1974; 19:257–267.

35. Jelinek JE. Cutaneous markers of diabetes mellitus and the role of microangiopathy. In: Jelinek JE, ed. The skin in diabetes. Philadelphia: Lea & Febiger; 1986; 58.

36. Bauer M, Levan NE. Diabetic dermangiopathy. A spectrum including pretibial pigmented patches and necrobiosis lipoidica diabeticorum. Br J Dermatol. 1970; 83:528–535.

37. Lithner F. Cutaneous reactions of the extremities of diabetics to local thermal trauma. Acta Med Scand. 1975; 198:319–325.

38. Binkley GW, Giraldo B, Stoughton RB. Diabetic dermopathy—a clinical study. Cutis. 1967; 3:955–958.

39. Fisher ER, Danowski TS. Histologic, histochemical, and electron microscopic features of the shin spots of diabetes mellitus. Am J Clin Pathol. 1968; 50:547–554.

40. Melin H. An atrophic circumscribed skin lesion in the lower extremities of diabetics. Acta Med Scand. 1964; 176(Suppl 423):1–75.

41. Danowski TX, Sabeh G, Sarver ME, et al. Shin spots and diabetes mellitus. JAMA. 1968; 251:570–575.

42. Murphy RA. Skin lesions in diabetic patients: the "spotted leg" syndrome. Lahey Clin Found Bull. 1965; 14:10–14.

43. Lithner F. Purpura, pigmentation and yellow nails of the lower extremities in diabetes. Acta Med Scand. 1976; 199:203–208.

44. Ditzel J. Functional microangiopathy in diabetes mellitus. Diabetes. 1968; 17:388–397.

45. Gitelson S, Wertheimer-Kaplinski N. Color of the face in diabetes mellitus. Observations on a group of patients in Jerusalem. Diabetes. 1965; 14:201–208.

46. Landau J, Davis E. The small blood vessels of the conjunctiva and nailbed in diabetes mellitus. Lancet. 1960; 2:731–734.

47. Grassi W, Gasparini M, Cervini C. Nailfold computed videomicroscopy in morpho-functional assessment of diabetic microangiopathy. Acta Diabetol Lat. 1985; 22:223–228.

48. Lithner F. Cutaneous erythema, with or without necrosis, localized to the legs and feet—a lesion

in elderly diabetics. Acta Med Scand. 1974; 196:333–342.

49. Lithner F, Hietala SO. Skeletal lesions of the feet in diabetics and their relationship to cutaneous erythema with or without necrosis of the feet. Acta Med Scand. 1976; 200:155–161.

50. Oimomi M, Maeda Y, Hata F, et al. Glycosylation levels of nail proteins in diabetic patients with retinopathy and neuropathy. Kobe J Med Sci. 1985; 31:183–188.

51. Rocca F, Pereyra E. Phylctenar lesions in the feet of diabetic patients. Diabetes. 1963; 12:220–222.

52. Allen GE, Hadden DR. Bullous lesions of the skin in diabetes (bullous diabeticorum). Br J Dermatol. 1970; 82:216–220.

53. Cantwell AR, Martz W. Idiopathic bullae in diabetics. Bullosis diabeticorum. Arch Dermatol. 1967; 96:42–44.

54. Kurwa A, Roberts P, Whitehead R. Concurrence of bullous and atrophic skin lesions in diabetes mellitus. Arch Dermatol. 1971; 103:670–675.

55. James WD, Odom RB, Goette DK. Bullous eruption of diabetes mellitus. A case with positive immunofluorescence microscopy findings. Arch Dermatol. 1980; 116:1191–1192.

56. Bernstein JE, Medinica M, Soltani K, et al. Bullous eruption of diabetes mellitus. Arch Dermatol. 1979; 115:324–325.

57. Muller SA. Dermatologic disorders associated with diabetes mellitus. Mayo Clin Proc. 1966; 41:689–703.

58. Ellenberg M. Diabetic complications without manifest diabetes. JAMA. 1963; 1983:926–930.

59. Wilson Jones E. Necrobiosis lipoidica presenting on the face and scalp. Trans St. Johns Hosp Dermatol Soc. 1971; 57:202.

60. Ackerman AB. Histologic diagnosis of inflammatory skin diseases. A method by pattern analysis. Philadelphia: Lea & Febiger; 1978; 424–431.

61. Eldor S, Diaz EG, Naparstek E. Treatment of diabetic necrobiosis with aspirin and dipyridamole (letter to the editor). N Engl J Med. 1978; 298:1033.

62. Fjellner B. Treatment of diabetic necrobiosis with aspirin and dipyridamole (letter to the editor.) N Engl J Med. 1978; 299:1366.

63. Unge G, Tornling G. Treatment of diabetic necrobiosis with dipyridamole (letter to the editor). N Engl J Med. 1978; 299:1366.

64. Stratham B, Finlay AY, Marks R. A randomized double-blind comparison of aspirin-dipyridamole combination versus a placebo in the treatment of necrobiosis lipoidica. Acta Derm Venereol. 1981; 61:270–271.

65. Martin MM. Involvement of autonomic nerve fibres in diabetic neuropathy. Lancet. 1953; 264:560–565.

66. Kennedy WR, Sakuta M, Sutherland D, et al. Quantitation of the sweating deficiency in diabetes mellitus. Ann Neurol. 1984; 15:482–488.

67. Brown MJ, Asbury AK. Diabetic neuropathy. Ann Neurol. 1984; 15:2–12.

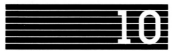

Management of Neuropathic Ulceration with the Total Contact Cast

MARK MYERSON, M.D.
AND KELLY WILSON, R.P.T.

The total contact cast is an effective means of managing neuropathic ulceration on the sole of the foot. Although other forms of treatment are available for managing diabetic plantar ulceration, the total contact cast is reliable, cost-effective, and associated with minimal morbidity to the patient. The rationale behind the total contact cast has been well documented:

1. The cast reduces pressure over the wound site and redistributes the weight-bearing load over the entire plantar surface of the foot and distal leg.
2. The pressure reduction is furthered by foam padding placed directly over the ulcer.
3. Immobilization of the limb decreases the spread of local infection and limits the stress on granulation tissue and skin edges, simultaneously protecting the foot from further trauma.
4. Reduction of swelling occurs after 24 to 48 hours in a cast and the interstitial fluid pressure diminishes, with improved microcirculation.
5. The need for patient compliance is reduced with regard to weight-bearing, dressing changes, and physical therapeutic measures for the foot.
6. The cast is applied on an outpatient basis and patients remain ambulatory, allowing them to return to work.

Decision making in treatment neuropathic ulceration is a team effort. It depends on successful communication and interaction among the physician, cast technician, physical therapist, and footwear specialist. Postcast care should be directed toward providing safe and effective footwear for the patient once healing has occurred. Furthermore, any patient factors that can be identified as having precipitated the ulceration must be addressed. Patient education is critical and represents an integral part of the treatment process. Modification of the patient's environment, shoewear, gait patterns, activities and, especially, daily care of the feet increases the chance of success with the cast treatment. All plantar ulcers can be treated with this technique. Although ulceration under the metatarsal heads are most frequently encountered, ulcers in the forefoot, midfoot, and hindfoot are also amenable to this type of treatment.

Certain patients are not suitable candidates for this treatment. Active and profuse drainage associated with infection should be treated first. This often involves the debridement of necrotic tissue and appropriate wound care with whirlpool and antibiotic therapy. After 2 to 3 days, when drainage has ceased, application can commence. In these patients the cast is changed more frequently during the first few weeks, until the wound shows good healing. Osteomyelitis is not a contraindication to cast treatment but, because it is generally associated with draining wounds or sinuses, these might require initial debridement.

Patients need to comply with restricted weight-bearing for the first 24 hours after casting with crutches, a walker, or a wheelchair. Significant edema of the foot and ankle should be controlled before casting is initiated. This can take days or weeks, particularly if the edema is chronic, but we have used a cyclic, intermittent, external extremity compression pump successfully to decrease edema within hours. This is used just prior to cast application. In patients with moderate edema the cast must be changed after 1 or 2 days, because swelling is mobilized extremely rapidly once the cast has been applied. Severe complications of casting with ulceration and infection can occur when attention is not paid to this. Although patients lack protective sensation they can comply with simple instructions regarding a loose cast, and should be nonweight-bearing until a new, snug-fitting cast can be applied.

APPLYING THE CAST

Wound Preparation

Fabrication of the total contact cast begins with wound preparation. The wound is first debrided of necrotic tissue, particularly in the depths of the ulcer (Fig. 10-1). The wound edges are trimmed and shaved, removing callus to provide a smooth transition from the wound to the adjacent surrounding skin border, because the over-

hanging hypertrophic callus harbors pathogens. Epithelialization can occur more rapidly if the crater is removed. This invariably causes bleeding, but is necessary.

The wound is then cleansed with an appropriate antibacterial solution such as Betadine and a sterile dressing is applied. Usually no more than one or two sterile 2 × 2-inch gauze pads are used. This decreases the bulk of the dressing over the ulcer and prevents excessive pressure build-up underneath the affected area.

Drainage should be minimal. If drainage is excessive the cast is changed more frequently or other methods are used to initiate treatment. The plaster itself acts to absorb excess drainage. Even the dressings are wet when the casts are changed. Repeated cast treatment need not be interrupted.

Protective Padding

Prior to applying the cast, strategic areas are protected with padding to guard against additional skin breakdown and maceration (Fig. 10-2):

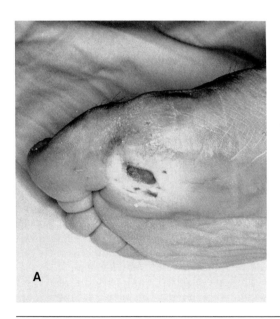

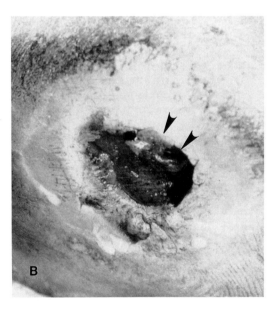

FIGURE 10–1 ■ A, This ulcer under the first metatarsal head had been present for 3 years and an amputation of the foot had been recommended to the patient. Note the heaped-up callus around the ulcer. B, Prior to casting the edges of the ulcer must be debrided so that a smooth transition is present between the bed of the ulcer and the adjacent skin. The margins of one side of the ulcer still have to be shaved down (*arrows*).

1. Cotton padding is applied between the toes to avoid their rubbing inside the cast.
2. A 4-inch stockinette is applied from the knee to the toes. The end of the stockinette is folded back over the top of the toes and taped with minimum amounts of 1-inch paper tape. Wrinkling of the stockinette here should be avoided, but is not usually a problem, because additional padding is applied over the toes later on. The stockinette is cut transversely along the anterior ankle to avoid any wrinkling in this area. It is preferable to overlap the stockinette wherever possible to avoid pressure build-up or friction directly beneath the area of wrinkling. In these areas the stockinette is also taped into position.
3. A low-density, 1/2-inch thick foam, such as Sci-foam, is then applied over the toes and extended to cover any bony prominence, such as the first and fifth metatarsal heads and the malleoli. The proximal edge of the foam must be bevelled to provide a smooth transition to the adjacent skin. To minimize pressure over the ulcer, Sci-foam is also applied directly over the wound using 1/8-inch cut out pads, which are also bevelled. The malleoli are protected with either the Sci-foam or adhesive-backed felt. A 1-1/2- to 2-inch wide strip is also applied over the dorsum of the foot from the edge of the Sci-foam distally; this extends proximally up the leg to pad the anterior tibial crest.
4. The cast is applied with the patient in a prone position. Two persons are needed to apply the cast. The assistant holds the leg with the knee in 90° of flexion and the ankle in 5° of dorsiflexion. The amount of ankle dorsiflexion, however, might depend on the type of rocker to be applied to the bottom of the cast.
5. The padding and stockinette are checked for wrinkles or shifts in position and final corrections are made.

Plaster and Cast Application

The leg is now ready for plaster application. Inner layers of the shell are critical. Care is taken to avoid wrinkling of the plaster or tenting over bony prominences. The first layer of plaster is applied loosely so that it can be molded to conform exactly to the crevices and folds of the leg, foot, and ankle. The shell of the cast can be made out of standard plaster but elasticized plaster is preferred, because it adheres more closely to the folds and contours of the ankle and foot. When using standard plaster tucking is essential to avoid wrinkling during application. With elastic plaster tucking is not necessary but there is a tendency to overstretch the plaster and this should be avoided, particularly over bony prominences. Both types of plaster, however, are safe to use.

Plaster is applied from 1 inch distal to the fibular head to the toes, and should cover the foam by approximately 1 inch. Two rolls of 4-inch wide plaster is adequate for a three-layer inner shell, but an additional roll might be necessary on a large leg. The plaster is further molded to conform to the leg and the entire foot until it begins to harden.

Two rolls of 3- or 4-inch standard plaster are now applied from the distal third of the leg to cover the foot and reinforce the inner shell. This is also applied loosely, although wrinkling is not as much of a problem in these superficial layers. This plaster is again smoothed and contoured until firm.

Creating a rocker bottom on the cast is ideal, and this can be done in a number of ways. A walking heel is one alternative. This can be applied over a 1/4-inch piece of plywood. Patients bear weight on the heel, which protects the cast from breakdown. A rocker sole is preferred, however, and is built into the cast itself. Plaster is layered onto the bottom of the cast from the heel distally to an area just proximal to the metatarsal heads. It is tapered down toward the toes so that on weight-bearing the toe of the cast is approximately 1-1/2 inches off the floor. The patient's gait is easier, because a more natural roll and cadence are achieved during ambulation. This provides a broader area of weight-bearing during the stance phase and improves proprioception. Unfortunately, both methods increase the thickness of the cast. If the cast is applied with the ankle in 5° of dorsiflexion, the thickness of the cast is reduced. This is an important consideration, because the leg length discrepancy created with the cast can be a problem.

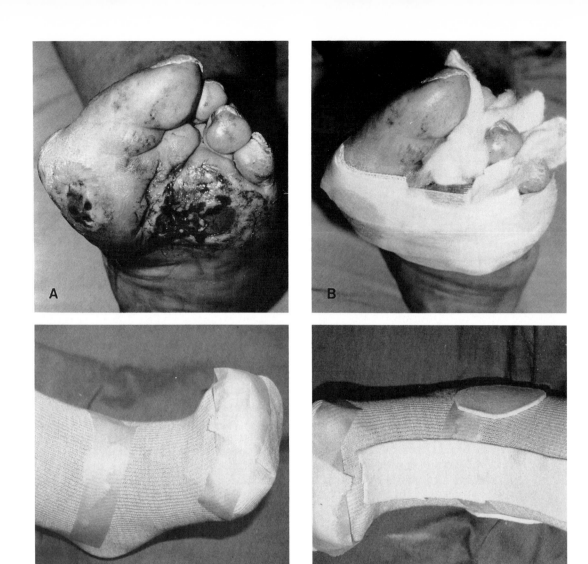

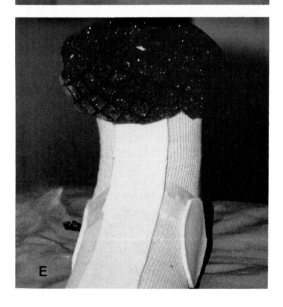

FIGURE 10–2 ■ A, The edges of the ulceration on the forefoot have been debrided and no active infection or excessive drainage is present. B, Cotton is applied between the toes and Betadine gauze pads are placed over the ulcer and taped to the skin. C, A single layer of stockinette is applied, enclosing the toes and cut over the ankle to eliminate folds or creases. D, Adhesive-backed felt is applied to the malleoli and along the tibial crest over the dorsum of the foot. E, Adhesive foam padding (Sci-foam) is applied to cover the toes.

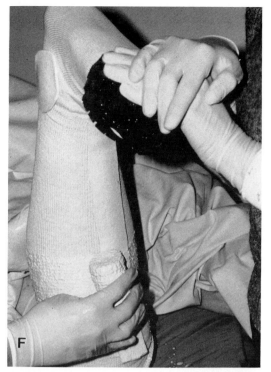

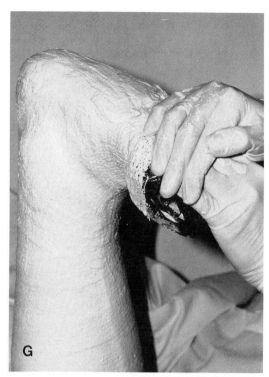

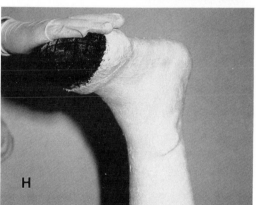

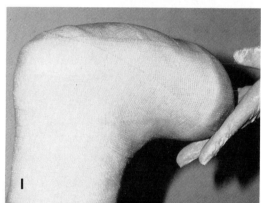

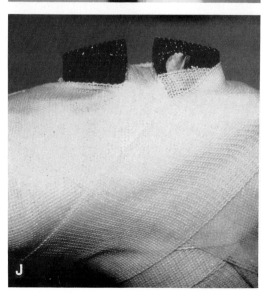

F, The cast is applied with the patient prone, with an assistant holding the foot in a plantigrade position. The first roll is elasticized plaster and is rolled on without any tension or tucking. *G,* The first layers or inner shell extends from the Sci-foam padding distally to within 2 inches of the stockinette proximally. *H,* Plaster is now rolled and tucked, again maintaining the ankle in neutral or 5° of dorsiflexion. *I,* The final layer consists of fiber glass, applied on the foot to create a rocker bottom. *J,* A heel can be incorporated into the cast as an alternative to a rocker sole but it tends to be higher and causes more of a leg length discrepancy.

The cast is finally reinforced with fiber glass. The roll is applied after turning down the edge of the stockinette over the plaster edge and enclosing the toes. This is the only protection for the toes. At least three layers are applied in this location.

The patient is instructed to be nonweight-bearing for 24 hours and to resume full weight-bearing activities thereafter (Fig. 10-3).

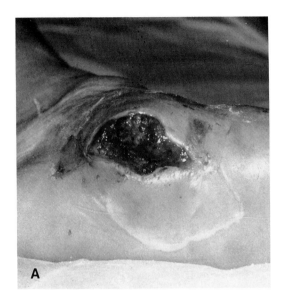
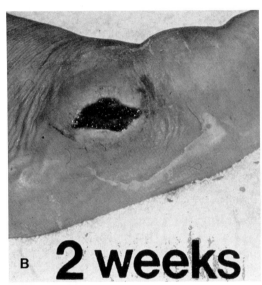
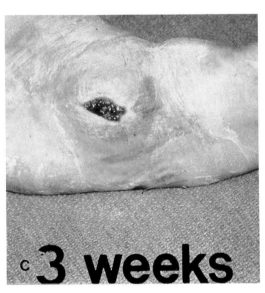
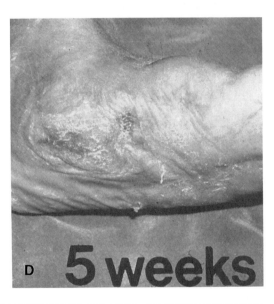

FIGURE 10–3 ■ *A,* A massive abscess was drained from the foot for the seventh time in this patient, who had an underlying neuropathic arthropathy of the midfoot. Once the bed of the ulcer was clean, cast treatment was begun. Healing was present within 5 weeks of commencing casting. *B,* After 2 weeks. *C,* After 3 weeks. *D,* After 5 weeks. Patients should not be allowed to return to the same harmful environment once healing of the ulcer occurs. Prior to unrestricted weight-bearing, a total contact plastizote mold was made for the patient while still in the cast so that the transition into shoes was protected.

ADDITIONAL CONSIDERATIONS

Some problems can develop with the use of this technique. A well-trained cast technician, however, can anticipate these during patient evaluation, because it is during this phase that most major complications can be recognized.

Studies of this technique have shown that, in the first phase of cast treatments for neuropathic ulceration, only 3 of 73 patients had complications requiring more than 1 week of interrupted casting. Of these three patients, two developed an abscess and the third developed a superficial heel ulcer. Casts were discontinued temporarily and were re-applied 2 weeks after appropriate wound care and antibiotics were instituted. Other complications do not require interrupting the cast treatment. These include skin irritation and small, noninfected, grade I ulceration on the posterior aspect of the heel or over a bony prominence, such as the tibia, malleoli, or foot. These are easily taken care of with Scifoam padding applied directly to the stockinette over the area of skin breakdown. Generally, close follow-up, attention to patient education, and proper instruction ensure a satisfactory result.

The healing of neurotrophic ulceration of the foot is probably the easiest part of the treatment for this immense problem. Once healing has occurred, the greater challenge is to maintain the skin interface and to prevent recurrent breakdown. It is important to focus on correcting the events that preceded the ulceration. These patients tend to be noncompliant, and it is only through repeated patient education and reinforcement that these precipitating factors can be minimized. Even so, they are rarely eliminated.

After consideration is given to healing the ulcer, the entire problem is also addressed with regard to patient education, protective footwear, orthoses, molded shoes, rocker bottom soles, metatarsal bars and pads, and possible prophylactic surgery. Claw toes, prominent metatarsal heads, and bone on the plantar aspect of the foot might require surgical treatment to prevent recurrent breakdown.

Recurrent ulcers respond rapidly to a short period of repeat casting. With proper education patients can identify signs of early tissue breakdown and the progress of ulceration can be halted with a short series of casts. When ulcers continue to recur or pressure is not relieved, surgery must be considered.

BIBLIOGRAPHY

1. Alon G, Azaria M, Stein H. Diabeticc ulcer healing using high voltage TENS [abstract]. Phys Ther. 1986; 66:775.
2. Baker LL, Chambers R, Merchant L, et al. The effects of electrical stimulation on cutaneous oxygen supply in normal older adults and diabetic patients [abstract]. Phys Ther. 1986; 66:749.
3. Bauman JH, Girling JP, Brand PW. Plantar pressures and trophic ulceration. J Bone Joint Surg. 1963; 45B:652–673.
4. Bauman JH, Girling JP, Brand PW. Plantar pressures and trophic uleration: evaluation of footwear. J Bone Joint Surg. 1963; 45B:652–673.
5. Birke JA, Sims S, Buford WL. Walking casts: effect on plantar foot pressures. J Rehabil Res Dev. 1985; 22:18–22.
6. Bohannon RW, Pfaller BA. Documentation of wound surface area from tracings of wound perimeters: clinical report on three techniques. Phys Ther. 1983; 63:1622–1624.
7. Boulton AJM, Franks CI, Betts RP, et al. Reduction of abnormal foot pressures in diabetic neuropathy using a new polymer insole material. Diabetes Care. 1984; 7:42–46.
8. Boulton AJM, Bowker JH. The diabetic foot. In: Olefsky JM, Sherwin RS, eds. Diabetes mellitus: management and complications. New York: Churchill Livingston; 255–275.
9. Boulton AJM, Kubrusly D, Dowker JH, et al. Impaired vibratory perception and diabetic foot ulceration. Diabetic Med. 1986; 3:335–337.
10. Broadstone VL. Foot care in the diabetic patient. J Ky Med Assoc. 1986; 84:162–165.
11. Cameron B. Experimental acceleration of wound healing. Am J Orthop. 1961; 3:336–343.
12. Coleman WC, Brand PW, Birke JA. The total contact cast: a therapy for plantar ulceration on insensitive feet. J Am Podiatr Med Assoc. 1984; 74:548–552.
13. Ctercteko GC, Dhanendran M, Hutton WC, et al. Vertical forces acting on the feet of diabetic patients with neuropathic ulceration. Br J Surg. 1981; 68:609–614.
14. Duckworth T, Boulton AJM, Betts RP, et al. Plantar pressure measurements and the prevention of ulceration in the diabetic foot. J Bone Joint Surg. 1985; 67B:79–85.
15. Fischer BH. Treatment of ulcers on the legs with hyperbaric oxygen. J Dermatol Surg. 1975; 1:55–58.
16. Gault WR, Gatens PF, Jr. Use of low intensity direct current in management of ischemic skin ulcers. Phys Ther. 1976; 56:265–269.
17. Helm PA, Walker SC, Pullium G. Total contact casting in diabetic patients with neuropathic foot ulcerations. Arch Phys Med Rehabil. 1984; 65:691–693.
18. Holstein P, Larsen K, Sager P. Decompression with

aid of insoles in treatment of diabetic neuropathic ulcers. Acta Orthop Scand. 1976; 47:463–468.

19. Jacobs RL, Karmody AM, Wirth C, et al. The team approach in salvage of the diabetic foot. Surg Annu. 1977; 9:231–264.

20. Kalker AJ, Kolodny HD, Cavuoto JW. The evaluation and treatment of diabetic foot ulcers. J Am Podiatr Med Assoc. 1982; 72:491–496.

21. Kelly PJ, Conventry MB. Neurotrophic ulcers of the feet: review of 47 cases. JAMA. 1958; 168:388–393.

22. Larsen K, Christiansen JS, Ebskov B. Prevention and treatment of ulcerations of feet in unilaterally amputated diabetic patients. Acta Orthop Scand. 1982; 53:481–485.

23. Livingston R, Jacobs RL, Karmody A. Plantar abscess in the diabetic patient. Foot Ankle. 1985; 5:205–213.

24. Louie TJ, Bartlett GJ, Tally FP, et al. Aerobic and anaerobic bacteria in diabetic foot ulcers. Ann Intern Med. 1976; 85:461–463.

25. Oakley W, Catterall RCF, Martin MM. Aetiology and management of lesions of the feet in diabetics. Br Med J. 1956; 2:953–957.

26. Pring DJ, Casiebanca N. Simple plantar ulcers treated by below-knee plaster and molded double-rocker plaster shoe: a comparative study. Lepr Rev. 1982; 53:261–264.

27. Sapico FL, Bessman AN. Foot infection in the elderly diabetic. Geriatric Med. 1986; 5:42–48.

28. Silvino N, Evanski PM, Waugh TR. The Harris and Beath footprinting mat: diagnostic validity and clinical use. Clin Orthop. 1980; 151:265–269.

29. Sinacore DR. Total contact casting in the treatment of diabetic neuropathic ulcers. In: Levin, ME, O'Neal LW, eds. The diabetic foot. 4th ed. St. Louis: CV Mosby, in press.

30. Stokes IAF, Faris IB, Hutton WC. The neuropathic ulcer and loads on the foot in diabetic patients. Acta Ortho Scand. 1975; 46:839–847.

31. Tappin JW, Pollard J, Beckett EA. Method of measuring "shearing" forces on the sole of the foot. Clin Phys Physiol Meas. 1980; 1:83–85.

32. Wagner FW. Treatment of the diabetic foot. Compr Ther. 1984; 10:29–38.

33. Walker SC, Helm PA, Pullium G. Chronic diabetic neuropathic foot ulcerations and total contact casting: healing effectiveness and outcome predictability. Arch Phys Med Rehabil. 1985; 66:574.

11 Diabetic Arthropathy

G. JAMES SAMMARCO, M.D.

The effects of diabetes result from metabolic disturbances involving all body systems. Of paramount importance in the foot is the basic metabolism of the soft tissues. Control of the disease and of cell function lessens the degree of the resultant injury. This includes control of blood sugar levels through insulin injection, medication, diet, and weight control, as well as through exercise, hygiene, ankle-foot orthoses, arch supports, modified and custom shoes, and surgery. All are important in preventing and controlling regional foot disease and deformity. If an infection is present in the foot or ankle, controlling the blood sugar level is difficult. This lack of control is associated with abnormal metabolic processes in the foot and makes it difficult to control the infection, a "catch 22" situation. Proper antibiotics, immobilization, and meticulous control of the blood sugar level are necessary to control infection. Control of the disease also helps in managing its neuropathic manifestations including neurotrophic ulcers, polyneuropathy, and autonomic neuropathy.

Foot deformity usually occurs as a result of normal loads or minor trauma in a foot with polyneuropathy and disease of the autonomic nervous system. In the presence of stiff, glycosylated tissues and small vessel arterial disease, this permits rapid progression of deformity, with the patient often unaware of its occurrence. In addition, many diabetics with asensory feet ignore or deny the development of deformity, with or without neurotrophic ulcers. Often the best treatment consists of allowing the foot to collapse and then molding a shoe around the deformity. With the help of orthotics or total contact shoes, load sparing is permitted and hopefully ulcers are prevented or allowed to heal, but this is not always possible.

Because the first symptoms of the presence of a neuropathic joint are redness and swelling in the foot, the patient often notices a painless swelling without ulcers. It is therefore important that patients be taught self-examination and to note these symptoms. Good hygiene should be practiced. Patients should watch for signs during the daily routine of cleaning the feet and should wear shoes large enough to accommodate the foot, and an orthotic when necessary. When obtaining a new orthotic for the first time patients should be advised that they might require going up in size or out a width in their shoe to accommodate it.

Surgical treatment of infection is discussed elsewhere (Chapters 8 and 12), but it is important to ensure that ulcers are eliminated or well controlled. The foot is placed in a short leg cast, which relieves pressure beneath the ulcer. If an ulcer does not heal after application of several casts, the surgeon should consider associated poor circulation and infection, including osteomyelitis. Doppler tests on the foot and toes help evaluate the vascular status and aid in predicting the successful outcome of surgery.

THE RATIONALE FOR SURGERY

Unfortunately, there is no such thing as a non-weight bearing foot.

Under certain conditions the foot might be so deformed or vascularity so compromised as to indicate that amputation is the best course for stabilizing the extremity and preventing further deformity and infection. After it has been ascertained that circulation is adequate and control of diabetes is satisfactory, it is necessary to determine the need for stability, particularly if the foot has become deformed in a short time. The best immediate treatment is immobilization and a short leg cast. It is impossible to keep the patient with an asensory foot completely nonweight-bearing, but this should be attempted for at least 1 month. A second or third cast can be applied with partial weight-bearing for an additional 2 months. The cast should be padded around bony prominences to prevent ulceration. If deformity progresses rapidly in the cast or ulcers form following its removal, surgery should be considered, including open reduction and arthrodesis. Frequent examination and serial radiographs often show rapid destruction, particularly in the midfoot.

The polyneuropathy of diabetes progresses from distal to proximal and the first deformity is often seen in the toes. Because much of this deformity can be accommodated by shoe modification, surgical stabilization is reserved for severe clawing or transfer lesions resulting from dislocated contracted toes or displaced neuropathic fractures of the metatarsals. The functional length of the foot begins at the heel and ends at the toes with toe-off. A stiff foot with claw toes permits functional shortening, allowing only the metatarsals to bear weight at toe-off. If the midfoot collapses as a result of Lisfranc's or Chopart's fracture-dislocation, the resultant rocker bottom deformity permits the functional length of the foot to shorten even more or to transfer loads to beneath a single metatarsal head. Valgus or varus of the hindfoot with associated ankle equinus rapidly limits activities of daily living and can lead to gross ulcer formation, severe infection, and below-the-knee amputation. Bony prominences result from the dislocations, producing areas of increased normal and shear forces in the sole of the midfoot.

Stabilizing the foot and maintaining the functional length and architecture permits loads to be carried over a broad plantar area. The position of the foot must remain directly beneath the ankle and tibia in normal weight-bearing alignment. Without immobilizing the foot during this period of rapid deformity, unrestricted motion of the fracture site results in increased vascularity, which accompanies attempts at fracture healing and may lead to rapid resorption of bone at the fracture site—bone atrophy. Contracture of the soft tissues and tissue stiffness, which are part of diabetes, produce a deformed, stiff foot. This complicates conservative treatment inasmuch as no cast, molded appliance, or orthotic can completely relieve pressure from these prominent areas.[1-3]

TECHNICAL ASPECTS

Following the decision that surgery is necessary, the diabetes must be brought under control and the vascular status of the foot documented as satisfactory. This often requires consultation with a vascular surgeon and the determination of acceptable vascular indices in the toes, with use of arterial digital doppler in addition to critical clinical evaluation. The edema that accompanies both acute and chronic fracture-dislocations must be reduced to a minimum. Radiographs are obtained to determine whether changes in the bone are primarily lytic or hypertrophic, an important consideration because active bone resorption hinders arthrodesis, even in the presence of bone grafting. Internal fixation is inadequate because of severely osteoporotic bone. Hypertrophic or near-normal bone presents a more favorable situation because compression screws can gain purchase and function appropriately. Often, simple excision of osteophytes or bony prominences is all that is required. Such bony prominences can be the result of a stable but subluxed joint, as is commonly found in Lisfranc's fracture-dislocation at the first metatarsal, medial cuneiform, or fifth metatarsal cuboid joint. Debulking of such joints, the so-called "bumpectomy," is often all that is necessary. Ostectomy of part or all of a bone is considered for recurrent ulceration as a result of bony prominence, osteomyelitis, or circulatory compromise of soft tissue. If a metatarsal head is resected it is important to stabilize the remaining toe so that proximal and dorsal migration does not occur.

Resection of the entire ray might be chosen to avoid this postoperative occurrence, which often results in further deformity of a displaced clawed toe. Ray amputation should also be considered when it is thought that other approaches will be ineffective.

Ostectomy and osteotomy with arthrodesis can be considered in suitable candidates who have had early but rapid progression of a deformity, such as Lisfranc's or Chopart's fracture-dislocation and normal or hypertrophic bone. The joint is reduced, held in position with or without bone graft using compression techniques, and immobilized for a prolonged period until healing is complete. It is important to realize that, in the absence of normal nerve function, immobilization for 8 months to 1 year might be required.

Care in handling the soft tissues is important. Healed ulcers on the sole provide poor healing tissue. It is recommended that incisions not be made through these healed ulcers. The skin and soft tissues of the diabetic are altered physiologically, being thicker and stiffer than in nondiabetics. Retraction with small instruments should be gentle and hemostasis controlled with electrocautery. A thigh tourniquet is preferred if severe atherosclerosis is absent and if the patient has not had previous vascular bypass surgery. Incisions are placed on the dorsal, medial, or lateral aspects of the foot, avoiding areas of high pressure that occur beneath the heel and metatarsal heads and areas of increased pressure that occur as a result of deformity, such as over the tips of the toes, tarsometatarsal or intertarsal joints, and ankle malleoli. Soft tissue closures are made with interrupted absorbable 3-0 suture and the skin closed with monofilament 4-0 nylon suture, which is removed 3 weeks postoperatively.

Experience has shown that sitting during surgery provides comfort and control for the surgeon. For forefoot and midfoot surgery, the patient lies supine with the operating table flexed 40° at the knee. To accommodate the placement of guide pins during hindfoot and ankle surgery it is sometimes helpful to have the patient in the lateral decubitus position using the "beanbag." This position allows easy access to the subtalar joint and lateral ankle. The natural tendency for the leg to rest in external rotation allows access

to the medial foot and ankle structures. An image intensifier and compatible operating table are recommended to check the position of guide wires and screws. The ipsilateral hip is prepared, because bone graft is often used in midfoot, hindfoot, and ankle arthrodeses. Cannulated compression screws made of titanium, 5.5 and 7.5 mm, are preferred because of their computerized tomography (CT) and magnetic resonance imaging (MRI) compatibility. The Achilles tendon is usually contracted in midfoot and hindfoot deformity and operative plans should include its lengthening as part of the procedure. Midfoot, hindfoot, and ankle surgeries are closed over a suction drain. A high-speed air motor dissecting tool (e.g., Midas Rex) is used for ease in resecting sclerotic joint surfaces and shaping the joints for arthrodesis.

Postoperative care following stabilizing surgery includes application of a bulky dressing and cast. Splints are placed on the posterior and anterior aspects of the foot and leg as an alternative to a bivalved short leg cast. Within the first few days the dressing drains and splints are removed and a short leg cast is applied. Weight-bearing ambulation is limited to toe touching for the first few months. One reason for failure of surgery in the neuropathic foot is failure to protect the foot and ankle in a cast, with limited weight-bearing, until healing is complete. In the operative treatment of neuropathic fracture-dislocations of the midfoot it is common for the period of cast immobilization to exceed 6 months—not necessarily because healing is not occurring, but because the osteoporosis and delayed healing resulting from the disease allow motion of the arthrodesis site within the cast even with internal fixation. Permitting early motion out of the cast after partially destabilizing the joint to reduce the fracture-dislocation would allow the same forces that produced the deformity to act again, leading to recurrences.

In my experience cast immobilization for midfoot and hindfoot surgery is usually for more than 8 months, after which an ankle-foot orthosis or prescription shoe is prescribed. Ambulation is permitted as soon as the patient can manage. Cast changes are made at weekly and biweekly intervals for the first month with toe touching only and with 10% weight-bearing. Cast changes are performed thereafter at monthly intervals until early healing is evident, and 25% weight-bearing is permitted. After 4 months or more a removable ankle-foot orthosis with a variable ankle gatch (Donjoy R.O.M. Walker) to permit some motion is prescribed. This is worn at all times, but permits the patient to remove the cast to carry out personal hygiene measures. Partial weight-bearing is gradually increased to 50% weight-bearing. The postoperative course is monitored clinically and radiographically to determine whether position is maintained and healing progressing satisfactorily. Use of a wheelchair, walker, crutches, and ultimately a cane represent a natural progression in ambulatory aids. A supervised rehabilitation program is instituted preoperatively and early in the postoperative period so that flexibility of the lower extremities can be maintained as the patient becomes more independent. An ankle-foot orthosis is prescribed to protect the foot and ankle after complete healing.

REGIONAL SURGERY

The goal of foot surgery is to obtain a functional, stable, plantigrade foot. To do this the foot must be aligned beneath the ankle and leg. If permitted to heal in a varus or valgus position progressive deformity continues, often leading to ulceration beneath the prominent metatarsal heads, tarsal bones, or ankle malleoli.

Forefoot

Deformities of the forefoot can be divided into those associated with the hallux, lesser toes, and metatarsals.

THE HALLUX

Deformities of the hallux include fracture or fracture-dislocation through the interphalangeal joint, which often results in ulceration beneath the proximal phalangeal condyle. If circulation is adequate following ulcer healing and control of infection, an open reduction of the dislocated joint with axial placement of wires or screws is indicated. Excessive loads on the forefoot at toe-

off and the lack of sensation can lead to noncompliance, particularly in younger patients. The patient might feel that the ulcer is trivial and can heal simply by avoiding walking on that area. Attempts to carry out arthrodesis of this joint are usually futile (Fig. 11-1). It is recommended that open reduction be performed through a dorsal incision with internal fixation, either screws or pins. If the arthrodesis is not achieved but the joint remains reduced with a fibrous ankylosis and the ulcer does not recur, the surgery is considered successful. Excision of the offending plantar portions of the condyles and a stable joint with pseudoarthrosis permit loads to be transferred to the distal hallux tuft rather than remain beneath the proximal phalanx.

Deformity of the metatarsophalangeal joint of the hallux includes bunion, hallux valgus or rigidus, metatarsus primus varus, stress fracture, and dislocation (Fig. 11-2). Most of these deformities are treated with shoe modification and orthoses. The severity of the deformity is important in determining the need for correction. Recurrent ulcer formation resulting from neuropathy must be healed. Because of the stiffness of the tissues it is recommended that severe hallux valgus deformity be corrected by Keller bunionectomy (Fig. 11-3). During this procedure excision of the osteophytes is also performed. This tends to destabilize the joint and requires axial pin fixation to maintain alignment for at least 6 weeks postoperatively. A short leg weight-bearing cast is applied postoperatively to support the foot until soft tissue healing has stabilized the joint. A stiff-soled shoe and orthosis with a semi-rigid extension beneath the hallux is prescribed following healing.

Hallux extensus with fixed flexion deformity at the interphalangeal joint is treated with a Keller bunionectomy, resecting just enough of the proximal phalanx to permit appropriate reduction while performing a proximal phalangeal condylectomy to align the interphalangeal joint. Meticulous attention is paid to the handling of soft tissues and a minimal dissection is performed. The use of a high-speed oscillating microsaw is used to help reduce soft tissue trauma. Arthrodesis of the metatarsophalangeal joint of the hallux is difficult to achieve, but the pseudoarthrosis that results from the Keller

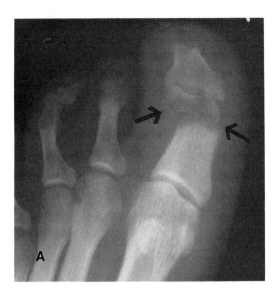
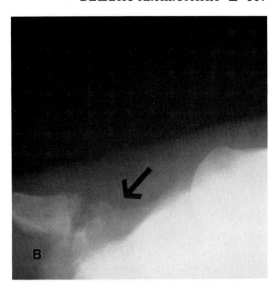

FIGURE 11–1. ■ Radiographs of a foot with a neuropathic interphalangeal joint of the hallux. *A,* Fracture of the proximal phalanx (*arrows*) allowed the distal toe to sublux dorsally. An ulcer formed beneath the joint. No osteomyelitis was found. *B,* Open reduction through a dorsal incision and pin fixation (*arrow*) for 2 months allowed a stable fibrous ankylosis to develop, thereby avoiding amputation. Satisfactory function, cosmesis, and patient acceptance were achieved.

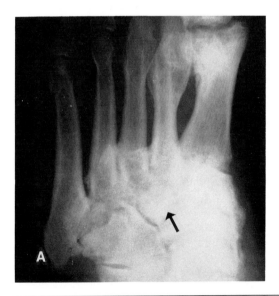
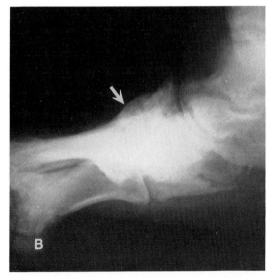

FIGURE 11–2. ■ Radiographs of a foot with a neuropathic first metatarsophalangeal joint, hallux rigidus. *A,* Metatarsus elevatus has occurred secondary to a concomitant Charcot fracture-dislocation of Lisfranc's joint (*arrow*), causing a transfer lesion beneath the second and third metatarsals and resulting in stress fractures. *B,* All forefoot lesions healed during immobilization following open reduction of the Lisfranc's fracture-dislocation. No subsequent ulcers occurred for 13 years following surgery, and the patient remained employed as a full-time maintenance worker.

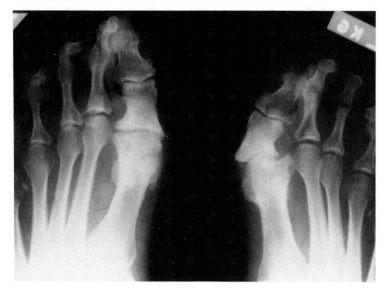

FIGURE 11-3. ■ Radiographs of both feet 5 years after Keller bunionectomies for Charcot joints and fixed hammertoe correction. The 60-year-old patient could wear nonprescription shoes, with full insole semirigid accommodative orthoses. Bunions and ulcers did not recur.

bunionectomy is satisfactory in maintaining position, load-bearing, and cosmesis. Ulceration beneath the metatarsal head of the hallux often occurs as a result of imbalance in load-bearing in the forefoot, lack of education, or patient noncompliance with respect to periods of time permitted for standing and walking. It might occur in spite of the use of foot orthotics. A sesamoidectomy through a medial incision can be performed after debridement and healing of the ulcer. A foot orthosis and patient education are always part of the postoperative regimen.

LESSER TOES

Fixed deformity of the lesser toes with ulcer formation is related to collapse of the arch and resultant forefoot valgus, muscle imbalance, and contracture of tissues. Evaluation of circulation is most important. Doppler analysis of the toes is helpful in determining whether circulation is adequate. Ulcers that might be present must be a result of neuropathy and not vascular insufficiency. No tourniquet is used. Often no anesthetic is required. However, anesthesia can be general or consist of regional ankle block. A local anesthetic is also recommended if it does not compromise an otherwise satisfactory circulation.

A dorsal incision is used and surgery is performed occasionally with loupe magnification. The extensor hood is divided. Mal-

let toe or hammertoe deformity is corrected by phalangeal condylectomy of the middle or proximal phalanx, respectively (Fig. 11-3). Meticulous care is taken to protect soft tissues, and only enough bone is removed with a microsaw to permit the toes to be extended easily. No tension is permitted on the toe that would allow circulatory compromise. An extensor tenotomy and dorsal capsulotomy of the metatarsophalangeal joint are performed through the proximal end of the incision to reduce the extended metatarsophalangeal joint.

It is also necessary to divide the collateral ligaments. A percutaneous 0.045-mm Kirschner wire is passed axially through the toe into the metatarsal neck. The postoperative dressing is not placed between the toes to avoid external pressure on the digital arteries. A wooden clog is used. The pin remains in place for at least 6 weeks, after which the toes are held with a foam rubber toe comb. Showers are permitted when the soft tissues have healed and the sutures removed, but soaking the foot is not allowed until the pins have been removed. Recurrence can occur.

DISLOCATIONS OF THE METATARSOPHALANGEAL JOINTS

Dislocations of the metatarsophalangeal joints often accompany fixed hammertoe deformity. If this occurs, the dorsal longitudinal incision along the ray is extended and an open reduction is performed. Excision of the proximal portion of the proximal phalanx might be necessary. These dislocations often have a thick plantar callus formation beneath the metatarsal head, with or without ulceration. Reducing the dorsally dislocated phalanx raises the metatarsal head relative to the toe and other metatarsals and helps reduce the fat pads beneath the metatarsal heads. This decreases the bony prominence on the plantar surface of the foot and reduces the pressure beneath the metatarsal head. Enough proximal phalanx is resected so as to reduce the dislocation without tension of the soft tissues. It is often necessary to remove part or all of the metatarsal head. If the soft tissues are stiff and the metatarsal head prominent, an osteotomy of the metatarsal neck might be all that is needed to relieve pressure. If osteophyte formation in the metatarsal has become prominent these should also be excised. Ray amputation through a dorsal incision is discussed elsewhere (Chapter 12).

Midfoot

Fracture-dislocations of the tarsometatarsal joints (Lisfranc's joint) can include part or all of the joint.[2,3] If symptoms of redness and swelling in the midfoot occur and radiography and CT scanning reveal evidence of fracture in the absence of joint displacement or spreading of the metatarsals proximally, cast immobilization is recommended

(Fig. 11-4). The cast should be well molded beneath the arch to help maintain structural and architectural continuity while the fracture heals. The metatarsals themselves can spread at their bases or become disrupted at one or all of the tarsometatarsal joints (Fig. 11-5). Shortly after fracture, atrophy or massive resorption of the bones surrounding the joint can occur. Nonweight-bearing cast immobilization during this period is essential so that gross dislocation does not occur prior to onset of fracture healing. The atrophic period can last up to 1 year. Cast changes are required regularly because edema in the foot fluctuates as healing progresses.

ACUTE FRACTURE-DISLOCATION

Stabilizing surgery has two purposes. In the early stages it aids in stabilization of the fracture, thereby preventing dislocation as healing occurs[4] (Fig. 11-6). It can also prevent further dislocation of the remaining portion of the tarsometatarsal joints if only one or two rays have begun to sublux. A grossly atrophic joint cannot be stabilized through internal fixation, because pins and screws are ineffective for compression. It is necessary to wait until callus formation has occurred. At this time reduction and stabilization of the joint permit healing of the foot, with a well-maintained medial longitudinal arch and lateral pillar stability.

First metatarsal subluxation often occurs medially, with the lesser metatarsals drifting

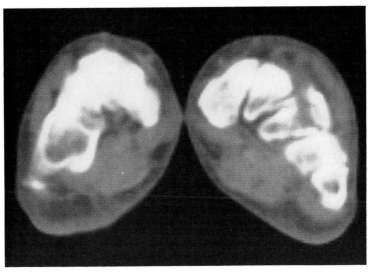

FIGURE 11–4. ■ Axial CT scan of a foot with Lisfranc's (Charcot's) fracture (*right*). The cut is made through the cuneiforms. The patient had painless redness and swelling, seen as soft tissue engorgement when compared to the opposite normal side.

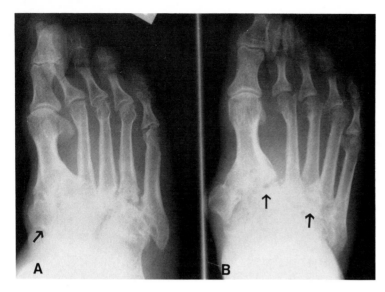

FIGURE 11–5. ■ Oblique (A) and anteroposterio (B) radiographs of a foot with Lisfranc's (Charcot) fracture-dislocation. The first ray has migrated medially and the lesser metatarsals have migrated laterally (B, *right arrow*). Note the healed pathologic fractures of the second and third metatarsal necks.

laterally (Fig. 11-7). First metatarsal medial cuneiform dislocation, with or without associated intercuneiform joints, is approached through a medial incision extending from the navicular to the midshaft. This exposes the first and second rays. Retraction of the tibialis anterior tendon, a deforming force, exposes the first metatarsal medial cuneiform joint. The first and second metatarsals and the second metatarsal middle cuneiform joint are exposed dorsomedially; the dorsalis pedis artery is protected. The articular surfaces are excised with an osteotome and curettes or a high-speed air motor dissecting tool. Stabilization is achieved with compression screws, which can be removed after the fracture heals (Fig. 11-2). The medial arch is held in appropriate alignment with guide wires and checked with the image intensifier at surgery. Cannulated compression screw fixation with 4.0- or 5.5-mm cancellous lag screws is performed. The wound is closed over drains.

In a complete dislocation of Lisfranc's joint, with good-quality bone present, a dorsal curvilinear incision is made over the dislocation and open reduction is performed. All articular surfaces are excised including the first through fifth metatarsal and the cuneiform and intercuneiform joints. The calcaneus and cuboid alignment tends to remain intact. It is difficult to obtain fusion

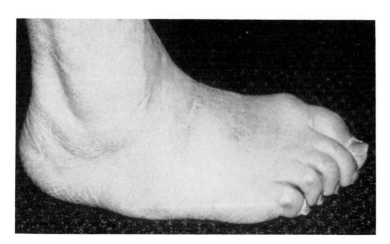

FIGURE 11–6. ■ A foot 12 years after open reduction and internal fixation of an acute Lisfranc's fracture-dislocation. This white male diabetic is now 65 years old and wears only an extra-depth shoe. No sequelae have occurred.

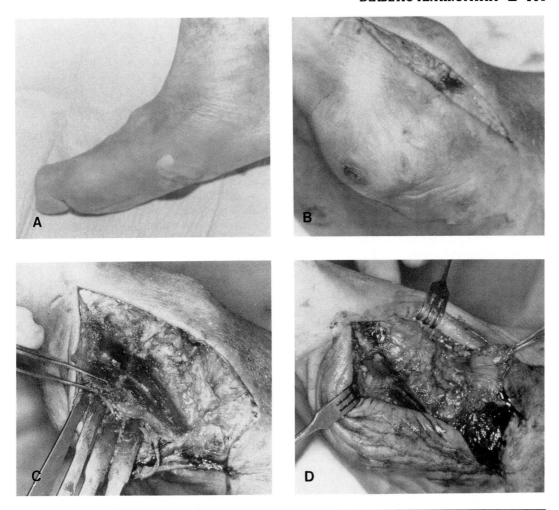

FIGURE 11–7. ■ First metatarsal medial cuneiform subluxation. *A,* A foot with dorsal subluxation of the first metatarsal. A recurrent neurotrophic ulcer is present beneath the arthritic medial cuneiform. A rocker bottom deformity has occurred. Through a medial incision (*B*) the joint is debulked (*C*). *D,* A wedge resection of the joint with screw fixation allows recreation of the arch. The foot is held in a cast until healing occurs. No recurrence of deformity or ulcer had occurred 3 years after surgery. The patient wears a semirigid accommodative orthotic.

of the fifth metatarsal and cuboid until the medial portion of Lisfranc's joint fuses. After reduction, guide wires are placed through the metatarsals in their reduced position and checked with the image intensifier. Cannulated screws are passed from the metatarsals into the tarsal bones or from the cuneiforms or cuboid into the metatarsals, whichever is technically easier for the particular patient. The ipsilateral iliac crest is prepared for surgery, because bone excision

can leave gaps at the joints and a graft is often needed to augment the arthrodesis. Closure over drains is done with absorbable 3-0 sutures in the subcutaneous tissue and 4-0 monofilament nylon sutures in the skin. Cast immobilization with a compression dressing is applied. The drain is removed in 48 hours and the cast is changed in 1 week. At that time the foot position is observed and radiographs are taken to ensure that alignment is maintained. Cast changes are made weekly, biweekly, and monthly thereafter until healing is evident on radiographs. Following this, an ankle-foot orthosis that supports the longitudinal arch of the foot is prescribed.

CHRONIC FRACTURE-DISLOCATION

Chronic fracture-dislocations of tarsometatarsal joints present a special problem.[5,6,7] All metatarsals can be dislocated as a unit, or the lateral four metatarsals might be split from the medial ray in a severe valgus deformity. A chronic complete dislocation is often associated with ulcers beneath the tarsal bones. If the medial cuneiform rides with the first metatarsal, the ulcer can occur beneath the middle cuneiform or cuboid. Ulcers should be healed prior to surgery.

A curvilinear dorsal transverse incision is made and immobilization of the soft tissues performed. The neurocirculatory bundle in the first intermetatarsal space is mobilized without stripping the nerves and artery, with its venae comitantes and supporting connective tissue. The proximal metatarsal joints are dissected first, because these lie dorsally and proximally over the tarsal bones. Resection of the proximal metatarsals might be necessary to visualize the tarsal bones. Reduction might require excision of a large portion of the cuneiform and cuboid bones. Anatomic alignment of intermetatarsal diastasis need not be fully achieved, because scarred, stiff, soft tissue often prevents this. The use of cannulated compression screws maintains alignment. Metatarsal and tarsal bone that has been removed to obtain a reduction of the dislocation is prepared and used for a bone graft. Additional material for a bone graft is obtained from the ipsilateral iliac crest.

Because these fracture-dislocations are associated with a rocker bottom foot, equinus of the hindfoot with contracture of the Achilles tendon is present. An Achilles tendon lengthening through a 4-cm incision medial and anterior to the Achilles tendon is performed by Z-plasty lengthening. Compression screws can be inserted from the metatarsals into the tarsal bones. If retrograde screw placement is not possible because of the size of the metatarsal or the inability to insert the screw through the wound, a lag screw is inserted through the posterior

calcaneus into the metatarsal (Fig. 11-8).

A compression dressing with split cast immobilization following closure is applied (see above). In patients with adequate vascularity, healing can be expected within 1 year. Cast immobilization for the first several months until early healing is evident radiographically is followed by the use of a cast-brace with a gatched ankle (e.g., Don Joy R.O.M. Walker), which permits ankle motion. When healing is complete a molded foot-ankle orthosis that maintains the arch is prescribed. A rehabilitation program is also included in the regimen.

Chronic deformity of a single ray can be present, such as the metatarsus elevatus, with a prominent mature callus at the first metatarsal medial cuneiform joint under which repeated ulceration occurs. These patients can have planovalgus of the hindfoot. For patients whose hindfoot is aligned and stable, an osteotomy and arthrodesis of the first metatarsal cuneiform joint is performed. The surgery includes excising periarticular ossification from the joint (i.e., bumpectomy), while at the same time performing an arthrodesis of the first metatarsal-medial cuneiform joint with a plantar-based wedge-shaped osteotomy to restore the medial longitudinal arch. The Achilles tendon is lengthened, if necessary, to permit ankle dorsiflexion since it is usually contracted. Compression screws maintain the restored position. The regimen described above for postoperative care is followed.

As the patient begins to bear weight on a healing midfoot fracture-dislocation, loads are again carried on the forefoot. It is not uncommon for stress fractures to develop in the distal metatarsals. Because the foot is immobilized in a plaster cast, these fractures are not significantly displaced and are not painful. Sequential radiographs demonstrate the natural course of healing.

Intertarsal and Chopart's Joint Fracture-Dislocations

As with Lisfranc's joint, the intertarsal joints, Chopart's joint,[8] and talonavicular and calcaneocuboid joints can also fracture and dislocate, creating a rocker bottom foot. The talonavicular joint subluxes so that the navicular rides dorsally and laterally to the

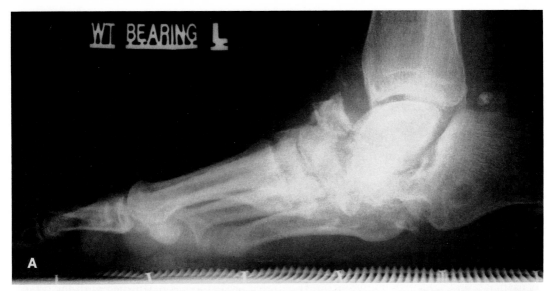

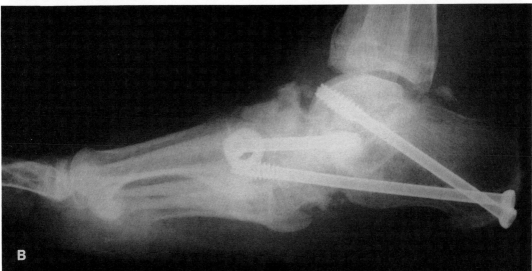

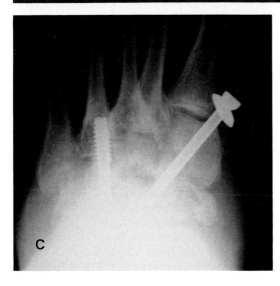

FIGURE 11–8. ■ Intertarsal fracture dislocation. *A,* Lateral radiograph of a foot in a diabetic with a 5-month history of painless swelling and redness. Collapse of the arch with rocker bottom deformity and ulcer formation beneath the midfoot were uncontrolled despite cast immobilization with restricted weight-bearing. *B* and *C,* X-rays showing the postoperative result of triple arthrodesis combined with midfoot fusion. Note the length and placement of the screws required to stabilize the midfoot. After 9 months, the patient was fitted with a full insole semirigid orthosis and extradepth shoe.

talus. The calcaneocuboid joint can sublux dorsally or remain intact, with dislocation occurring at the lateral tarsometatarsal joints, slipping dorsally and laterally. The foot appears thickened, short, and flat, with abduction in the forefoot. Ulceration beneath the cuboid or head of the navicular is not uncommon because valgus and equinus of the hindfoot can accompany the condition.

ACUTE FRACTURE-DISLOCATION

In the acute condition, provided the bone is not in its resorptive state, an open reduction with internal fixation using compression screws can be performed in selected cases (Fig. 11-9). Preservation of the neurovascular bundle that lies between the tibialis anterior and extensor hallucis longus tendons is important. Minimal resection of articular surfaces and the use of compression screws augmented by iliac bone graft are recommended. Healing occurs in 8 to 12 months.

CHRONIC DISLOCATION

If the dislocation has been present for some time, resection of part of the cuboid and cuneiforms might be required to achieve reduction. Large cannulated compression screws provide the compression necessary to achieve fusion (Fig. 11-7). This is augmented by bone graft and held immobilized until complete arthrodesis has occurred. An Achilles tendon lengthening is necessary using the Z-plasty technique through a 4-cm incision anteromedial to the Achilles tendon.

Subtalar Joint

The subtalar joint can sublux medially or laterally in the neurotrophic foot.[9] In lateral dislocations the foot develops planovalgus and heel cord contracture, and ulcers form beneath the talar head or medial malleolus. This can be associated with pathologic fracture through the talar neck. In medial dislocations paralysis of the peroneals permit unopposed activity of the tibialis posterior and long flexors in the toes, creating an equinovarus contracture with ulceration over the lateral foot or ankle with an unstable ankle.

Rapid onset of valgus deformity in the hindfoot in the absence of bone atrophy and with satisfactory circulation is treated by subtalar or triple arthrodesis. An 8-cm lateral incision is made at the dorsolateral aspect of the foot at the level of the subtalar joint. Because the bone here is dense and the deformity fixed, soft tissue dissection is required to mobilize the joint. If the forefoot cannot be pronated to recreate the arch, a triple arthrodesis is necessary. Contracted peroneal tendons are lengthened. Large cannulated compression screws are placed from the calcaneus into the talar dome through the posterior facet. Alignment is checked with the image intensifier. The subtalar joint is stabilized first. The resection of sclerotic articular surfaces is performed with the aid of a high-speed air motor dissecting tool. An Achilles tendon lengthening is performed. A staple is used to compress the calcaneocuboid joint. To approach the talonavicular joint a 5-cm medial incision is made, extending far enough distally so that a compression screw can be passed through the anteromedial navicular body into the neck and body of the talus. The wounds are closed over drains. A cast boot walker is used after 4 months to mobilize the ankle joint.

A medial dislocation of the subtalar joint is accompanied by equinovarus and adductus deformity.[2,3] A 12-cm medial incision is made beginning at the medial cuneiform and extending posteriorly beneath the medial malleolus and curving proximally (Fig. 11-10). The hindfoot contracture is released at the subtalar joint. Neurocirculatory structures are identified in the posteromedial compartment of the ankle, along with the surrounding soft tissue, to protect them. Z-plasty lengthenings of the Achilles tendon, tibialis posterior, flexor hallucis longus, and flexor digitorum longus are performed, as necessary. The subtalar joint is approached from the medial side. Enough talus and calcaneus are resected to permit reduction without tension on the soft tissues. Occasionally, deformity is severe enough to prevent reduction without excision of large amounts of the talus and calcaneus. It might be necessary to perform a subtotal talectomy, leaving only part of the dome, but this is enough to permit some ankle motion and spare additional stress on a healing triple arthrodesis. If a pathologic fracture of the talus is present, with resorption of a portion of the talar neck and head, it can be filled with bone graft. Cancellous lag screws hold the reduction, which is checked at surgery with the image intensifier. Alignment in the hindfoot is important, because excessive varus and valgus can lead to recurrent deformity and ulceration.

Ankle

Neuropathic arthropathy of the ankle is often a difficult diagnosis. A sprain or fracture can lead to the development of a progressive, painless deformity with gross edema, surprising both the patient and physician. Recommended treatment for pathologic fracture without deformity in the diabetic includes immobilization, frequent cast changes, and regular radiographic monitoring for periods of up to 8 months. Only toe touching is allowed at first. Once early healing is in evidence, partial weight-bearing is permitted with a walker or crutches. If displacement begins to occur open reduction must be considered. For the ankle to develop neuropathic changes, a loss of sensation and the potential for arthropathy must exist distally in the foot, because polyneuropathy progresses distally to proximally. Immobilization following open reduction is prolonged, for up to 8 months, with limited weight-bearing. An ankle-foot orthosis is worn when activity resumes. A SACH heel or rocker bottom on the sole of an extra-depth shoe also helps dissipate loads beneath the foot.

If subluxation of the joint occurs in spite of immobilization or open reduction, ankle arthrodesis might be indicated after hypertrophic bone begins to form. Many types of ankle arthrodesis have been proposed. My preference for neuropathic joints involves a lateral approach with osteotomy of the fibula and the use of bone graft between the talus and tibia. The fibula is not completely detached but soft tissue is allowed to remain attached to the distal, lateral, and posterior borders. The articular surface is removed from the dome of the talus and tibial plafond. A second incision is made anteromedially to remove additional cartilage from the medial malleolus and talar dome. Autogenous iliac bone graft is used in conjunction with large compression screws placed medially and laterally. A screw placed from the posterior tibia into the talar neck can also aid in stabilizing the joints, the positions of which are checked with the X-ray image intensifier.

Cast immobilization is prolonged, for up to 1 year. Delayed union and nonunion in procedures of the hindfoot are not uncommon. Failure of a complete arthrodesis, a pseudoarthrosis, is not failure of surgery if the joint is stable, maintains circulation, and provides a means through which activities of daily living can continue. If deformity is irreducible a partial talectomy can be performed, removing only enough bone to reduce the joint (Fig. 11-11). The leg must be held immobile for several months to permit maturing of the scar and soft tissues to stabilize the ankle. An orthosis is then worn with shoe modifications as described above.

Stabilizing neuropathic arthropathy is an important aspect of the treatment of diabetes. Underlying disease, including diabetes, concomitant infection, neurologic conditions, and patients' perception of their condition are important in treatment, because it is prolonged and requires close cooperation of the patient and the entire treatment team. Clinical preoperative preparation of the foot is a prior consideration, because it must be free of ulcers and infection. Circulation must be adequate, including that in the toes. Reconstruction of the foot and stabilization of joints maintain the functional length and stability of the foot and ankle and help keep the patient independently ambulatory. Deformity of the foot can develop slowly or rapidly, and usually progresses distally to proximally. Surgery must be delayed if the fracture healing process is in the lytic phase. Hypertrophic bones are better stock on which to use compression screws.

Surgical correction includes excision of osteophytes, debulking of joints (bumpectomy), resection of bones (ostectomy), osteotomy, arthrodesis, and amputation. The treatment of soft tissues is important. Minimal edema should be present preoperatively. The skin must be handled delicately and incision placement designed to permit primary healing. Postoperative care includes the use of bulky dressings, splints, and

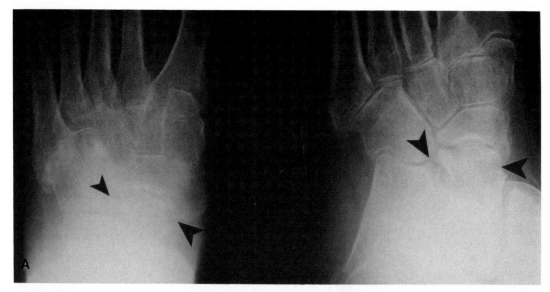

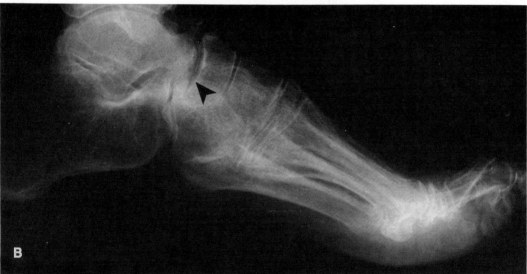

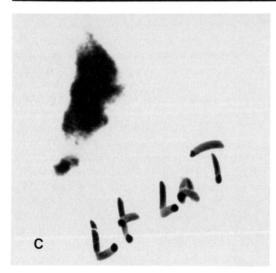

FIGURE 11–9. ■ Acute disruption of Chopart's joint. *A* and *B*, Radiographs (non-weight-bearing) of a diabetic foot 2 months after painless onset of redness and swelling in the midfoot. Earlier radiographs were normal. Talonavicular collapse is now seen (*arrows*). Clinical collapse of the arch during weight-bearing became evident despite cast immobilization. *C*, Bone scan revealing reaction in midfoot and hindfoot. This should not be confused with osteomyelitis. Redness and edema decreased with elevation for several days.

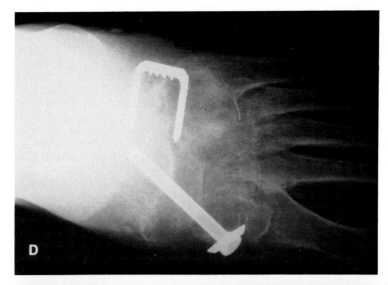

D and E, Triple arthrodesis stabilized the hindfoot. The patient now wears only a full insole semi-rigid orthotic and extra-depth shoes. She has undergone a diabetic education program and has had no recurrence of deformity or additional fractures in the 2 years since surgery.

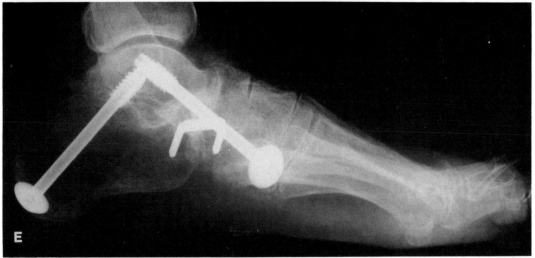

split casts, as well as frequent cast changes and ultimately an ankle-foot orthosis, arch supports, and prescription shoes. Early ambulation is encouraged, with minimal weight-bearing. During the later stages of healing a cast boot with a variable ankle gatch to permit motion is used.

Failure of complete arthrodesis is not failure of surgery, because it permits the foot to remain stable through a pseudoarthrosis. Surgery on the forefoot is designed to maintain functional length and permit a plantigrade foot. Along with amputation, this reduces ulceration by eliminating rubbing on footwear. Metatarsophalangeal joints can be treated by such procedures as the Keller bunionectomy, capsulotomy, and joint resection of the lesser rays. Arthrodesis might not be successful in the forefoot. Ulcers of the midfoot are treated by debulking of bone and, in selected cases, by open reduction of dislocated joints with arthrodesis. Chopart's joint and the subtalar joint require major reconstruction with the use of specialized techniques, internal compression, and prolonged immobilization. Resection of part or all of certain tarsal bones to achieve reduction is sometimes necessary. Open reduction of neuropathic ankle fractures might be necessary in the acute fracture, but must be accompanied by prolonged immobilization of several months and by close follow-

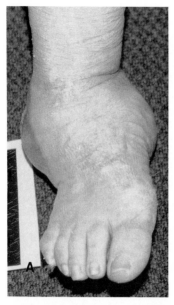

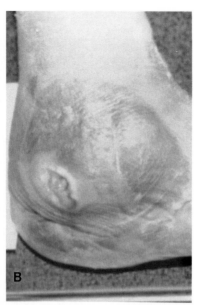

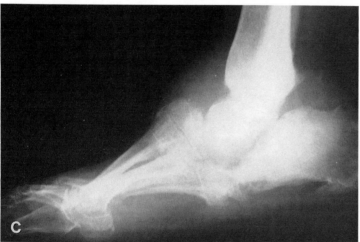

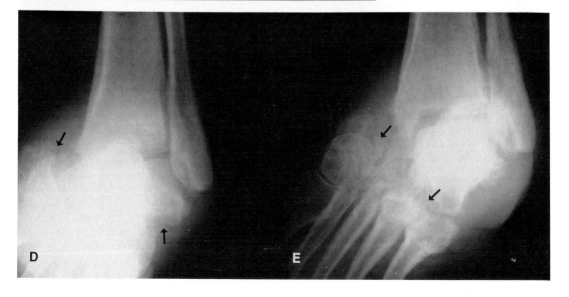

FIGURE 11-10 ■ A foot with progressive medial peritalar dislocation in a 65-year-old woman with a 20-year history of diabetes. *A* and *B*, A neuropathic ulcer is present from bearing weight directly on the lateral malleolus, and fixed varus contracture of the hindfoot is present. The patient refused amputation. Nonweight-bearing cast immobilization for 6 months failed to improve the position of the foot but healed the ulcer. *C*, *D*, and *E*, Radiographs of medial dislocation of the foot on the talus (*arrows*). The talar head has disintegrated. Chopart's joint has dislocated dorsally and the calcaneus is in equinus. *F*, (opposite page) Operative photograph of medial exposure of the foot and ankle. The medial flexor and Achilles tendons were lengthened. The neurovascular bundle was dissected free and protected during the triple arthrodesis. A partial talectomy was performed to accommodate reduction. The ankle joint was not resected to allow motion.

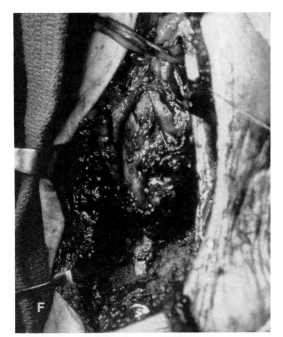

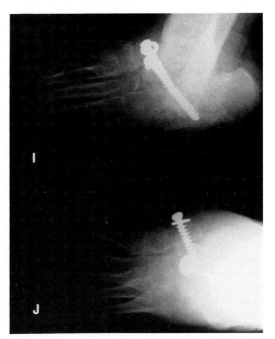

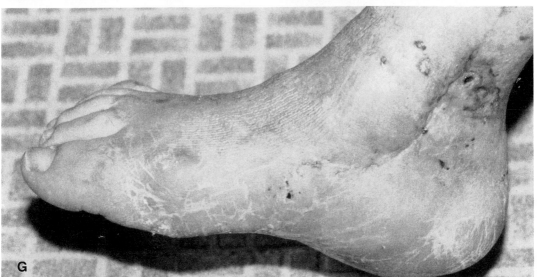

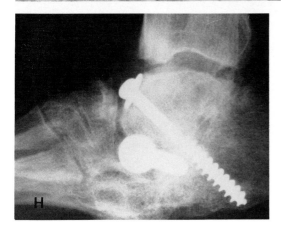

G, The foot 1 year postoperatively. The arch is stabilized, equinus corrected, hindfoot stabilized, and ulcer healed. H, I, and J, Radiographs showing fusion of the hindfoot. The patient now wears a semi-rigid full insole accommodative orthosis in extra-depth shoes. No recurrence of deformity, additional fractures or dislocations, or ulcers have developed in the 4 years since surgical stabilization.

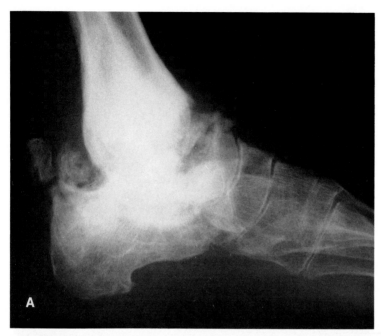

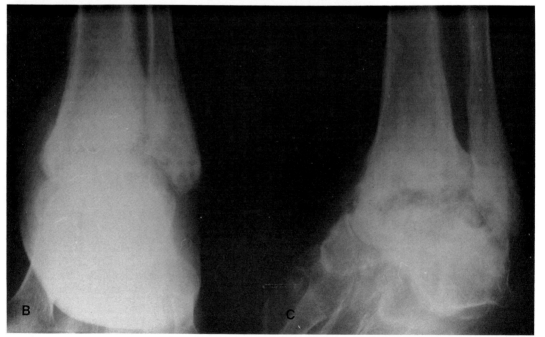

FIGURE 11–11 ■ *A, B,* and *C,* Radiographs of the foot of a 45-year-old female diabetic wth neuropathic ankle and subtalar joint destruction. Varus hindfoot deformity occurred despite cast immobilization for several months. Attempted reduction of a talar neck fracture had failed. The patient refused amputation.

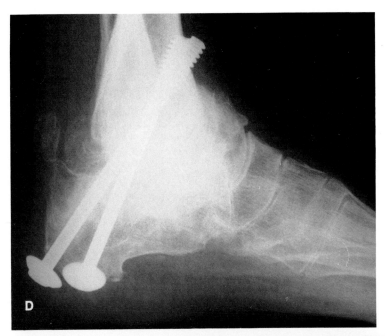

D, E, and *F,* Radiographs taken 6 months following ankle and subtalar arthrodesis with bone graft. The arthrodesis is healed. The deformity has not recurred nor have additional fractures or ulcers. The patient wears an ankle-foot orthosis.

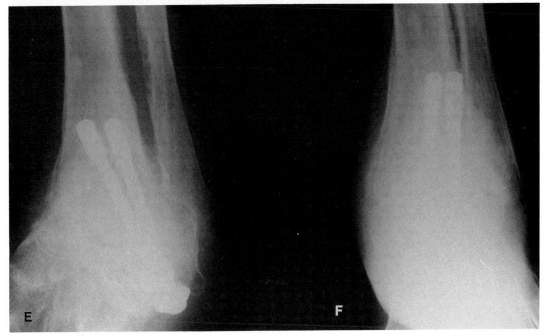

up in an ankle-foot orthosis. Ankle arthrodesis requires bone grafting, compression screws, and prolonged immobilization.

The primary objective in the treatment of the foot in diabetes, a chronic disabling disease, is to maintain independent ambulation with the use of a plantigrade, functional foot. Appropriate alignment of weight-bearing structures with an orthosis and minimal shoe modification is the goal of surgery.

References

1. Myerson M. Surgery of the foot in diabetics. Presented at the Fifth Annual Meeting of the American Orthopaedic Foot and Ankle Society. Symposium on the Diabetic Foot. Sun Valley, Idaho, August 1989.
2. Sammarco GJ. Stabilizing the neuropathic hindfoot. Presented at the Fifth Annual Meeting of the American Orthopaedic Foot and Ankle Society. Symposium on the Diabetic Foot. Sun Valley, Idaho, August 1989.
3. Sammarco GJ. Stabilizing the Neuroarthritic Foot. Presented in Instructional Course Treatment of the Diabetic Foot at the American Academy of Orthopaedic Surgeons meeting. New Orleans, Louisiana, February, 1990.
4. Cohn BT, Brahms MA. Diabetic arthropathy of the first metatarsal cuneiform joint. Introduction of a new surgical fusion technique. Orthop Rev. 1987; 16:465–470.
5. Angrick M, Denner F. Beitrag zur diabetischen arthropathie. Beitr Orthop Traumatol. 1988; 35:263–268.
6. Cleveland M. Surgical fusion of unstable joints due to neuropathic disturbance. Am J Surg. 1939; 43:580–584.
7. Connolly JF, Jacobsen FS. Rapid bone destruction after a stress fracture in a diabetic (Charcot) foot. Nebr Med J. 1985; 438–440.
8. Lesko P, Maurer RC. Talonavicular dislocations and midfoot arthropathy in neuropathic diabetic feet. Clin Orthop Rel Res. 1986; 240:226–231.
9. Heiple KG, Cammarn MR. Diabetic neuroarthropathy with spontaneous peritalar fracture dislocation. J Bone Joint Surg. 1966; 48A:1177–1181.

12 Amputations

MARK S. MYERSON, M.D.

The impact of diabetes and peripheral vascular disease in the general population is staggering. It is estimated that vascular disease is approximately 30 times more common in diabetics than in the general nondiabetic population.[1-3] Similarly, the incidence of gangrene has been found to be 70 times more common in diabetics than in nondiabetics.[3] The incidence of diabetes-related amputations has been estimated to be 10 in 100,000 population in Sweden,[4] and 7 in 100,000 in Denmark.[5] In the United States, however, data have shown that the incidence of amputation in diabetes is higher, with an annual rate of 60 in 100,000,[6] and this is probably closer to 100 in 100,000 in patients over the age of 65.[7,8] In an excellent review, it was calculated that this would account for 30,200 amputations annually in the United States.[6] Davidson and colleagues have showed that, in a well-organized program of diabetic education and prevention, the amputation rate could be decreased from 14 in 1,000 to 6.7 in 1,000 patients.[9] The cost of these amputations is enormous, amounting to approximately $200 million annually, because the average length of hospitalization is 30 days.

In addition to the obvious morbidity from the amputation itself, the mortality rates for diabetic patients who have had amputation for gangrene are increased. Additionally, the percentage of patients requiring a second amputation in the contralateral leg at 5 years ranges from 50%,[10] 51%,[11] 57%,[12] 61%,[13] and 66%.[14] As with morbidity data, the statistics regarding mortality after amputation are also consistent, ranging from 40 to 57% within 3 years and from 50 to 75% within 5 years.[12,15-19] These data suggest that in spite of technologic advances in the medical and surgical management of diabetes and diabetic gangrene, no substantial improvement appears to have occurred in the 3- to 5-year mortality figures.

Over the past 40 years, the principles of amputation surgery in diabetes have been changing. The incidence of above-knee amputations has decreased, whereas that of below-knee and partial foot amputations has been escalating.[15,20,21] This has largely been a result of careful preoperative planning, improved selection criteria for the level of amputation and, perhaps most important of all, improved patient education and the institution of other preventative programs.[9,22]

This chapter defines the principles of diabetic amputation surgery, emphasizing the role of careful preoperative evaluation. The indications for surgery, preoperative planning, and specific treatment programs to enhance the outcome of surgery are stressed. General surgical principles are presented, including the specific levels of amputation in the foot and ankle, with indications and operative technique for each. Discussions of postoperative care and prosthetic rehabilitation and appropriate footwear for each level of amputation are also included.

INDICATIONS

Ablative surgery for the diabetic foot is performed for uncontrolled infection and uncorrectable deformity. A third category of surgery in the diabetic foot is aimed at protecting the foot at risk. Such prophylac-

173

tic operations are seldom ablative and are not discussed here.

Infecton and deformity are associated, in most clinical situations, often because it is some component of deformity that has precipitated the infection. Minor injury, continuous trauma to a plantar callosity, or irritation from a fungal infection are all events that would normally be tolerated in a non-diabetic. In diabetics, a moderate vascular impairment, which would otherwise be asymptomatic, might not be able to support a gross infection, which requires more blood than the impaired vessels can supply. Therefore, a neuropathic ulcer or minor infection from an ingrown toenail could be disastrous, because the natural history of these relatively minor conditions is an inexorable spread of the infection, rapidly producing extensive abscess formation and tissue necrosis, and necessitating amputation. No single cause is responsible in most cases of breakdown leading to amputation. These diabetic lesions are a result of a combination of neuropathy and infection, with or without vascular insufficiency.

This is important, because infection and disturbances of the microcirculation were formerly thought to be the primary factors in the causation of diabetic foot lesions. It is currently believed, however, that sepsis is a complication of neuropathic lesions and not actually a causative factor. In addition, structural changes in the microcirculation are often present in the diabetic foot, but are not in themselves the primary infection.[23,24] The distinction between these two underlying causes, neuropathy and occlusive arterial disease, is important early in the surgical management of the diabetic foot.

Two classes of diabetics are candidates for amputation—those with adequate circulation and those with arterial insufficiency. Any rest pain is a contraindication to partial foot amputations. Often, though, a nonhealing ulcer or a localized form of gangrene is found that is unresponsive to local measures. The management of this large group of patients with arterial insufficiency has been discussed in previous chapters. Pulses are not palpable in these patients, and other signs of ischemia are commonly present. It is important that the association between these lesions and ischemia be recognized, because these limbs can be salvaged with arterial re-

construction, permitting amputations at a more distal level than would otherwise have been possible without revascularization.

PREOPERATIVE EVALUATION

Clinical Examination

Diabetic foot infections are only one manifestation of a serious systemic disorder. Many patients have co-existing cardiac, renal, vascular, ophthalmologic, and social disorders that need attention prior to surgery. Although surgeons cannot be expected to evaluate all these problems, as the team leader they should coordinate the work-up of the patient in a logical and orderly fashion to enhance the outcome of surgery.

The foot is examined systematically, with attention to the extent of infection, other areas of the foot at risk, the neurovascular status, analysis of the plantar weight-bearing surfaces, and evaluation of the opposite foot. The essential points on examination—other than obvious infection, ulcer, fissures, and gangrene—are the color, temperature, and nutritional state of the skin. The fullness of the veins, circulatory impairment, wasting of the intrinsic muscles, and a complete neurologic evaluation are other integral components of the examination. The essence of the preoperative evaluation is a systematic approach to the foot at risk. This decreases the potential for operative failure, enhances recovery, and results in a healed, functional, plantigrade foot.

The most important factor is selection of the level of amputation that is likely to result in recovery consistent with these criteria. In amputations resulting from trauma, tumor, or congenital anomalies, the decision for level selection is not difficult and length is preserved at the most appropriate level consistent with prosthetic rehabilitation. In diabetic and vascular amputations, however, no well-defined and universally accepted criteria exist. No single level at which amputation should consistently be performed can be defined, and each case must be modified to suit individual needs. This is determined by functional considerations, presence of infection, status of the circulation, and age and patient activity level. Because many reports on amputation surgery are contradictory, selecting the appropriate level can be confusing. A number of patients are still treated with above-knee amputation, when a more distal level might have been possible. Conversely, many patients undergo a second amputation at a more proximal level because the wound does not heal from the more distally based amputation. It is often difficult to determine the most appropriate level for amputation.

Determining the Level of Amputation

From a functional standpoint, amputation below the knee is far superior to the above-knee amputation, because preservation of the knee joint improves prosthetic rehabilitation. Over the past few decades this has led to increasing numbers of distal-level amputations. Although such patients have improved function and shorter rehabilitation periods, it has also led to increasing numbers of operative failures.[18,25]

Many tests have been devised to facilitate decision making for amputation. None of these are absolute, but each should supplement clinical, pathologic, anatomic, and prosthetic considerations. A decision regarding the optimal level for amputation should therefore be made at the completion of the work-up prior to surgery.

The status of the arterial circulation is the major determinant of wound healing and should be relied on to assist in determining the level of amputation. Various tests are currently used to determine the status of the arterial circulation, including the major arterial tree, smaller vessels, capillaries, and skin. In one report patients were evaluated preoperatively by the history and physical examination alone, without resorting to special tests. Determination of peripheral pulses, venous filling time, color return, and the general appearance of the limbs was relied on.[26] This 5-year study indicated that the history of onset of the ischemic lesion, the physical findings, and the ultimate prognosis are factors that allow "conservative" amputations. These were either above- or below-knee amputations, however, and the criteria are not accurate enough to determine the levels for amputation in the foot and ankle.

Arteriography has traditionally been the technique of choice for evaluating the patency of the peripheral vasculature. Angiography might not accurately reflect the ability of the limb to heal, however, because it measures the status of the larger arteries and arterioles and not the skin capillaries, which are also important in healing. Furthermore, involvement of the major vessels is usually patchy and, if these vessels are gradually occluded, a collateral blood supply develops that could support an adequate peripheral circulation. Therefore, the absence of pulses in major extremity vessels does not necessarily indicate severe ischemia. Below-knee amputations might therefore heal, even when the femoral artery is obstructed. This has the same implications for arteriography, because conservative amputations might still heal in spite of arteriographic occlusion.[18,27] Some authors therefore have not advocated the use of arteriography in selecting a level for amputation, citing a failure rate of healing of only 12% when amputations are routinely done below the knee.[28] Other authors have cited an accuracy of 71% in determining the correct level when arteriography was routinely used.[29]

Of the various measures available to assess the circulatory status, the most economic, efficient, and reliable means are the Doppler ultrasound and the ischemic index. Transcutaneous Doppler ultrasound can be used to measure arterial flow patterns and to assess quantitative blockage of the arterial tree.[30–34] Brachial systolic pressures are obtained simultaneously at various points along the leg, foot, and distally to the toes, and each lower extremity pressure is divided by the brachial artery pressure to calculate the ischemic index. Wagner has reported on a series of 277 cases of infected or gangrenous feet in which the predictive value of the index was used successfully in 93% of diabetic and 98% of nondiabetic patients.[34] Experience with this method reveals no failures when the index was greater than 1.0. An ischemic index of 0.45 is used as the cut-off point in diabetic amputation surgery. This is combined with other criteria, including the presence or absence of infection, to determine the level of amputation.

Despite the success of the use of segmental blood pressure measurements, these methods have been criticized because they measure the status of the larger arteries and arterioles, and not the skin capillaries, which are also important in healing. The Doppler effect might also be unreliable in the presence of obstructed vessels. Other methods that measure the blood flow to the skin directly or indirectly might be more accurate for selecting the level of amputation compatible with healing.

Cutaneous temperature has been correlated with skin blood flow using venous occlusion plethysmography.[35-37] The evaluation of skin temperature by palpation is inaccurate. Many commercial skin thermistors and thermocouples are available that are accurate enough for determining the level of amputation.[37] Skin temperature measurements can be used in various ways. Golbranson[37] has reported a direct correlation between healing and skin temperature above 32° C, in which all amputations performed with a skin temperature below 30.5° C failed. If the difference between the skin and room temperature was greater than 5° C, the amputation usually healed.[37]

Another method is the xenon washout technique.[38,39] Xenon in isotope form penetrates the skin when applied to it and is subsequently cleared only by the bloodstream. The blood flow rate can therefore be correlated with the rate of disappearance of radioactivity.

In some patients with extensive peripheral vascular disease or sclerosis of the vessels measurement of the Doppler index is impossible, because the vessel walls cannot be compressed. In these patients it is important to listen for pulsatile flow with the Doppler. If pulsatile flow is audible, it is supplemented with the examination using cutaneous thermistor. A final decision on amputation level is made based on the overall skin condition and the presence or absence of infection.

Management of Infection

Many factors mitigate against a successful outcome in diabetic amputation surgery. The diseased foot is only one manifestation of a severe systemic disorder and the patient needs to be thoroughly prepared for surgery. The most important factor in decision making is the correct timing of surgery. This can be successfully achieved once infection has been brought under control and well demarcated. Although most amputation surgery in the diabetic foot is associated with infection, surgery should never be performed in an attempt to gain control of advancing sepsis.

Prior to any definitive ablative surgery, infection must be controlled.[40-42] The success of amputation surgery depends on adequate control of the local ischemic and infective processes. Unless tissue is aggressively debrided viable tissue is further harmed, probably because of septic thrombosis extending through normal tissue.

Any necrotizing process and active infection should be stabilized by surgical drainage, bed rest, elevation, warm compresses, and antibiotics. This is best accomplished by a team equipped to deal with these patients in the hospital although, with the current restrictions placed on prolonged hospitalization, this can be achieved by carefully supervised home care.

Over the years philosophies have changed regarding the exact timing of surgery. Generally, surgical procedures should be delayed until the infection and patient's general nutritional status have improved. Increased operative success in the past decade is attributed to delaying surgical treatment while simultaneously maximizing the patient's overall health status.[43,44] In reviewing these reports, however, it should be noted that delaying the definitive surgical procedure might give results because certain patients will no longer be candidates for lesser amputations. These patients, who might be treated by local resection, could also fail by underestimating the severity of the disease process.[43]

Following debridement, ulcers and gangrenous lesions are cultured and broad-spectrum antibiotics are given until the results of the culture and sensitivities are obtained. The nature of the infection has no specific prognostic value, provided the patient has been placed on appropriate antibiotics. Patients are placed on strict bed rest, the extremity elevated, and warm compresses applied. Warm compresses have been used to treat superficial skin and wound infections for centuries. Since the introduction of antibiotics, however, these measures have largely been ignored. Experience with warm compresses has shown them to be an excellent adjunct to immobilization, parenteral antibiotic therapy, and surgical debridement for incision and drainage of deeper abscesses. A warm (95 to 105° F), moist towel is wrapped around the foot. Three layers of commercially available, thin, impermeable plastic are applied, followed by two layers of plastic-lined disposable absorbent pads. The compress is completely changed every 12 hours for a maximum of 4 days. The rationale is to induce active hyperemia, retaining body heat and moisture in the dressing and increasing blood flow to the skin and subcutaneous tissues.

Once the cellulitis and wet gangrenous process are under control, minimal mechanical debridement needs to be performed. Instead, wet-to-dry dressings with iodides are applied in the hope that the gangrene becomes dry and demarcates. Iodides that can be prepared as an aqueous solution of 0.5% potassium iodide[45,46] have been shown to be effective in the management of gangrene. The tri-iodide complex releases free iodine, an antimicrobial agent.

Nutritional Assessment

The patient's general metabolic and nutritional status should always be considered impaired. It has been shown that the preoperative white blood count, temperature, and fasting blood sugar level are significantly correlated with operative success or failures.[43] All patients should receive appropriate nutritional support. Studies have shown that, in randomly surveyed hospital populations, pre-existing malnutrition is unrecognized and untreated and is often compounded during hospitalization. Many diabetic patients become malnourished prior to hospitalization because of the catabolic effects of the sepsis. The basal energy expenditure of a 70-kg male is approximately 1800 k cal, but energy requirements increase by about 40% during periods of severe infection. These catabolic losses are often worsened during hospitalization as a result of the routine of repeatedly starving patients prior to each operative procedure.

Indices are available to assess the extent of nutritional depletion quantitatively. Visceral protein depletion, a simple test, can be estimated by determining the serum albumin level and the presence of an anergic state can be determined by measuring the total lymphocyte count. Severe nutritional depletion is indicated by an albumin concentration of less than 3.0 and by a total lymphocyte count (the percentage of lymphocytes multiplied by the white blood cell count) of less than 1000. Providing an optimal nutritional environment for the patient preoperatively and postoperatively enhances healing. This is best achieved by a team effort, in which sophisticated pharmacologic therapy is provided to boost the patient's metabolic status.

The definitive surgical procedure should *not* be performed in an effort to "get ahead" of the infective process. This should be carried out when the precipitating local infection has been stabilized. During this conservative phase of treatment, the patient is assessed by the entire diabetic foot team, including specialists in orthopedic surgery, infectious disease, vascular surgery, and nutrition.

OPERATIVE TECHNIQUE AND GENERAL SURGICAL PRINCIPLES

Anesthesia

General anesthesia is not necessary for diabetic amputation surgery, and I perform almost all foot and ankle procedures under local or regional anesthesia. I have found that, in most amputations of the foot, even the Syme's amputation, regional anesthesia is sufficient. Most diabetic patients have a profound peripheral neuropathy that in itself facilitates extensive debridement without any anesthesia. These patients might also have significant cardiorespiratory and renal problems, which could be contraindications to the use of general anesthesia.

It has been reported that successful partial amputation of the foot can only be performed under general or spinal anesthesia,[47] but experience has shown that many local amputations of the foot can be performed using regional anesthesia. A contraindication to the use of local anesthesia is the presence of active infection or gangrene. Local acidosis can also inactivate the anesthetic. The use of local or regional anesthesia should not compromise the surgical procedure, particularly in the presence of pus, in which case thorough debridement and adequate drainage must be carried out.

The anesthetic is administered in a standard fashion using a combination of 10 ml of 1% plain lidocaine and 10 ml of 0.5% plain bupivicaine. The posterior tibial nerve, deep peroneal nerve, and superficial peroneal nerves are all infiltrated.[48]

Surgical Technique

A general principle of amputation surgery is to maximize the length of the limb, and this also applies to the foot. This concept has evolved over the past few decades, so that more feet are now being saved. Surgeons are now tempted to perform partial foot amputations on patients who might do as well with a more proximal amputation level. Some limited forefoot amputations might not always do well, and this has prompted some surgeons to perform routine transmetatarsal rather than ray amputations.

In spite of this, maximum foot length is preserved whenever possible. In each patient the operative procedure is tailored to the disease process and by the limitations imposed by infection, pre-existing deformity, and age and activity level. The use of aggressive local amputation surgery can lead to unusual and unorthodox-appearing amputations. Provided a smooth, plantigrade, weight-bearing surface of the forefoot or midfoot remnant is maintained, however, the functional result can be satisfactory.[21]

Conservative amputations succeed in many patients. The incidence of lesions affecting the opposite limb is about 30% within 3 years of the onset of the first.[15,21] For patients with one above-knee amputation and one partial foot amputation, their rehabilitation and prosthetic recovery is markedly improved.

Preservation of length is particularly applicable in patients with intact circulation. In such patients infection is associated with abscess formation and wet gangrene. Although ischemia can be present, the major problem is the metabolic disturbance against a background of peripheral neuropathy.[49] A relatively minor fungal infection, an abrasion, the presence of thick callosities, or injudicious attempts to cut the toenails can precipitate the infection, culminating in local gangrene.[50] In a second group of diabetics gangrene is caused by ischemia and, instead of a florid infection, the affected part is dry and associated with a necrotic process that has been present for a few weeks. Although preservation of length in this group of patients is also important, amputation should only be considered after arterial reconstruction.

Amputation in diabetics with marginal circulation should be performed using plastic surgery principles. The soft tissues are always friable and incisions are made with minimal subcutaneous dissection. Although surgery is performed meticulously it can be accomplished without concern for precise anatomic landmarks. At no time is the skin or soft tissue firmly grasped with forceps. Skin hooks and rakes are used whenever possible and overzealous skin retraction should be avoided. Bone cuts are made with sharp instruments or a power saw. Bone edges are bevelled with a rongeur and rasp. All infected or gangrenous tissue is radically debrided. This applies particularly to more avascular tissue, such as tendons, plantar fascia, and bone.

If local skin is insufficient for coverage, rather than shortening the foot further by resecting more bone to facilitate closure, the wound is covered by a split-thickness skin graft, provided it is not on the weight-bearing plantar surface. Split-thickness skin grafts from a proximal donor site or pinch grafts from the amputated part can be used. All incisions are closed loosely using minimal subcutaneous sutures and nylon sutures for skin. A small catheter is placed in the subcutaneous tissues, which is then closed loosely for irrigation. Postoperatively the bed of the wound is irrigated continuously with an antibiotic solution.

USE OF THE TOURNIQUET

I prefer not to use a tourniquet during diabetic amputation surgery. Instead, all bleeders are clamped immediately with small hemostats and then cauterized. Post- tourniquet metabolic changes occur and can compromise an already tenuous extremity. Wagner has noted that the incidence of complications related to wound healing appears to be the same whether a tourniquet is used.[34] It was also noted, however, that, in above-knee amputees, a 50% increase in postoperative complications was seen when a tourniquet was used. Wagner therefore recommended that a tourniquet not be used for above-knee amputation.

This is not an absolute. The tourniquet can be inflated for a short period prior to actual removal of the affected part. If a tourniquet is used it is inflated after elevating the limb, but not with exsanguinating it. Use of an Esmarch bandage is contraindicated, particularly in the presence of infection.

WOUND CLOSURE

I attempt to close all wounds primarily but without tension. All incisions are closed loosely using minimal subcutaneous sutures and nonabsorbable sutures such as monofilament nylon are used for skin.

If the wound cannot be closed it heals by secondary intention or it can be covered with a split-thickness graft, obtained as a pinch graft at a later stage. Split-thickness grafts can also be obtained with a dermatome and meshed for immediate application from the amputated part. Application of pinch grafts can stimulate granulations, which in turn can be covered with additional grafts later.

DRAINS

Drains should always be used. Kritter[51] has stated that candidates for major amputation can be treated by local radical surgery of gangrenous lesions of the foot, followed by successful healing using a continuous drain system. These Kritter drains are placed subcutaneously through the dorsum of the foot into the operative site. During closure suction is placed on the catheters to maintain their patency. The wounds are closed loosely using skin sutures only. This prevents necrosis of the wound edges, which are marginally ischemic. Once the wound has been closed, the catheters are irrigated with a continuous infusion; lactated Ringer's solution is preferred. The irrigating fluid exits between the sutures to dilute bacteria and hematoma and to wash out debris.

Amputation Levels of the Foot and Ankle

TOE AMPUTATIONS

"Few patients will go on to full healing after simple toe amputation" (Fig. 12-1).[52] Hunter has shown that diabetics should not be treated differently from nondiabetics when considering the level of amputation, even with minor toe amputations.[52] Simple removal of the toes is not recommended, however, unless vascular surgery has been successful in improving the circulation to the forefoot before amputation. Transmetatarsal amputation is a more suitable and conservative operation.

For the toe amputation to be successful, though, gangrene must be well localized to the tip of the toe and adequate perfusion of the foot as determined by the Doppler index must be present. Intraoperative bleeding can be used as a guide to sufficient blood supply.[33] Skin vessels in flaps are observed and, if bleeding occurs within 3 minutes following release of the tourniquet, 80% of these wounds are considered healed. If blood flow does not start by 3 minutes a more proximal level of amputation should be considered.[41]

The lesser toes should be amputated through the proximal phalanx, although any level through the phalanges or joints can be used (Fig. 12-2). A prerequisite is that the flaps be long enough to close without tension. Flaps can be of any design (e.g., fish-mouth, long plantar, long dorsal, or side-to-side), but should be individualized. Prior to closure the flap should be pulled to close it to determine whether it closes without tension. Bony prominences are rounded off and resected to prevent pressure. Similarly, dog ears need to be trimmed.

AMPUTATIONS OF THE HALLUX

The lesser toes can be removed without loss of function. The same applies to the hallux, although amputations of the hallux cause a problem with push-off in rapid walking. Therefore, the hallux is approached differently to preserve some length, even if only a small stump is left (Fig. 12-3).

Acute and chronic osteomyelitis of the

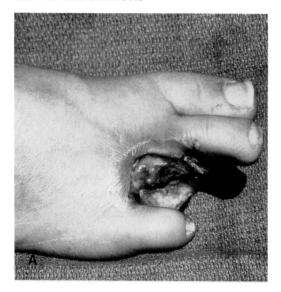

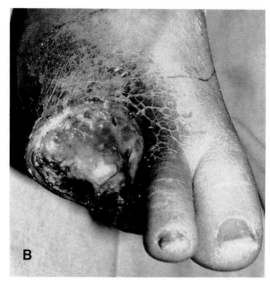

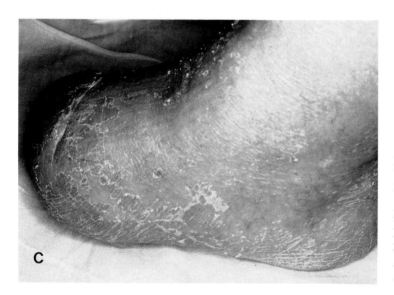

FIGURE 12-1 ■ *A,* This patient is a 50-year-old, insulin-dependent female who presented with a 3-month history of a painless draining lesion of the fourth toe. *B,* The toe was amputated at the metatarsophalangeal joint, followed by dry gangrene of the third toe. Vascular evaluation revealed no palpable pulses distal to the ankle and the Doppler ischemic index at the midfoot was 0.2. *C,* The patient underwent a popliteal to dorsalis pedis bypass graft and the foot was salvaged with a successful transmetatarsal amputation.

hallux are approached by a radical debridement of the toe. All infected bone is removed, leaving a flail soft tissue stump. The bone should be excised through a single longitudinal incision medially, dorsally, or laterally. This incision is determined by the position of the draining sinus. The wound is packed open and left to granulate in. Patients usually prefer a shortened, floppy hallux rather than an amputated one.

METATARSAL RAY RESECTION

When carefully performed metatarsal ray resection is an excellent procedure because it can be fashioned in any manner, removing portions of infected metatarsals. Isolated middle metatarsal or ray resection (second, third, fourth) or a partial lateral amputation of the forefoot can also be performed, with good results (Fig. 12-4). A functional foot remains after removal of all

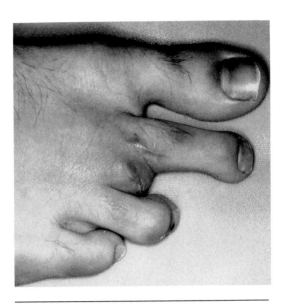

FIGURE 12–2 ■ This amputation of the third toe was performed for dry gangrene, which was localized to the tip. Note the small stump of the third toe remnant, because the amputation was performed through the base of the proximal phalanx. Short toes prevent medial and lateral drift of the adjacent toes and, if possible, should be preserved.

the lesser toes and an oblique resection of the lateral metatarsals. If the medial forefoot remnant is long enough these amputations function well, so that it is not necessary to resort to a more proximal level of amputation.

Partial amputations are worth the effort and can be fashioned to meet the constraints of forefoot anatomy and infection (Fig. 12-5). Generally, lateral ray resection is more successful. Medial resections of the first or first and second metatarsals have been performed successfully, but are less commonly indicated. Some do not recommend ray resections on the medial side of the foot and proceed directly to transmetatarsal amputations (Figs. 12-6 and 12-7).[20,52]

METATARSAL HEAD RESECTION

Diabetic patients with ulcerative lesions on the plantar aspect of the forefoot might not require a metatarsal ray resection. In any forefoot ablative surgery it is important to provide a well-distributed, weight-bearing plantar surface of the forefoot. In some patients who have had single or multiple metatarsal head resections the weight is redistributed to the adjacent metatarsal head, and could cause further ulceration. Under these circumstances, treatment of the mal perforant ulcers can be approached by resection of all the metatarsal heads. This procedure was originally described by Hoffman for use in those with rheumatoid arthritis, and it is also helpful in managing the diabetic foot.[53] It relieves major pressure areas under the forefoot that are likely to cause future ulcers. Simultaneously, it decompresses the forefoot in the presence of large ulcerations (Fig. 12-8).[53,54]

Surgery can be performed in the presence of plantar ulceration. A transverse dorsal incision at the level of the metatarsal neck is used. In the presence of claw toes the extensor tendons should be cut. Some preserve the extensor tendons, which could produce recurrent clawing of the lesser toes. The metatarsal heads are approached sequentially at the level of the metatarsal neck. An oscillating saw blade should be used rather than a bone cutter. The bone edges need to be smoothed and cut obliquely through the metatarsal neck, providing a beveled, weight-bearing surface on the plantar aspect of the foot. In the presence of active ulceration a Betadine sponge is used to debride the plantar ulcer aggressively once the metatarsal heads have been amputated. The sponge is vigorously pulled backward and forward through the ulcer, removing all debris and contaminated tissue. The dorsal wound is closed loosely over a small Kritter drain, as described above (Fig. 12-9).

TRANSMETATARSAL AMPUTATION

The transmetatarsal amputation has been popularized by McKitrick and associates.[40] The rationale for this procedure is that a distally based amputation has a greater likelihood of success than removal of a single gangrenous toe. Additionally, this protects the patient against subsequent ulceration and involvement of the remaining toes and metatarsal heads. Wheelock and colleagues have reported two groups of diabetic patients who are candidates for this amputation.[55] One

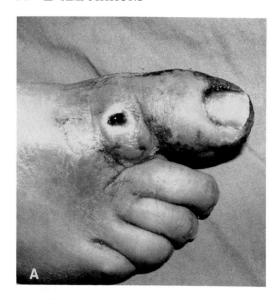

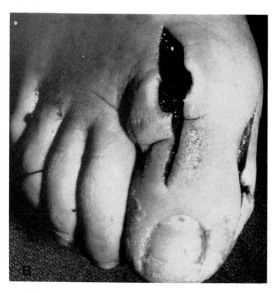

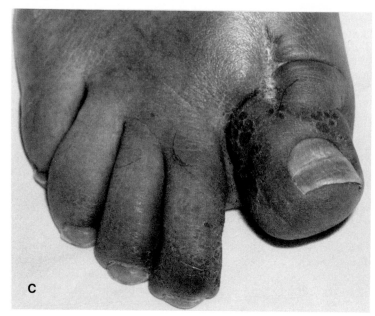

FIGURE 12–3 ■ *A,* This patient presented with a 6-month history of a draining sinus over the dorsal and medial aspects of the hallux. Radiographs showed chronic osteomyelitis of the hallux phalanges. *B,* Rather than perform an amputation of the hallux, the sinuses were drained through longitudinal incisions. As a rule, one incision is optimal to prevent sloughing of the intervening skin bridge. *C,* The wounds have healed and, in spite of a short stubby hallux, this patient functions well.

group consists of patients with a good blood supply but who have diabetic neuropathy and severe infection. The goal is to reconstruct the foot after severe infection in the forefoot. In the other group, with arterial insufficiency, multiple areas of skin necrosis are present and healing is more difficult. The indication for performing this procedure is gangrene of all or part of one or more toes, localized and not involving the dorsal or plantar aspects of the foot.[40] Both the wound

and infection should be controlled prior to surgery. If the gangrene is well localized to the distal toes, the procedure is likely to be successful if adequate Doppler ischemic indices are determined. If the gangrene has extended onto a small area on the medial or lateral aspect of the foot, this is excised without jeopardizing the final result. Local areas of distal and dorsal infection can also be excised. These can be left to granulate in or can be covered with a split-thickness graft.

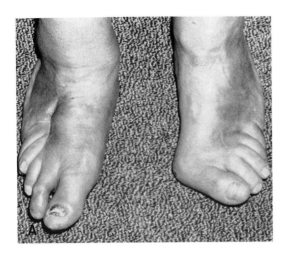

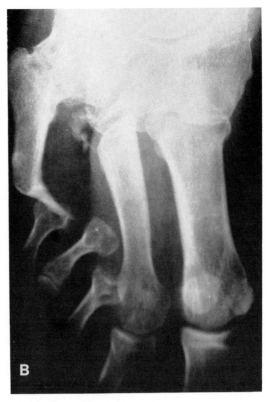

FIGURE 12–4 ■ *A*, This patient underwent resection of the third and fourth metatarsals on separate occasions. Resection of the fifth metatarsal head was performed at a later stage and the patient continued to function well in spite of the odd shape and appearance of the foot. *B*, Radiograph showing resected metatarsals.

The incision is carefully planned. A long plantar flap is preferable. The dorsal skin incision is made directly overlying the level of the metatarsal necks or the level at which the proposed bone cuts are to be made. On the medial and lateral edges the incision extends vertically midway between the dorsal and plantar skin, and then extends distally to the end of the plantar flap. On the plantar aspect of the foot the incision is made transversely 1 cm proximal to the metatarsal phalangeal joint crease. No undermining or dissection of the dorsal flap is carried out and the incision is deepened directly onto bone. The plantar flap is created as thickly as possible. The metatarsals are cut with an oscillating saw obliquely angled 15 to 20° against the horizontal axis. The plantar edge of the metatarsal shaft should be beveled to a curved lower edge. Hemostasis is obtained throughout using small hemostats and no electrocautery. Closure is made over a Kritter drain with loose sutures in the skin and subcutaneous tissue only.

LISFRANC'S AND CHOPART'S LEVEL AMPUTATIONS

Chopart's and Lisfranc's level amputations have not always been successful because of persistent postoperative equinus deformity (Fig. 12-10). This results in distal plantar ulceration. Nevertheless, in some instances preserving length of the foot at Lisfranc's level is indicated. Patients do not depend on prostheses at this level, as with a Syme's amputation. This amputation is also more likely to heal than a transmetatarsal amputation. It is indicated when more extensive necrosis and gangrene of the forefoot preclude transmetatarsal amputation.

The problems of equinus contracture and deformity are lessened by carefully planned surgery. An Achilles tendon lengthening, easily performed percutaneously, is essential in Chopart's amputation. Additionally, transfer of the extensor and anterior tibial tendons to the dorsum of the foot can minimize and prevent the deformity. A problem

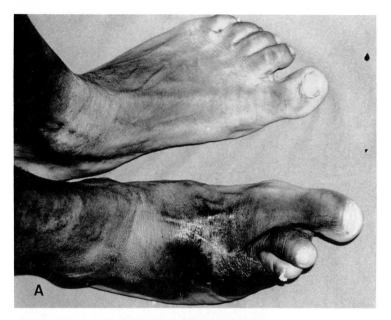

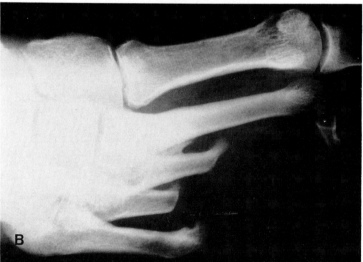

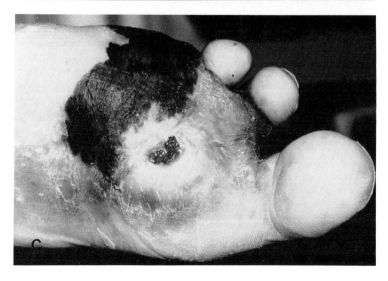

FIGURE 12–5 ■ *A*, and *B*, This partial foot amputation was successful until re-ulceration occurred. *C*, The patient was lost to follow-up and returned with continued ulceration under the second metatarsal head. A split-thickness skin graft had been carried out in the intervening period. This patient would have been better served by a short transmetatarsal or Lisfranc's amputation.

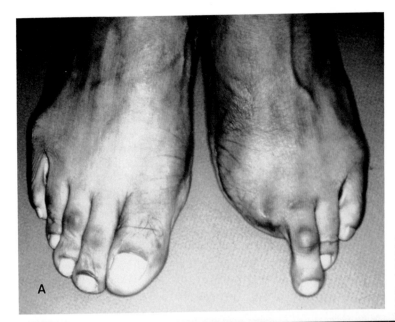

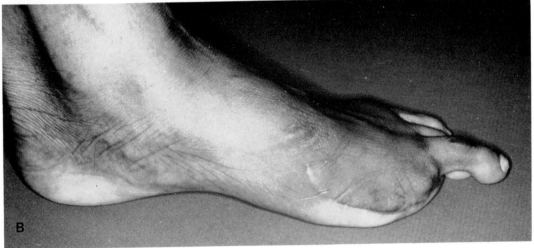

FIGURE 12-6 ■ *A* and *B*, Partial medial amputation of the hallux and second toe succeeded here and has been stable.

with transferring the extensor tendons is that it is done in a compromised host environment. Adding the tendon transfers could therefore compromise healing.

As with the transmetatarsal amputation, long plantar flaps are used. The length of the flap is one that joins the dorsal skin at the weight-bearing margins of the forefoot. Occasionally the plantar flap is compromised because of necrosis, and the design for closure is modified so that more of a fish-mouth-type flap closure is present. For Lisfranc's level the foot is disarticulated at the tarsometatarsal joints. As much soft tissue as possible, including the intrinsic mus-

cles, is preserved through subperiosteal dissection of the metatarsals. These local muscle pedicles are important in the presence of inadequate flaps distally, and provide extra bulk to the flap. When resecting the first and second metatarsals, the first dorsal and plantar interosseous muscles are carefully dissected to preserve the dorsalis pedis and major perforating branch. These muscles are sutured loosely to the adjacent periosteum. For Lisfranc's amputations the balance of the extrinsic flexor and extensor tendons must be preserved. The posterior tibial tendon insertion is preserved. With loss of the peroneal attachments the foot tends to drift

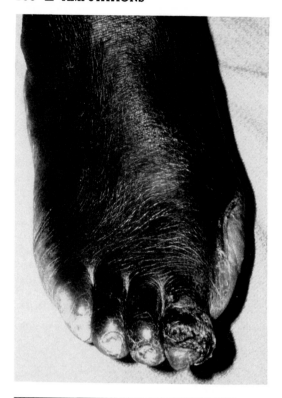

FIGURE 12–7 ■ Problems with medial ray resection include ulceration of the tip of the second toe. This can be avoided with proper attention to footwear and a soft orthosis to prevent rubbing against the medial edge of the second toe. This patient ultimately required a transmetatarsal amputation.

into varus. The anterior tibial tendon insertion can be preserved, although part of this is usually compromised by the resection of the first metatarsal. With loss of function of the extrinsic toe extensors the foot also develops an equinus contracture, but this is not as severe in Lisfranc's amputation as in Chopart's amputation. Both the varus and equinus deformities can be avoided by careful re-attachment of the long extensor tendons to the dorsolateral aspect of the foot. Experience has shown that insertion of these tendons into the lateral cuneiform is adequate.

In Chopart's amputations, the same principles of preserving the length of the plantar flap apply. An Achilles tendon lengthening is part of the procedure, because a postoperative equinus contracture is difficult to

prevent (Fig. 12-11). Varus deformity is not a problem, because the posterior tibial tendon insertion is sacrificed distally. The anterior tibial tendon is attached to the neck of the talus. This is sutured to the periosteal remnant at this site or passed through a 4.5-mm drill hole in the dorsolateral neck of the talus at 45° to the vertical axis.

Postoperatively, closure of the skin, drains, and irrigation are as described for the other amputations. The foot requires careful postoperative immobilization in dorsiflexion in a cast or a carefully molded splint.

Calcanectomy

The surgical approach to acute and chronic infections of the calcaneus presents consid-

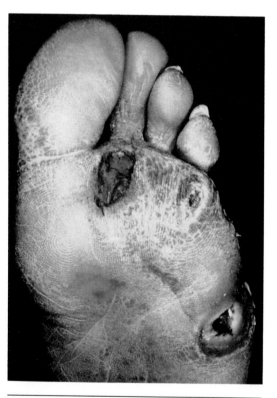

FIGURE 12–8 ■ This patient sustained repeated ulcerations under the metatarsal heads over a 1-year period. Resection of one head alone tends to cause a transfer of weight to the adjacent metatarsal head, with further ulceration. To avoid this problem, he was treated successfully by resecting all the metatarsal heads.

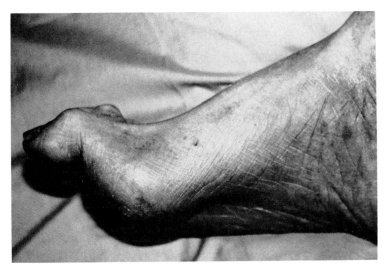

FIGURE 12-9 ■ This patient presented with chronic recurring ulceration of the forefoot. On each occasion the ulcers healed in a total contact cast but, with recurrent breakdown, resection of all the metatarsal heads was performed, with no recurrent ulceration over a 2-year period.

erable difficulty in the diabetic. Several authors have reported treatment of chronic osteomyelitis of the calcaneus caused by puncture wounds, trauma, and postsurgical and hematogenous infection.[56-60] Diabetic foot lesions with an exposed calcaneus re-

ceive aggressive wound care. Repeated pinch grafts are performed until the wound granulates in. In the few cases of calcaneal osteomyelitis extensive destruction of the bone has been present, and I have performed a total calcanectomy rather than repeated de-

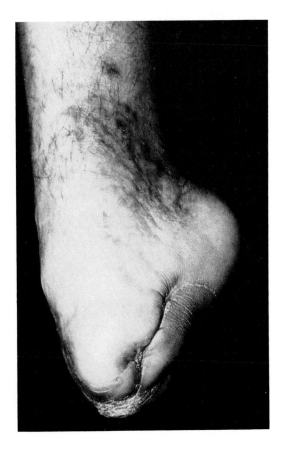

FIGURE 12-10 ■ Equinus contracture after this Lisfranc's amputation caused recurrent ulceration of the distal plantar stump. This problem can be avoided with an Achilles tendon lengthening and careful postoperative stabilization of the foot. This patient was finally treated 2 years following the amputation with an Achilles tendon lengthening, ankle capsulotomy, and application of a walking postoperative cast.

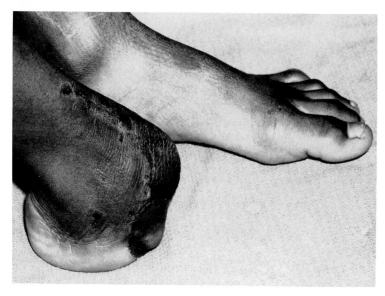

FIGURE 12–11 ■ This Chopart's amputation has been stable in spite of the anterior split-thickness skin grafts. The equinus position of the foot is not a result of contracture but of the position in which the patient is seated.

bridements (Fig. 12-12). These are likely to fail. A plantar longitudinal incision is used, through which the ulcer is excised as an ellipse. Infected tissue and pus are evacuated from the deep fascial space. The insertion of the Achilles tendon, the talocalcaneal interosseous ligaments, and the capsules of the subtalar and calcaneocuboid joints are divided. It is important to remove all debris and potentially infected tissue, followed by loose closure.

The wounds are managed postoperatively in the manner described by Gaenslen,[56] continuing irrigation for approximately 7 days. These wounds tend to continue draining for a long period. A total contact cast is applied as soon as the acute inflammatory phase has passed, even in the presence of drainage. An average of 7 weeks is required for drainage to cease and the wound to close. The alternative amputation for this problem is below the knee, because the Syme's amputation cannot be performed in the presence of draining lesions of the heel pad. Patients subsequently ambulate in a polypropylene splint with a plastizote and foam filler in the region of the heel defect.

The Syme's Amputation

The Syme's amputation has evolved since its introduction in 1843. Initial experience with this amputation in diabetic dysvascu-

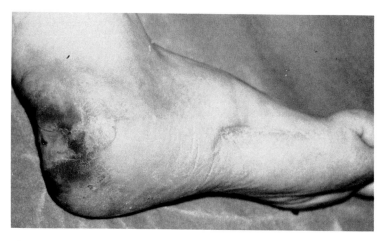

FIGURE 12–12 ■ This patient had undergone 14 previous operative debridements of the calcaneus and a free flap in an attempt to control the draining neurotrophic ulceration. Rather than perform any further debridements a total calcanectomy was carried out successfully, with delayed closure of the wound by secondary granulation in a total contact cast.

lar feet was unsatisfactory, and many of these amputations required a subsequent proximal amputation. Use of this type of amputation has been increasing. The success rate of the Syme's amputation is now about 95%.[31,61–64] The Syme's amputation has a number of attractive features. The longer length makes rehabilitation and prosthetic wear easier. With maturation of the stump patients can walk short distances without a prosthesis. This might be all that is required for some elderly patients.

The history of the Syme's amputation and its modifications in the past century parallel progress made in the field of diabetic amputation surgery. The use of intraoperative post-tourniquet bleeding was the first step toward improving the results of the operation. This was followed by successfully predicting the outcome of surgery using careful preoperative vascular assessment with Doppler ultrasound and the ischemic index. Close attention to detail is also important in obtaining a good result (Fig. 12-13). Further success has been achieved with the staging of this operation into two separate procedures.

Syme's two-stage amputation is indicated when extensive infection in the forefoot is present, whereas single-stage amputation is indicated for dry gangrene or chronic ulceration.[20] Candidates for this procedure must be able to bear weight in a prosthesis, the heel pad must be free of wounds, the Doppler systolic pressure at the ankle must be 70 mm Hg or more, the Doppler index should be greater than 0.45, no acute infection should be present in the ankle or more proximally, and intraoperative bleeding should occur in the skin flaps within 3 minutes after tourniquet release.[20]

Operative techniques have been described by Harris,[62] Spittler and co-workers,[64] and Warren and colleagues.[22] In the first stage of the amputation, an incision is made directly anterior to the ankle approximately 1.5 cm distal to the malleoli. This incision is deepened without any dissection of subcutaneous tissue planes. The tendons are incised and allowed to retract. The neurovascular bundle that lies posteromedially needs to be carefully preserved, because the posterior tibial artery supplies the entire flap. The Achilles tendon attachment is carefully divided from the calcaneus without perfo-

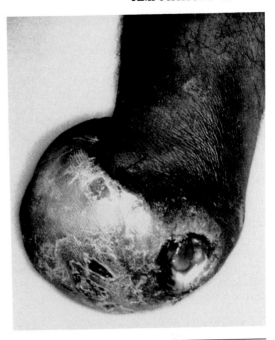

FIGURE 12–13 ■ This Syme's stump is imperfect and chronic ulceration necessitated a below-knee amputation. Care should be taken to place the heel flap so that the plantar surface of the flap is centered below the tibia and held there until healing has occurred. These ulcerations are also common with an unstable heel flap. A flaccid heel can be prevented by careful subperosteal dissection of the heel flap, which is then attached firmly to the cut surface of the bone. Once the heel flap has become unstable it cannot be corrected, and a below-knee amputation is required.

rating the skin. It is important to dissect the calcaneus beneath the periosteum to preserve the fascial septae and the heel pad. In this manner the heel is not too mobile and the flap adheres to the cancellous bone surfaces. During this stage no attempt is made to trim redundant skin or corners of the flaps. The wounds are closed in layers with thick absorbable sutures to preserve fascial layers and the skin is closed with nonabsorbable sutures without tension. A continuous irrigation drain is used. The wound is usually healed enough for the patient to commence walking in a well-padded cast 2 weeks postoperatively.

The second stage of the Syme's amputation is performed 6 weeks later. Medial and lateral incisions are made directly over the dog ears and the malleoli are osteotomized flush with the ankle joint, leaving the articular cartilage intact.

Syme's amputees often consider themselves to have no disability, but only an inconvenient shoe or prosthetic problem. The stump requires good care by the patient, but most patients have trouble-free lifetime use of this stump.[65] The stump is nearly as long as the normal leg and this, added to the potential for end-bearing, provides a stump that approaches a normal foot. It has been stated that this is the most serviceable of all the amputations of the leg.[62] Below-knee amputees cannot walk on their prosthesis all day without injuring the stump, because no specialized end-bearing skin surface is present. It is recommended that the Syme's amputation be used whenever possible.

POSTSURGICAL CARE

The limb is kept in a protected position postoperatively. Patients are required to remain at bed rest with the limb elevated for 3 weeks, avoiding the dependent position. The continuous irrigation drain system is left in place for 48 hours. Diabetic wounds take longer to heal and it is advisable to leave sutures in for about 3 to 4 weeks when uncertain about the status of healing. Systemic antibiotics are continued postoperatively until wounds are healed. Intravenous antibiotics are continued for approximately 10 days postoperatively, followed by oral medication as required. Once the wounds are healed partial weight-bearing is permitted, depending on the circumstances of the amputation and the appearance of the foot.

Patients are routinely fitted with a postoperative shoe or extra depth shoes with 1/4-inch plastizote insoles. If the foot is not ready for ambulation at this stage, even in a protected shoe, a plaster cast is used. When used, nonweight-bearing casts are applied initially for 2 weeks. The initial cast is changed in 4 days and the wound is inspected. After the second week a total contact cast is applied and the patient is permitted to ambulate. Some patients require ambulatory aids until independent, but most are fully weight-bearing after a few days in the cast. The cast is discontinued when maturation of the wound occurs.

Use of the total contact cast has helped postoperative management. It helps mobilize the patient rapidly, preventing many problems associated with prolonged bed rest. It also controls postoperative edema, distributes the load on the plantar surface of the foot, and supports the surgical wound. The presence of edema, local increases in temperature, and unhealed wound edges are all indications for continuing total contact cast treatment.

POSTOPERATIVE FOOTWEAR

Amputation surgery significantly alters the weight-bearing forces on the remaining foot during walking and standing. During stance phase, the load passes lateral to the center of the foot and then forward between the first and second metatarsal heads. This shifts directly under the hallux at the time of toe-off. Load-bearing in the forefoot is three times that of the hindfoot, and the hallux plays an important role in the distribution of these forces.[66-68]

In forefoot and midfoot amputations, a concentration of force occurs in the forefoot adjacent to the amputation site. This load on the plantar aspect during toe-off can be reduced by changing the shoe or sole, or both. A medial and lateral steel shank stiffens the sole, to which a tapered midfoot rocker is added. An orthotic device can also assist by decreasing the force on the forefoot. Orthoses are made of firmer densities of plastizote or polypropylene, supplemented by firm and softer plastizote distally.

A problem inherent in medial ray amputation is necrosis of the adjacent toe laterally. Loss of the hallux transfers the load laterally, causing callosity and ulceration over the tip of the remaining toe (or toes). This can be avoided by using an orthosis that incorporates a filler for the amputated hallux and provides appropriate metatarsal support and padding.

A healthy, long, transmetatarsal stump should present no problem for footwear. In some patients with shorter transmetatarsal amputations, however, loading the plantar aspect of the distal forefoot occurs. An ordinary shoe has a "break" at the level of the metatarsophalangeal joints, corresponding to the crease that occurs during the toe-off phase of gait. Patients with a shorter transmetatarsal stump might therefore have difficulty because the shoe break occurs at the end of the stump rather than distally, as the shoe is designed. The shoe leather forms irregular wrinkles, which dig into the top of the stump and produce ulceration. This can be avoided by fitting the shoe with a stiff steel shank medially and laterally to protect the forefoot. Rigidity itself, however, might allow the heel to piston out of the shoe during toe-off, but this can be prevented by adding a rocker bottom to the shoe sole. A 1/4-inch tapered rocker is recommended. This can later be increased to 1/2 inch if the forefoot requires further unloading.

Lisfranc's amputation stumps are usually long enough to suspend a shoe but, because of the tendency to develop an equinus deformity, shoe fitting is difficult. The wear on the plantar aspect of the distal foot can be prevented by stabilizing the ankle with a polypropylene ankle-foot orthosis. Chopart's amputations are too short to suspend a shoe, and these patients should be fitted with an ankle-foot orthosis or a Chopart's appliance. It was stated above that the Syme's amputation is durable and represents the most effective and serviceable amputation of the leg. The only drawback of this amputation is the large bulbous stump. The prosthesis must therefore be large to accommodate it, making it less attractive. Modifications of these prostheses are now available that are made from lighter materials, allowing a snug fit that is more acceptable.

References

1. Levin CM, Dealy FN. The surgical diabetic, a five-year survey. Ann Surg. 1935; 102:1029–39.
2. West KM. Epidemiology of diabetes and its vascular lesions. New York: Elsevier; 1978.
3. Bell ET. Incidence of gangrene of the extremities in nondiabetic and in diabetic persons. Arch Pathol. 1950; 49:469–473.
4. Christensen S. Lower extremity amputations in the county of Aallborg, 1961–1971: population study and follow-up. Acta Orthop Scand. 1976; 47:329–334.
5. Hierton T, James H. Lower extremity amputation in Upsala County 1947–1969: Incidence and prosthetic rehabilitation. Acta Orthop Scand. 1973; 44:573–582.
6. Most R, Sinnock P. The epidemiology of lower extremity amputations in diabetic individuals. Diabetes Care. 1983; 6:87–91.
7. The National Diabetes Data Group. Selected statistics on health and medical care of diabetics. 1980; a-3.
8. Diabetes data. Bethesda, MD: National Institutes of Health; 1977; NIH Publ. 79-1568.
9. Davidson JK, Alogna M, Goldsmith M, et al. Assessment of program effectiveness at Grady Memorial Hospital. In: Steiner S, Lawrence PA eds. Educating diabetic patients. New York: Springer; 1981; 329–348.
10. Hoar CS, Torres J. Evaluation of below-the-knee amputation in the treatment of diabetic gangrene. N Engl J Med. 1962; 266:440–443.
11. Sibert S. Amputations of the lower extremities in diabetes mellitus. A follow-up study of 294 cases. Diabetes. 1952; 1:297.
12. Cameron CC, Lennard-Jones JE, Robinson DM. Amputations in the diabetic: outcome and survival. Lancet. 1964; 2:605–607.
13. Ecker MD, Jacobs BS. Lower extremity amputations in diabetic patients. Diabetes. 1970; 19:189.
14. Goldner MG. The fate of the second leg in the diabetic amputee. Diabetes. 1960; 9:100.
15. Baddeley RM, Fulford JC. A trial of conservative amputations for lesions of the feet in diabetes mellitus. Br J Surg. 1965; 52:38–43.
16. Whitehouse FW, Jurgensen C, Block MA. The later life of the diabetic amputee. Another look at the fate of the second leg. Diabetes. 1968; 17:520–521.
17. Haimovici H. Peripheral arterial disease in diabetes mellitus. In: Ellenberg M, Rifkin H, eds. Diabetes mellitus: theory and practice. New York: McGraw-Hill; 1970.
18. Romano RL, Burgess EM. Level selection in lower extremity amputations. Clin Orthop. 1971; 74:177–184.
19. Huston CC, Bivins BA, Ernst CB, et al. Morbid implications of above-knee amputations. Report of a series and review of the literature. Arch Surg. 1980; 115:165–167.
20. Wagner FW Jr. Amputation at the foot and ankle: Current status. Clin Orthop. 1977; 122:62–69.
21. Singer A, Rossi G. Radical local surgery in diabetic gangrene. J Mt Sinai Hosp. 1968; 35:390–395.
22. Warren R, Thayer TR, Achenbach J, et al. The Syme amputation in peripheral arterial disease (West Roxbury and Framingham V.A. Hospitals). Surgery. 1955; 37:156.
23. Faris J, Duncan H. Vascular disease and vascular function in the lower limb in diabetes. Diabetes Res. 1984; 1:171–177.
24. Logerfo FW, Carson JE, Mannick MA. Improved results with femoropopliteal vein grafts for limb salvage. Arch Surg. 1977; 112:567.
25. Roon AJ, Moore WS, Goldstone J. Below-knee amputation: a modern approach. Am J Surg. 1977; 134:153–158.
26. Kelly PJ, Janes JJ. Criteria for determining the proper level of amputation in occlusive vascular disease. J Bone Joint Surg. 1957; 29A:883–891.
27. Warren R, Kihn RB. A survey of lower extremity amputations for ischemia. Surgery. 1968; 63:107.
28. Baddeley RM, Fulford JC. The use of arteriog-

raphy in conservative amputations for lesions of the feet in diabetes mellitus. Br J Surg. 1964; 51:658.

29. Pedersen HE, Lamont RL. Below-knee amputation for gangrene. South Med J. 1964; 57:820–825.

30. Barnes RB, Shanik GD, Slaymaker EE. An index of healing in below-knee amputation: leg blood pressure by Doppler ultrasound. Surgery. 1976; 79:13–20.

31. Carter SA. The relationship of distal systolic pressures to healing of skin lesion with arterial occlusive disease with special reference to diabetes mellitus. Scand J Clin Lab Invest. 1973; 31(Suppl 128):239–243.

32. Kazamias TM, Gander MP, Franklin DL. Blood pressure measurements with Doppler ultrasound flowmeter. J Appl Physiol. 1971; 30:585.

33. Wagner FW Jr, Buggs H. Use of Doppler ultrasound in determining healing levels in diabetic dysvascular lower extremity problems. In: Bergan JJ, Yao JST, eds., Gangrene and severe ischemia of the lower extremities. New York: Grune & Stratton; 1978; 131–138.

34. Wagner FW. The dysvascular foot. A system for diagnosis and treatment. Foot Ankle 1981; 2:64–122.

35. Peacock JH. A comparative study of the digital cutaneous temperatures and hand blood flows in the normal hand, primary Raynaud's disease and primary acrocyanosis. Clin Sci. 1959; 28:25–33.

36. Peacock JH. The effect of changes in local temperature on the blood flows of the normal hand, primary Raynaud's disease and primary acrocyanosis. Clin Sci. 1960; 19:505–512.

37. Golbranson FL. The use of skin temperature determinations in lower extremity amputation level selection. Foot Ankle. 1982; 3:170–173.

38. Moore WS. Determination of amputation level measurement of skin blood flow with Xe-133. Arch Surg. 1973; 107:798–802.

39. Kostuik JP, Wood D, Hornby R, et al. The measurement of skin blood flow in peripheral vascular disease by epicutaneous application of xenon-133. J Bone Joint Surg. 1976; 58A:833.

40. McKittrick LS, McKittrick JB, Risley TS. Transmetatarsal amputation for infection or gangrene in patients with diabetes mellitus. Ann Surg. 1949; 130:826.

41. Wagner FW Jr. The diabetic foot and amputations of the foot. In: Mann RA, ed. DuVries' surgery of the foot, 4th ed. St. Louis: CV Mosby; 1978; 341–380.

42. Wagner FW. The diabetic foot. Orthopaedics. 1987; 10:163–171.

43. Goodman J, Bessman AM, Teget B, et al. Risk factors in local surgical procedures for diabetic gangrene. Surg Gynecol Obstet. 1976; 143:587–591.

44. Sizer JS, Wheelock FC. Digital amputations in diabetic patients. Surgery. 1972; 72:1980.

45. Collens WS, Vlahos E, Dobkin GB, et al. Conservative management of gangrene in the diabetic patient. JAMA. 1962; 181:692.

46. Gershenfeld L. Bactericidal efficiency of iodine solutions. J Am Pharm Assoc. 1932; 21:894.

47. Singer A, Rossi G. Early results with 20 femoropopliteal vein by-pass grafts for severe peripheral ischemia. J Mt Sinai Hosp. 1968; 35:234.

48. Saraffian SK, Ibrahim IN, Brenhan JH. A method of ankle foot peripheral nerve block for mid and forefoot surgery. Foot Ankle. 1983; 4:86–90.

49. Rosenberg N, London IM. Excision and drainage for infections of the foot with gangrene in the diabetic. Arch Surg. 1956; 72:160.

50. Pratt TC. Gangrene and infection in the diabetic. Med Clin North Am. 1975; 49:987–1004.

51. Kritter AE. A technique for salvage of the infected diabetic gangrenous foot. Orthop Clin North Am. 1973; 4:21.

52. Hunter GA. Results of minor foot amputations for ischemia of the lower extremity in diabetics and non-diabetics. Can J Surg. 1975; 18:273–276.

53. Hoffman P. An operation for severe grades of contracted or clawed toes. Am J Orthop. 1911; 9:441–449.

54. Jacobs R. Hoffman procedure in the ulcerated diabetic neuropathic foot. Foot Ankle. 1982; 3:142–149.

55. Wheellock FC, McKittrick JB, Root HF. Evaluation of the transmetatarsal amputation in patients with diabetes mellitus. Surgery. 1957; 41:184.

56. Gaenslen FJ. Split-heel approach in osteomyelitis of the os calcis. J Bone Joint Surg. 1931; 13:759.

57. Broudy AS. The split heel technique in the management of calcaneal osteomyelitis. Clin Orthop. 1976; 119:202–206.

58. Antoniou D, Conner AN. Osteomyelitis of the calcaneus and talus. J Bone Joint Surg. 1974; 56A:338.

59. Martini M, Martini-Benkedache Y, Bekhechi T, et al. Treatment of chronic osteomyelitis of the calcaneus by resection of the calcaneus. A report of twenty cases. J Bone Joint Surg. 1974; 56A:542.

60. Eid AN. The treatment of chronic hematogenous osteomyelitis of the os calcis. Acta Orthop Scand. 1977; 48:712–717.

61. Catterall RCF. Syme's amputation by Joseph Lister after sixty-six years. J Bone Joint Surg. 1967; 49B:144.

62. Harris RI. Syme's amputation. The technical details essential for success. J Bone Joint Surg. 1956; 28B:614.

63. Rosenman LD. Syme amputation for ischemic disease in the foot. Am J Surg. 1969; 118:194.

64. Spittler AW, Brenner JS, Payne JW. Syme amputation performed in two stages. J Bone Joint Surg. 1954; 36A:37.

65. Baker GCW, Stableforth PG. Syme's amputation, a review of sixty-seven cases. J Bone Joint Surg. 1969; 51B:482.

66. Saunders JBCM, Inman VT. The major determinants in normal and pathologic gait. J Bone Joint Surg. 1953; 35A:543.

67. Grundy M, Tosh B, McLeigh RD, et al. An investigation of the centers of pressure under the foot with walking. J Bone Joint Surg. 1975; 57B:98.

68. Cavanaugh PR, Rodgers MM, Iiboshi A. Pressure distribution under symptom-free feet during barefoot standing. Foot Ankle. 1987; 7:262–276.

Suggested Readings

1. Harris RI. The history and development of Syme's amputation. Artif Limbs. 1961; 6:4.
2. Jacobs JE. Observations of neuropathic (charcot) joints occurring in diabetes mellitus. J Bone Joint Surg. 1958; 40A:1043–1057.
3. Jacobs RL, Karmody AM. The team approach in salvage of the diabetic foot. Surg Annu. 1977.
4. Mooney V, Wagner FW Jr. Neurocirculatory disorder of the foot. Clin Orthop. 1977; 122:53–61.
5. Srinivasan J. Symes amputations in insensitive feet. J Bone Joint Surg. 1973; 55A:558.
6. Wagner FW, Jr. A classification and treatment program for diabetic neuropathic, and dysvascular foot problems. In: The American Academy of Orthopaedic Surgeons Instructional Course Lectures, vol 28. St. Louis: CV Mosby; 1979; 143–165.

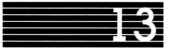

Prosthetics and Rehabilitation in the Diabetic Amputee

YEONGCHI WU, M.D.
JOEL PRESS, M.D.

Amputation of the lower extremity in diabetics because of soft tissue infection results not only in immediate impairment of locomotion and self-care, but also in psychosocial maladjustment. Amputation is more frequent in diabetic patients than in the general population. The exact number of patients with amputation is not known. According to the National Center for Health Statistics, an estimated 274,000 civilian noninstitutional patients had amputation of major limbs in 1971 in the United States. This number rose to 358,000 in 1977 and to 631,000 in 1981.[1,2] In 1984 the National Hospital Discharge Survey of 407 hospitals showed that an estimated 129,000 amputations were performed in acute care hospitals, including 41,000 toe or partial foot, 32,000 below-the-knee, and 33,000 above-the-knee amputations.[3]

With an increase in the elderly population and in the number of diabetics, the number of amputations caused by peripheral vascular disease is expected to rise steadily. The cost to the nation in providing care to diabetic amputees, in the time loss from work, and in the change of quality of life will continue to increase.

The goal of managing diabetic amputees is to minimize secondary medical and psychologic complications by helping patients gain their maximally attainable functional level as quickly as possible. The medical, psychosocial, and economic issues involved are complex, but good results can often be achieved by the well-coordinated efforts of a multidisciplinary team. All members of the specialized team contribute their particular knowledge and expertise to the overall re-habilitation of the patient. In addition, the importance of involving peer patients in counseling has been recognized by those in major amputee centers. The benefits of peer counseling include the reduction of psychologic maladjustment and the provision of consumer-oriented education to help attain rehabilitation goals.

GENERAL CONSIDERATIONS

For the past 20 or 30 years, selection of the proper amputation level using advanced preoperative evaluation techniques has improved the rate of primary wound healing and of the residual limbs capability to bear weight. The final functional level attained by any given patient depends not only on the presurgical evaluation and surgical management, but on postsurgical rehabilitation. Consideration of the patient as a whole in the rehabilitation process is essential to a successful outcome.

Three decades ago most (below knee: above knee ratio 0.81) lower extremity amputations were performed at an above-the-knee level.[4] Currently, many such amputations are at least attempted below the knee initially (below knee: above knee ratio 1.62).[5] This change is related to better understanding of the gait mechanism, to the importance of preserving the knee joint for an improved outcome, and to advances in medical and surgical management of the disease.

The principles of early postoperative care of the lower extremity amputee are similar, regardless of the type of amputation. These include improvement of the patient's general health and self-care independence, preparation of the stump for prosthetic fitting, and minimizing the emotional, social, and economic consequences that follow amputation. Prevention of secondary complications because of inadequate self-care, poor medical follow-up, and improper prosthetic fitting or footwear is emphasized.

In diabetic patients, foot deformity, insensitivity caused by peripheral neuropathy, impaired visual function, dysvascularity, infection, and gangrene are contributing factors for potential multiple limb amputation. With prophylactic programs, major limb amputations dropped 50% in centers in which better foot care had been instituted.[6] Total contact casting facilitates healing of chronic foot ulceration. Prevention of recurrence of such ulceration, however, requires proper footwear, and properly fitted footwear can promote healing of the foot ulcer. Prevention of trauma and chronic irritation from improperly fitting shoes is extremely important. Adequate foot hygiene, proper management of skin ulceration, and special footwear can often avert the need for amputation.

The diffuseness of atherosclerotic vascular disease is evidenced by a 33% incidence of contralateral lower limb loss within 5 years in patients undergoing lower extremity amputation.[7] Discontinuing smoking, weight control, and proper diet are also essential factors in total care, and can limit damage to an already impaired peripheral circulation. The most common causes of death in amputees are myocardial infarction and stroke.

A properly fitted lower extremity prosthesis can restore nearly normal gait, but amputees require a slightly greater energy cost to ambulate. Patients with a unilateral Syme's amputation (43%) or below-knee amputation (42%) have a relative energy cost higher than that of normal controls (40%).[8] Also, the relative energy cost for crutch walking is considerbly greater than that for walking with a below-knee prosthesis. More energy expenditure (65% more) is required at half the normal speed of ambulation for above-knee amputees as compared to that of normal controls.[9]

Therefore, from a practical standpoint, functional ambulation might not be a goal for patients with advanced cardiac disease or for geriatric patients with bilateral above-knee amputations. On the other hand, it is not unusual for a unilateral geriatric above-knee amputee with satisfactory general health to become a functional ambulator.

A 10-year follow-up of 1770 geriatric patients by Mazet and associates cited by Kerstein[7] showed that 66% of above-knee amputees given prostheses discard them within 6 months. The requirement for high-energy expenditure is probably the main reason for failure of functional ambulation in these patients. Improvements in prosthetic socket design, prosthetic components, and less frequent amputation at the above-knee level in the past 20 years have improved the overall functional outcome in amputees.

Over time, while wearing a prosthesis, skin irritation and excessive stump shrinkage can cause significant problems. Regular monthly follow-up is important to determine how reliable the patient is and to decide how often the patient should be scheduled for follow-up visits.

Rigid Dressing

The goal of stump care in the early postoperative period is to ensure primary wound healing. When the surgical wound has healed, graded pressure can be applied to the stump to facilitate maturation—that is, maximal stump shrinkage and pressure tolerance. Burgess[10,11] is credited for introducing the technique of immediate postsurgical fitting (IPSF) to the United States, which was developed by Berlemont of France in 1961 and adapted by Weiss of Poland in 1963. Immediate postsurgical fitting and ambulation can still be useful in skillful hands with wide experience in use of the technique, but others believe the approach to be difficult to monitor. Many prosthetists, especially when not working in the same facility, do not find it convenient to wait for the completion of surgery to apply the IPSF. This might be one of the main reasons that the IPSF has not been applied uniformly.[12]

The rigid dressing of the IPSF has the following advantages: (1) immobilizaton of soft tissue, which is important during the early stage of wound healing; (2) provision of a fixed volume in the cast to prevent edema;

and (3) protection of the stump from trauma. In a controlled study comparing three types of postoperative stump care procedures, including soft dressing, rigid dressing, and rigid dressing with pylon for weight-bearing, Mooney[13] concluded that immediate postsurgical weight bearing and ambulation can be a deterrent factor to wound healing and should be delayed for several weeks postoperatively. Many amputee specialists have modified the approach of immediate postoperative ambulation to that of "early" postoperative fitting. The early postoperative fitting consists of a thigh-high rigid dressing without an attached pylon for below-knee amputees.

The disadvantages of the conventional thigh-high rigid dressing, with or without a pylon, for below-knee amputees are the following: (1) inability to observe the stump condition during the early postoperative period and during weight-bearing training; (2) cumbersome removal and reapplication of the cast; (3) lack of continuing progressive stump compression for shrinkage; and (4) lack of active range of motion. Following stump healing and final removal of the thigh-high rigid dressing, the stump is managed with an elastic bandaging for shrinkage, which is an unreliable method of stump care. Skin breakdown along the tibial crest and the development of distal edema from improper bandaging have been common reasons for delayed prosthetic fitting.

Common Problems and Methods of Management

The need for total care of the amputee by the members of a multidisciplinary team is important. Before patients actually walk with a prosthesis, they must be in good physical condition. The most commonly seen problems in diabetic amputees are delayed wound healing, chronic ulceration of the contralateral limb, skin breakdown from inappropriate stump wrapping, flexion contracture of the hip and knee, stump edema, and upper extremity weakness with the inability to transfer or use crutches for walking. General deconditioning, anemia, and cardiac insufficiency are other limiting factors for participation in an active rehabilitation program. These problems prolong the rehabilitation process and increase medical expense.

DELAYED WOUND HEALING

Because of the involvement of small vessels, diabetic patients are prone to delayed wound healing. Proper selection of amputation levels improves primary healing of the surgical wound. At times, marginal skin necrosis along the incision line requires frequent debridement and use of a rigid dressing to reduce tissue tension and provide immobilization of the soft tissue.

Superficial open wounds are not a contraindication for prosthetic fitting. Often, weight-bearing with a rigid dressing or a preparatory prosthesis facilitates healing of the wide open superficial wound.[14]

FLEXION CONTRACTURE

Flexion and abduction contracture of the hip and flexion contracture of the knee are preventable complications commonly seen in elderly patients, often before amputation. Although poor positioning of the stump is blamed for this complication, pain in the stump and prolonged wheelchair usage resulting from delays in the rehabilitation process are the main predisposing factors. Lying in a supine position with elevation of the legs on pillows is a common cause of flexion contracture in patients and should be avoided.

When stump pain is present, the natural guarding response often leads to knee flexion contracture in patients with below-knee amputation. Immobilization of the healing soft tissue with the rigid dressing thereby reduces pain and can effectively prevent flexion contracture. Active and passive range-of-motion exercises of the hips and knees can effectively prevent this problem. This is an important aspect of the rehabilitation process during perioperative and preprosthetic care.

Flexion contractures of the hip or knee can cause difficulty in prosthetic fitting and ambulation. This can lead to unstable knee control, deviated gait pattern, and poor cosmetic appearance (Fig. 13-1).

SKIN BREAKDOWN

Pressure sores over bony prominences, especially the tibial tubercle of below-knee stumps, are commonly caused by elastic bandaging. Occasionally they result from

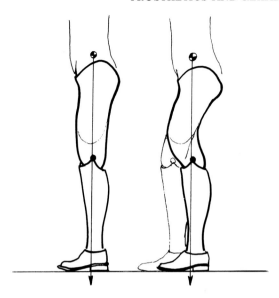

FIGURE 13-1 ■ Flexion contracture of the hip joint in an above-knee amputee requires special prosthetic socket alignment with poor cosmetic appearance and difficulty in prosthetic training and ambulation.

friction and pressure in the prosthetic socket. Application of the cast with inadequate cotton padding sometimes causes pressure sores along the tibial crest and tubercle or patella in below-knee amputees. This problem can be minimized by careful, frequent stump observation. Sharp bony edges should be eliminated at surgery.

STUMP EDEMA

The development of stump edema, rare with a rigid dressing, delays prosthetic fitting. Whenever possible rigid dressings should be used, because postoperative stump edema is uncommon with a rigid dressing. Poorly performed stump wrapping using elastic bandages can worsen edema and cause skin breakdown. For Syme's or below-knee amputees, stump edema is easily controlled and skin breakdown avoided with a removable below-knee rigid dressing.[15]

Elastic bandaging is a complicated and unreliable technique for diabetic patients with impaired sensation and poor vision. It has now been replaced by the removable rigid dressing for below-knee and Syme's amputees. In above-knee amputees the stump does not have a bony prominence, so a stump shrinker or elastic stockinette is often adequate and easier to apply than an elastic bandage.

VERRUCOUS HYPERPLASIA

The dermatologic problem of verrucous hyperplasia was common in the past when open-ended sockets were used routinely. Chronic venous congestion at the end of the stump causes verrucous hyperplasia. This condition should be treated with total contact fitting after control of possible infection and removal of hyperkeratotic tissue.

WEAKNESS OF THE UPPER EXTREMITIES

With one lower extremity missing, ambulation with canes, crutches, or a walker might be necessary. Thus, locomotion requires strong arms for substitution. Strengthening exercises for the upper extremities are therefore important from the preoperative period to the completion of rehabilitation training.

Inactivity before and after amputation causes generalized weakness. This can be prevented by continuous exercise in bed or in the wheelchair. Pull-up exercises in bed using the trapeze loop and or push-up exercises in the wheelchair are simple and useful techniques. Getting the patient up and into the wheelchair as soon as possible minimizes postoperative deconditioning from inactivity. Patients with orthostatic hypotension should use the tilt table and the reclining wheelchair for reconditioning. Active muscular activity during standing in the parallel bars sometimes can reduce the orthostatic hypotension, which is not controlled when using the tilt table.

CRUTCH WALKING AND TRANSFER TECHNIQUE

Most unilateral amputees should be able to ambulate with crutches. Crutch walking improves balance and facilitates prosthetic training. Ideally, training should begin during the preoperative period and continue after surgery, even before the prosthesis has been fitted. For patients with no potential for prosthetic or crutch ambulation, learning safe transfer techniques is essential.

ABOVE-KNEE AMPUTEES

Although the immediate rigid dressing is an ideal method of stump care, the complexity of applying and suspending the above-knee cast makes it impractical for clinical use. Postoperative care of the above-knee stump is commonly handled by an elastic shrinker. Because no bony prominences are over the above-knee residual limb, skin breakdown from elastic bandaging is seen infrequently. Adequate stump shrinkage prior to the prosthetic fitting can be a long process. Often, shrinkage is best achieved by fitting with a preparatory prosthesis, which can be done when the surgical wound tolerates weight-bearing.

For most diabetic amputees, an endoskeletal system is preferred. The vacuum-formed inner socket, held by an outer rigid frame to the endoskeletal pylon, can be easily remade to accommodate the change of stump size (Fig. 13-2). Various prosthetic components are available, including the stance phase control or stance-swing phase control knee mechanism, hydraulic knee unit, single or multiaxial foot, and solid ankle cushion heel, (SACH), and newer energy-storing feet. A prosthetic rotator is available for making it easier when crossing the leg, tying shoelaces, or placing the prosthesis in a more comfortable position during driving.

For more than 30 years, the quadrilateral socket design has been considered as the standard. Recently, many modifications were made in an attempt to improve the biomechanical deficiences of the socket, such as excessive femur abduction.[16,17] The most important common feature is the ischium containment inside the prosthetic socket. Shifting of the primary weight-bearing area medially in the ischium-containing socket (Fig. 13-3) causes less torque from body weight during stance phase than that of the conventional quadrilateral socket. In addition, the higher medial wall of the ischium-containing socket prevents the socket from moving laterally during stance phase. The pelvic band commonly used in the quadrilateral socket to hold the socket in is no longer needed.

The flexibility of the ischium-containing socket imparted by the anterior and posterior walls and along the proximal trim line improves the fitting comfort significantly.

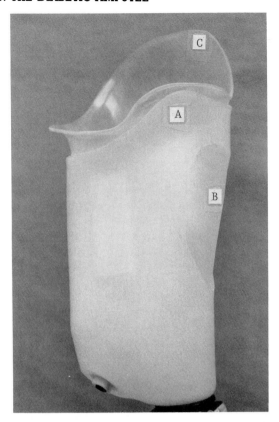

FIGURE 13-2 ■ Ideal above-the-knee socket design. *A,* Ischium containment. *B,* Flexible proximal trim line and portions of the anterior and posterior walls. *C,* Replaceable, flexible, inner socket.

Suspension of the prosthesis can be achieved by a suction socket or a silesian belt.

If amputees can ambulate on crutches, requiring less energy than using a prosthesis, they are considered as potential candidates for a preparatory prosthesis. This gives the staff a chance to evaluate the feasibility of functional ambulation further. Patients with moderate cardiovascular or pulmonary disease, balance disturbance, learning impairment, and bilateral above-knee amputations seem to be limited in their ability to be functional ambulators with prostheses.

BELOW-KNEE AMPUTEES

If we were to take the 1981 estimated figure for amputees—631,000—and the fig-

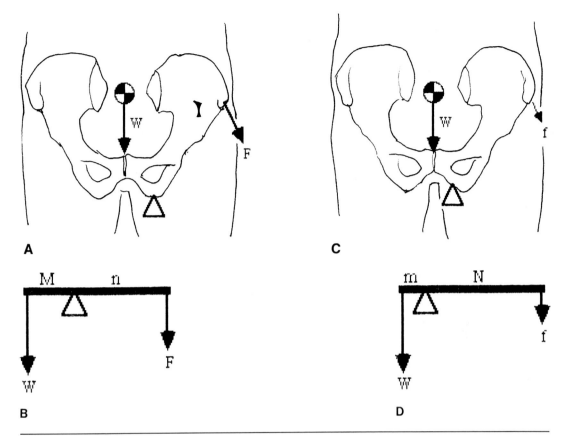

FIGURE 13–3 ■ Schematic representation of the biomechanical differences between the traditional quadrilateral (*A,B*) and ischium-containing sockets (*C,D*). Shifting of the primary weight-bearing point (fulcrum, △) medially reduces the torque from the body weight during the stance phase and thus requires less contraction of the hip abductors (f < F) for balance. (*W*, the force from the center of gravity; *M* or *m*, perpendicular distance between the force line of the center of gravity and the fulcrum; *N* or *n*, the perpendicular distance between the representative force of the hip abductors and the fulcrum; *F* or *f*, both represent forces of the hip abductors).

ure of 53.8%, of patients with below-knee amputation reported earlier,[5] there would be about 340,000 patients with below-knee amputation in the United States at any given time. Improved management of below-knee amputees can certainly benefit the majority of all amputees.

Removable Rigid Dressing

At Northwestern University, the "removable rigid dressing," (RRD) has been developed for postoperative and preprosthetic management of below-knee amputees. Our clinical experience with this technique for 10 years continues to show the following benefits:

Prevention of edema
Soft tissue immobilization to facilitate wound healing
Reduction of wound pain
Rapid stump shrinkage
Capability for frequent stump observation, elimination of skin breakdown commonly seen with the use of elastic bandaging
Simplicity of putting on and taking off
Development of skin tolerance to weight-bearing
Prevention of stump trauma

Use of the RRD shortens the rehabilitation process by facilitating stump shrinkage and by the complete elimination of skin breakdown commonly seen with the elastic bandaging technique.[14,18,19] The RRD can be applied at the completion of surgery or when the first thigh-high rigid dressing is removed for wound inspection. It can be used whenever the need for stump shrinkage exists, in the recent or former amputee.

COMPONENTS OF THE SYSTEM

The RRD system involves a below-knee plaster cast suspended by a stockinette to a supracondylar suspension cuff (Fig. 13-4). Underneath the below-knee plaster cast, sport tube socks are added to provide continuous controlled compression. The RRD therefore consists of four components—tube socks, a below-knee plaster cast, suspension stockinette, and supracondylar cuff.

Tube Socks. For most patients cotton tube socks, available nonprescription commercially and with the elastic band removed, can be used as stump socks. Unlike wool socks, cotton tube socks are cheaper and machine-washable. The tube sock leaves a clear sock mark on the skin that provides information about pressure distribution over the residual limb. Short tube socks are effective for providing localized compression in a bulbous stump so that shrinkage can be achieved more distally than proximally. For the large

stump, when the tube socks are not long or wide enough, Soft-socks* can be used.

Plaster Cast. The cast for the RRD is made only up to the knee level for easier removal and reapplication. The cast procedure differs slightly from that for IPSF for pressure relief. In IPSF, felt pads are used to bridge the bony areas, whereas with the RRD, cotton spacers are used to make an indentation in the cast for pressure relief. These tapered cotton paddings cover all the bony prominences, including the tibial tubercle, tibial crest, and fibular head, and any pressure-sensitive areas. Once the cast is made the spacers are discarded. A graded space between the cast and skin is formed to provide desirable pressure relief (Fig. 13-5).

The trim line of the plaster cast is higher anteriorly, up to midpatellar level, and lower posteriorly to allow knee flexion. It is wider proximally to ensure easy removal and reapplication. This is especially needed for a bulbous stump, in which the concave side needs additional padding so that the cast is not too tight at the top and can be reapplied after removal for wound inspection. If the cast is made too narrow proximally, it is cut on the back longitudinally to widen the opening for easier reapplication.

Suspension Stockinette. The suspension stockinette, made of 4-inch casting stocki-

---

*Available from Knit-Rite, Inc. from most prosthetic vendors.

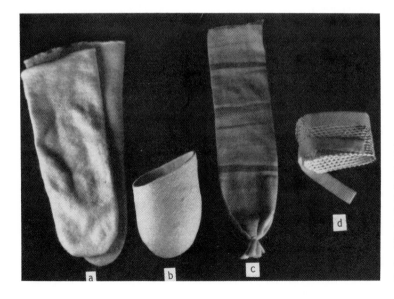

FIGURE 13–4 ■ Components of the removable rigid dressing. *A,* Stump socks. *B,* Below-the knee cast. *C,* Suspension stockinette. *D,* Supracondylar suspension cuff. (From Wu Y, Keagy RD, Krick JH, et al. J Bone Joint Surg. 1979; 61A:725.)

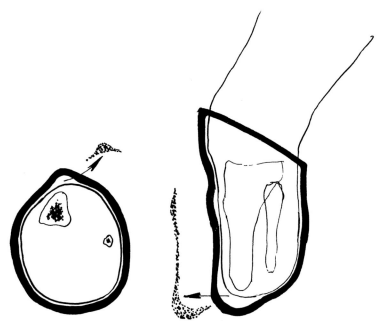

FIGURE 13–5 ■ Cotton paddings are used as spacers for pressure relief. The cotton paddings are discarded after the cast is made.

nette with one end tied, holds the cast to the suspension cuff.

Supracondylar Suspension Cuff. The suspension cuff is made of thermoplastic material. It has a Velcro closure to keep the cuff in place and a strip of Velcro hooks along the upper edge to secure the suspension stockinette. For the obese patient, with limited purchase over the femoral condyles because of tissue bulk, a fork strap with a waist belt can be used for suspension of the RRD cast.

APPLICATION

After the surgical wound has been properly dressed, the proper number of tube socks are applied layer by layer to avoid possible wrinkles. This is followed by the plaster cast, the suspension stockinette, and finally the supracondylar cuff. To make the application easier a semicircular mark is made on the cast and another on the supracondylar cuff, so the patient can match both marks to form a circle over the patella (Fig. 13-6). The system is worn continuously except for periodic stump observation and hygiene procedures, or when the prosthesis is being worn. A strap attached between the armrests for the RRD to push against is an effective static weight-bearing exercise while

the patient is in the wheel chair (Fig. 13-7A).

To achieve rapid and progressive stump shrinkage, when possible, additional socks are applied for a comfortable, snug fit. Localized cotton padding to the bulbous area under the last tube sock can ensure maintenance of local pressure and maximal shrinkage of the medial distal end. This can also be done by using short socks to provide localized distal compression without building up the thickness proximally.

It cannot be stated with certainty when the patient can start weight-bearing on the stump. In general, initiation of weight-bearing exercises is determined by the condition of wound healing, usually 7 to 14 days after surgery. Excessive, immediate, postoperative weight-bearing is likely to cause mechanical shearing from movement and to delay wound healing during the first 2 weeks after amputation.[13] Partial and steady weight-bearing without mechanical shearing on the stump using a wheelchair strap can, however, be beneficial.

EXERCISE PROGRAM

Because the RRD is removable, the time to start graded weight-bearing exercises can be decided based on wound healing (Fig. 13-

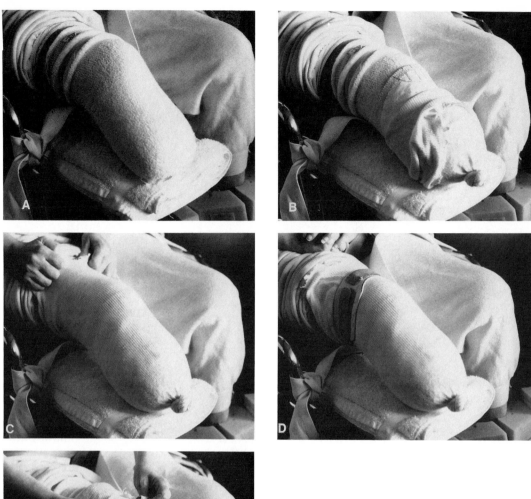

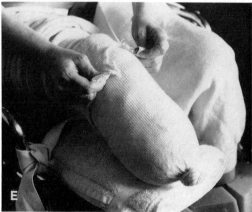

FIGURE 13–6 ■ Sequence of application of removable rigid dressing. *A*, Stump socks. *B*, Plaster cast, up to the patella. *C*, Suspension stockinette. *D*, Supracondylar cuff. *E*, Stockinette pulled and folded over the suspension cuff.

7). By observing the wound, the amount and duration of the next weight-bearing exercise can be planned.

The weight-bearing exercise can be done by standing on a padded car jack for unilateral amputees or on the tilt table for bilateral amputees. The degree of weight stress is controlled by the inclination of the tilt table and by the duration of standing. This progresses to the upright position and is followed by ambulation, with walking heels attached to the cast or preparatory prosthesis.

Walking with rigid dressings—using them as functional prostheses—is often preferred by obese and cardiac patients at home. These walking "stubbies" also assist the staff in evaluating candidates for prosthetic fitting.

The biomechanical benefit is apparent, because the obese patient can move forward to assume a standing position from sitting in the wheelchair without having to push up out of the wheelchair. This conserves energy and reduces the pressure exerted on the stumps when the patient is trying to stand.

The below-knee cast is changed whenever the stump has shrunk to the point at which too many tube socks are being used, usually about 10 to 14-ply of socks. The total number of casts needed depends on the speed of progressive stump shrinkage. Frequently, two or three casts might be required before the patient is ready to be fitted for a preparatory prosthesis.

Unlike the IPSF, the RRD, because it is removable, allows frequent stump observation without cast-cutting and cast reapplication. It also permits frequent addition of tube socks for fast shrinkage rather than cast changes.

By using cotton spacer padding, controlled pressure relief is achieved over bony prominences. Therefore, adding tube socks produces a compression force on soft tissues without causing pressure sores. If excessive pressure is noted, the cast can be softened from the outside with a hammer and pushed from the inside for relief over the desired area without remaking the cast.

Monitoring the stump response to weight-bearing is important during physical therapy. The RRD facilitates progressive weight-bearing within the safe tolerance range of the stump. Skin breakdown from excessive weight-bearing is minimized.[13] Unnecessary hesitation in application of early, graded, weight-bearing exercise can be avoided.

Delayed wound healing is not a contraindication for using the RRD or for prosthetic fitting. It is useful in facilitating wound healing by reducing stump edema and tissue tension. With frequent debridement of the necrotic tissue and adding socks for shrinkage, a superficial open wound can often be healed without a skin graft.[14]

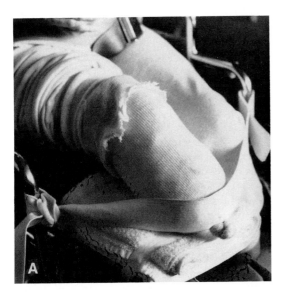

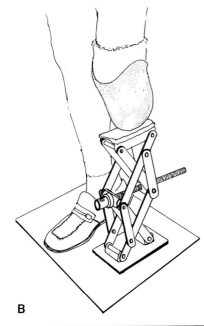

FIGURE 13–7 ■ A, A strap attached to the arm rests allows the patient to carry out weight-bearing exercise while in the wheelchair. (Modified from Wu Y, Krick HJ. Clin Prosthet Orthot. 1987; 11:33–44.) B, A car jack mounted onto plywood becomes an inexpensive adjustable stand for weight-bearing and balance exercises. (From Wu Y, Brncick MD, Krick JH et al. Bull Prosthet Res. 1984; 10–36:40–45.)

Preparatory and Definitive Prostheses

Once the stump is no longer bulbous and the wound tolerates weight-bearing exercises, a Scotchcast preparatory prosthesis can be made in less than 2 hours for early gait training.[20] A laminated socket using an endoskeletal system for the preparatory prosthesis is preferred. When the stump matures with marked shrinkage, the laminated socket alone can be replaced. A soft foam cover is provided for cosmesis when the patient is totally satisfied with fitting and alignment.

For most diabetic patients, the socket design is a patellar-tendon bearing total contact socket with supracondylar suspension. A soft insert is used routinely to provide an additional interface between the skin and socket.

Many prosthetic components are now available to meet the needs of amputees. For nonathletic diabetics, an expensive energy-storing foot might not be needed. Lightweight feet, such as the Carbon Copy II, the Seattle foot, and the Endolite foot are satisfactory. For inactive patients, the traditional lightweight geriatric SACH meets their requirements for limited indoor ambulation.

Lightweight construction reduces the problem of suspension. For most nonobese patients a supracondylar suspension is adequate. Except for obese patients, a waistbelt or supracondylar strap is seldom used.

The patient must be instructed in the importance of proper stump care as well as in the care of the prosthesis, soft insert, and stump socks. Although wool socks were used in the past, cotton stump socks are less expensive and machine-washable. The patient should change socks daily, and, if necessary, several times a day to keep the stump from sitting in a moist environment. When too many socks are needed the number of socks can be reduced by adding liners on the soft insert. A nylon sheath is sometimes used to reduce friction on the skin and to permit easier prosthetic donning.

It is not uncommon for the stump to continue to shrink after long prosthetic use. If the patient experiences "bell clapping" in the socket, stump socks can be added to improve the total contact. A thin plastic bag with trapped air can also be used in the soft insert to increase distal total contact.

SYME'S AMPUTEES

The Syme's amputation, developed in 1943 for traumatic foot injury, is a one-stage procedure that includes resection of both the medial and lateral malleoli at a level slightly above the articular surface. This extensive one-stage procedure often results in significant problems with primary wound healing. In 1978, Wagner[21] described a two-stage procedure; ankle disarticulation is done initially and the heel pad is brought forward to cover the wound. The entire surgical area is protected by a nonweight-bearing cast for 6 weeks to permit the blood supply to become established. Immobilization of the soft tissue permits the heel pad to be stabilized onto the distal residual limb. During the second-stage operation, the malleoli are removed through elliptic incisions. This improves the degree of primary wound healing and minimizes the bulbous stump for a more cosmetic prosthetic fitting.

With the two-stage procedure, a modified below-knee removable rigid dressing can be applied. This Syme's removable rigid dressing allows earlier controlled weight-bearing and stump observation. The procedure of making a Syme's removable rigid dressing involves the following:

1. Measure the maximal circumference of the heel pad and determine the level of similar circumference proximally.
2. Fill in the concave space with cotton padding (used as a spacer) so no area proximal to the end of the residual limb is narrower than the circumference of the heel pad.
3. Use cotton padding over the tibial crest as a spacer (similar to that of the BK removable rigid dressing) for controlled pressure relief between the residual limb and the plaster cast to be made (Fig. 13-8).
4. Apply layers of plaster as for a walking cast and attach a rubber heel for weight-bearing, as desired.
5. Remove the cast when set and discard the cotton padding over the tibial crest and concave areas above the end of the stump.
6. Plaster a section of stockinette to the proximal end for suspension.
7. Attach the stockinette to the supracondylar suspension cuff; this part is identical with that of below-knee removable rigid dressing.

Application of the Syme's dressing is similar to that of the BK removable rigid dress-

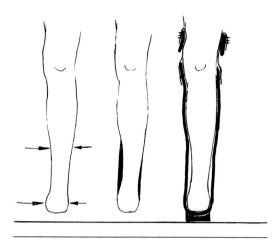

FIGURE 13–8 ■ Syme's removable rigid dressing. A stovepipe-like walking cast is removable and permits progressive stump shrinkage by adding socks. The distal tibial area without total contact can be covered with an elastic stockinette to prevent edema.

ing. Development of slight edema in the concave areas is controlled by use of elastic stockinette. In our experience, mild degree of edema in this area has not caused any significant problems. With a narrow distal stump, the Syme's prosthesis can be made without a medial opening to improve cosmetic results.

OTHER AMPUTEES

Transtarsal-Tarsometatarsal Amputees

If possible, transtarsal amputations, including Chopart's, Boyd's, and Pirogoff's amputations, should be avoided, because the residual limbs are very difficult to fit successfully. From the viewpoint of the physiatrist, the stump deformity caused by muscle imbalance, lack of space for construction of a functional ankle joint for the artificial foot, and potential skin breakdown from high localized pressure over the anterior distal corner during heel strike make it difficult to fit and protect the stump.

Amputation at the tarsometatarsal junction (Lisfranc's amputation) should not be done because of the inevitable inversion-equinus deformity. It is our opinion that it always results in prosthetic failure and poor functional outcome.

Transmetatarsal and Partial Foot Amputees

Amputations involving the forefoot or toes, ray resection, or transmetatarsal level require only foam filler in the shoe. Shoe modification with the addition of an extended steel shank or rocker sole to reduce pressure over the dorsal surface of the foot might be all that is necessary.

References

1. La Blanc MA. Patient population and other estimates of prosthetics and orthotics in the USA. Clin Prosthet Orthot. 1973; 27:83.
2. United States Department of Health and Human Services. Vital and Health Statistics: prevalence of selected chronic conditions—United States, 1979–1981, Series 10, 1986; 155:29–32.
3. United States Department of Health and Human Services. Detailed diagnosis and procedures for patients discharged from short-stay hospitals, United States, 1984, Series 13, 1986.
4. Glattly HW. A statistical study of 12,000 new amputees. South Med J. 1964; 57:1373.
5. Kay HW, Newman JD. Relative incidence of new amputations. Statistical comparisons of 6,000 new amputations. Orthot Prosthet. 1975; 29:3.
6. Runyan JW Jr. The Memphis chronic disease program. JAMA. 1975; 231:264–267.
7. Kerstein MD, Zimmer MA, Dugdale FE, et al. Rehabilitation after bilateral lower extremity amputation. Arch Phys Med Rehabil. 1975; 56:309.
8. Waters RL, Perry JP, Antonelli D, et al. Energy cost of walking of amputees: the influence of level of amputation. J Bone Joint Surg. 1976; 58A:42–46.
9. Traugh GH, Corcoran PJ, Reyer RL. Energy expenditure of ambulation in patients with above-knee amputations. Arch Phys Med Rehabil. 1975; 56:67–71.
10. Burgess EM, Romano RI. The management of lower extremity amputees using immediate post-surgical prostheses. Clin Orthop. 1968; 57:137–146.
11. Burgess EM, Romano RI, Zettl JH. The management of lower extremity amputations. Washington, DC: Veterans Administration, Department of Medicine and Surgery, Prosthetic and Sensory Aids Service, 1969; Technical report TR10-6.
12. Baker WH, Barnes RW, Shurr DC. The healing of below-knee amputation. A comparison of soft and plaster dressings. Am J Surg. 1977; 133:716–718.
13. Mooney V, Harvey JP Jr, McBride E, et al. Com-

parison of postoperative stump management: plaster vs. soft dressings. J Bone Joint Surg. 1971; 53:241–249.

14. Wu Y, Krick H. Removable rigid dressing for below-knee amputees. Clin Prosthet Orthot. 1987; 11:33–44.

15. Mueller MJ. Comparison of removable rigid dressing and elastic bandages in preprosthetic management of patients with below-knee amputations. Phys Ther. 1982; 62:1438–1441.

16. Long IA. Normal shape-normal alignment (NSNA) above knee prosthesis. Clin Prosthet Orthot. 1985; 9:9–14.

17. Sabolich J. Contoured adducted trochanteric-controlled alignment method (CAT-CAM): introduction and basic principles. Clin Prosthet Orthot. 1985; 9:15–26.

18. Wu Y, Flanigan DP. Rehabilitation of the lower-extremity amputee with emphasis on a removable below-knee rigid dressing. In: Bergan, JJ, Yao ST, eds. New York: Grune & Stratton, 1978; 435–453.

19. Wu Y, Keagy RD, Krick JH, et al. An innovative removable rigid dressing technique for below-the-knee amputation. J Bone Joint Surg. 1979; 61A:724–729.

20. Wu Y, Brncick MD, Krick JH, et al. Scotchcast P.V.C. interim prosthesis for below knee amputees. Bull Prosthet Res. 1981; 10:360.

21. Wagner FW Jr. Syme's amputation for ischemia of the toes and forefoot. In: Bergan JJ, Yao ST eds. Gangrene and severe ischemia of the lower extremities. New York: Grune & Stratton, 1978, 419–434.

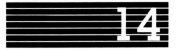

Orthotic and Pedorthic Management of the Diabetic Foot

BARRY C. ULLMAN, C. PED.
MICHAEL BRNCICK, C.P.O.

MECHANICAL EVALUATION OF THE DIABETIC FOOT

A difficult problem facing the physician and allied medical professional is how to manage the diabetic foot mechanically, especially the foot with a neurotrophic lesion or arthropathy. Not every patient is a surgical candidate nor will they respond to drug therapy. Moreover, it is not possible to keep a patient in a total contact cast or at bed rest indefinitely. At some point, patients must ambulate with some form of shoe or foot covering protecting their feet so they can participate in activities of daily living.

Frequently the diabetic with a foot problem is referred to the orthotist or pedorthist with instructions to relieve pressure, help manage a neurotrophic ulcer, or accommodate a Charcot foot. The goal is to keep the patient ambulating while limiting the risk of further damage to the foot. The patient can seldom be of assistance, because the impaired sensation, common in diabetic feet, diminishes the patient's incentive to seek help. In fact, it is this lack of feeling pain—impaired sensation—that makes even a basic evaluation of the patient's problem difficult. It is necessary to evaluate complaints without requiring the patient to say "where it hurts the most." Mechanical evaluation techniques are more useful in determining areas of high and low pressure and areas of tissue stress in response to floor reaction.

When conducting a mechanical evaluation of the diabetic foot, we frequently look for floor-reactive forces, which tend to be injurious when applied to the foot repetitively. The patient with impaired sensation

cannot feel the effect of these disruptive forces until damage has actually occurred. The material in this chapter can help determine what is causing a problem or predict where a problem is most likely to occur on the diabetic foot.

Three basic forms of floor reaction testing are currently available that provide information useful to the practitioner. The most advanced technique is an electronic one, with computer refinement, but view systems and imprint systems are currently more widely available and affordable.

Most electronic systems now in use are produced in Europe. These systems are based primarily on a force plate or Pedobarograph principle. Both systems are computerized and not only record forces crossing the contact area, but also interpret, enhance, and reproduce the data in printed and televisual form. Although this is perhaps the most accurate type of floor reaction testing, it is also the most expensive, and presently is probably most useful in the large hospital or clinic setting, or as a research tool. Problems of calibration and standardization have yet to be resolved. It is expected that within the near future these monitors will become more affordable and useful. In fact, several new systems are being developed in Europe at this time. It is expected that these newer systems will be available in about 2 years and at a lower cost than current models.

View systems have been used in research for about 50 years and recently have become available to clinicians. Typically, these systems include a stand with an opening filled with glass plates, which are underlaid with a mirror placed at an angle. Using refracted or polarized light, an image of the plantar surface of the foot can be viewed at various stages of weight-bearing. Areas of relatively high or low pressure can be determined and the weight-bearing pattern can be followed during the stance phase of walking. A permanent record can be obtained by filming the foot in motion or by photographing the foot at a particular instant in the stance phase of gait.

Perhaps the most commonly used and cost-effective system of recording floor reaction is the floor reaction imprint (Fig. 14-1). Several types are available, varying from self-contained automatic inking systems, from France, to carbon imprint systems, to self-contained imprinters from Germany requiring inking, to inked mats from England, (e.g., the Harris mat system).

All the systems available share a common feature—they provide a reasonably accurate image of the floor reaction forces acting on the foot during the stance phase of gait. The image is presented in relative terms, because no mechanical imprint systems now available can measure the forces on the foot directly. The imprints usually show areas of high and low pressure, with some of the systems also able to show shear forces. Interpretation of the image produced is left to the physician or technician. Generally, the image provides sufficient information for formulation of an orthotic or pedorthic device.

Another system available for gathering information is a thermograph, a heat evaluation device. This is made of a heat-sensitive imaging material, or thermistor. In-shoe

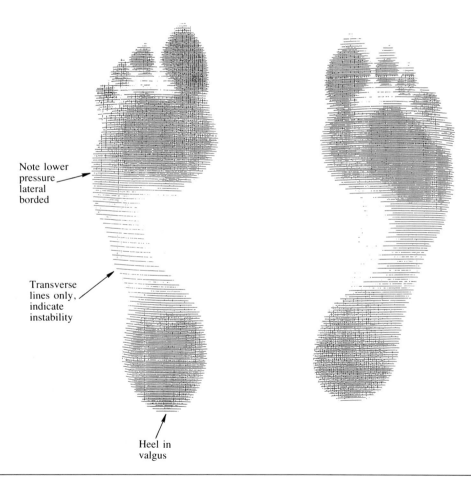

Note lower
pressure
lateral
borded

Transverse
lines only,
indicate
instability

Heel in
valgus

FIGURE 14–1 ■ Foot within the range of normal. Note the instability of the left foot with heel valgus.

pressure testing has been done, but with mixed results. It is expected that usable computerized systems will be available in the future to monitor surface temperatures in various areas of the foot during gait and over prolonged periods of time.

Interpretation of Results

The type of test used for evaluating foot and floor forces depends on the type of information desired. Because the most commonly used mechanical evaluation system is the floor reaction imprint, it is important to review the information that is generated by this relatively simple and inexpensive device.

Attention is given to areas of high or low pressure or to a sharp variation from high to low pressure across a relatively small distance. An area of high pressure might be caused by an imbalance in the foot, typically in the metatarsal area, frequently as a result of pronation or supination. High pressure can be caused by a plantar callus or old scar tissue. Ulceration can result from repetitive stress under the high-pressure area or at the edge of the high-pressure area be-

cause of shear stress. High pressure is the easiest to see, because it is usually presented as an intensely dark area (Figs. 14-2 and 14-3).

Low pressure is revealed by areas of light imprint or no imprint at all. A cavus foot can reveal dark areas beneath the heel and metatarsal head areas while showing no contact in the midfoot. This type of incongruity often contributes to foot problems in the normal foot with normal sensation. In the neurotrophic foot, however, lack of contact with the floor combined with areas of high plantar pressure can have disastrous effects (Fig. 14-4).

When carrying out floor reaction tests it is important to record both static and dynamic imprints to determine the major differences between static and dynamic stance. Once areas of high and low pressure and shear stress have been identified, the data can be interpreted.

It is helpful to view the floor reaction imprint clinically as a topographic map of the plantar foot surface. Areas of high pressure are likened to hills or mountains, low pressure areas are valleys or canyons, and edges

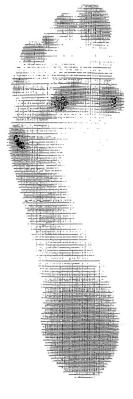 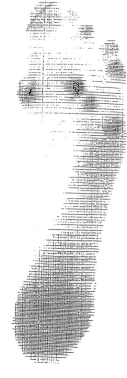

FIGURE 14-2 ■ Extremely high pressure under first, third, and fifth metatarsal heads, with fat pad atrophy.

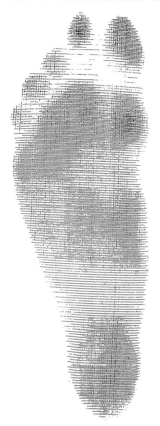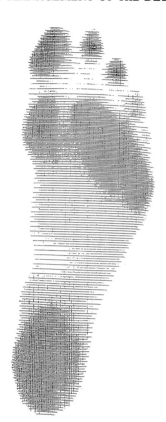

FIGURE 14–3 ■ Pes planus with pronation.

where pressure changes abruptly from high to low are cliffs representing a dangerous area. As pressure increases so does the height of the perceived hill, and this is accompanied by an increase in risk. This simple comparison can help the test results to be represented as a visual image and can aid in planning the proper treatment.

The goal is reduction of the areas of high and low pressure to the point where the perceived topographic view is one of gently rolling hills and valleys rather than steep mountains and canyons. Reducing the pressure reduces the risk of tissue breakdown.

IDENTIFYING HAZARDS

Unexplained lines of shear stress or areas of high pressure can represent foreign bodies in the foot or a hazard under the foot, such as a stocking seam. Several unusual conditions can contribute to abnormal mechanical stress in diabetic feet. It is not uncommon to find an ulceration caused by the seam of a sock located under a high-pressure area.

The patient's shoes and orthoses should be thoroughly inspected as part of the clinical examination. Patients have been known to develop ulcers from a dog hair embedded in their Plastazote* foot orthoses. Nails and glass fragments can also perforate shoes, creating a high-pressure area for which there is no immediate explanation. Items as innocent as the distal end of a sock liner can set up a shear stress line that can result in tissue breakdown, even with an orthosis in place as an interface.

CLINICAL APPLICATION

Two basic approaches can be used in the management of the diabetic foot. These paths constantly overlap if the patient is managed properly. Proper medical treatment, drug therapy, and diet control yield limited results when the mechanics of the patient's feet are left unbalanced and out of control. Similarly, mechanical management fails if the patient's body chemistry is uncontrolled or

---

*Plastazote is a registered trademark of BXL, Ltd.

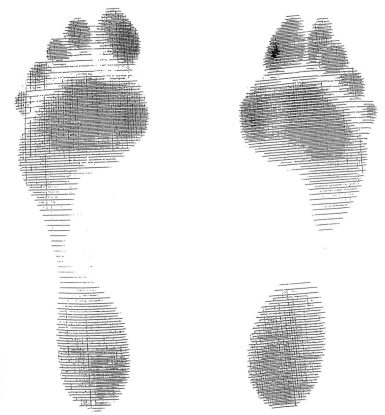

FIGURE 14–4 ■ Cavus foot. Note the instability of the right foot, with resultant pronation at toe-off.

the presence of infection is not recognized and treated.

The ideal patient profile is one whose ulceration has been healed medically or with a total contact cast and whose diabetes is medically under control. Often, however, patients whose disease process might not be under adequate control present with a large, untreated, neurotrophic ulcer. The advantages of a diabetic treatment team become obvious when we find the patient seeing a practitioner whose knowledge and experience is limited to one part of the body or one area of treatment. It is easier to be successful in keeping a healed ulcer closed than to attempt healing the ulcer using mechanical devices.

It is unrealistic, however, to expect every patient to present with a healed ulcer. Many patients are not candidates for total contact cast treatment and many do not respond promptly to the various medical regimens currently available. To treat the neurotrophic foot, the orthotic or pedorthic clinician must develop a workable plan for mechanical management based on a series of proven orthotic and pedorthic techniques. Some problems might be so complex as to require innovative measures when treatment is begun and periodically as treatment progresses.

Options of Mechanical Treatment

Total contact casting on the ulcerated or Charcot foot is an ideal initial mechanical treatment. Whether or not the patient is a candidate for such casts, the next option is some form of footwear, foot orthosis, or both. The degree to which this form of treatment is carried out depends on the patient's general health, history, and condition of the foot.

The patient without history of foot ulceration, no present lesions, and whose diabetes is under control might only require a well-fitted shoe with some form of protective insole. Concern increases in the patient with a history of ulceration or who has current lesions.

The grade 1 foot[1] does well when placed in an extra-deep shoe using a molded foot orthosis fabricated from some combination of polyethylene foams. This combination works well to maintain the healed ulcer and generally allows a superficial ulcer to heal readily. The important factors here are relief of surface pressure and fitting the patient with proper footwear to reduce the risk of further involvement.

If the ulcer is deeper the problem becomes more involved and the solution more complex. Using synergistic foot orthotic systems, combined with extra-deep shoes to which modifications have been made, becomes more desirable for relieving pressure on the ulcer and redistributing weight-bearing.

The patient might present with plantar fragility, which dictates the need for management of a bony lesion. In the case of a Charcot joint with a plantar projection, a custom-molded shoe with a molded polyethylene foam insert is often a successful mechanical approach. When the abnormality involves the hindfoot or the ankle, the use of an ankle-foot orthosis (hybrid) becomes necessary. A patient with a Charcot ankle and associated active or potential plantar ulceration requires the combination of a well-planned ankle-foot orthosis, including a foot orthotic component that efficiently distributes the forces when walking.

Occasionally, deformities are severe enough to require a custom-made shoe with the ankle-foot orthosis built in as part of the shoe. This provides some degree of total contact along with the stability inherent to each component.

ORTHOTIC MANAGEMENT

When an orthosis is required, the question becomes "Do we use the orthosis for support and limitation of motion, or do we seek to achieve these goals and limit the axial load—that is, reduce weight-bearing?"

Selection of Technique

Most diabetic foot problems can be managed with some combination of foot orthosis and footwear, with or without footwear modifications. When the problem indicates the need for something more than a well-fitted shoe, a decision must be made to accommodate the problem or to control it. Often, in the case of the neurotrophic foot, the forefoot must be accommodated while attempting to control the hindfoot.

This particular problem has generated the need for such techniques as multidensity systems that use orthotic synergy.[†] An example might be the diabetic with ulcerations under the first interphalangeal joint and the first metatarsophalangeal joint that are secondary to a valgus hindfoot deformity. Pressure under the ulcers must be relieved and the forefoot accommodated, but treatment is not complete unless the hindfoot valgus problem is controlled. Use of a low-density polyethylene foam, such as Plastazote soft, would relieve plantar pressure but the foot would remain in valgus. By combining a material such as medium-density Plastazote with a firmer material, such as UCOkork[*], one can accommodate with the top layer while providing some control with the stronger base material.

When the hindfoot cannot be stabilized with footwear, a foot orthosis, or footwear modifications, and this contributes to ulceration in the forefoot, the need to consider an ankle-foot orthosis (AFO) becomes apparent. The following factors need to be considered before proceeding with the AFO:

1. Do the ankle- and sub-talar joints require a longer lever arm to control them?
2. Will the limitation of motion exercised by the orthosis contribute to healing?
3. Can the patient's tissues tolerate the forces applied by the AFO?
4. Will patients accept the "apparatus load" or will they see this as being too much for what they perceive as a "minor problem"?

Criteria to be met before proceeding with an axial load resistance AFO include the following:

1. Can the patient tolerate proximal weight-bearing as opposed to distal weight-bearing?
2. Is load reduction of the plantar surface

---

[*]UCOkork is a registered trademark of UCO International.

[†]Orthotic Synergy—A cooperation between different materials to create a multidensity system with improved characteristics over a single density material.

of the foot going to give us the result we are looking for?

Selection of Materials

FOOT ORTHOSES

When selecting materials for foot orthoses in the management of diabetic feet, inert materials are always preferable. If an open ulceration is present, the orthotic material must not be able to react with the tissue or draining fluids.

Polyethylene

Among the preferred materials for foot orthoses are those in the polyethylene family. For those orthoses requiring control, high-molecular-weight and ultrahigh-molecular-weight polyethylenes lend themselves well to orthotic work. With working temperatures in the 350°F (177° C) range, these plastics are easy to fabricate, can be vacuum-formed, can be fused to foamed polyethylenes, are easy to adjust, and provide a degree of semirigid to rigid control. If more strength or rigidity is required, polyethylene and polypropylene copolymers might be more desirable.

Care should be used when applying these rigid materials to the diabetic foot because of the tendency for tissue breakdown resulting from pressure against a prominence. If used, the rigid polyethylenes should be combined with a polyethylene foam liner to decrease direct pressure on the skin.

Polyethylene Foam. The family of polyethylene foams is extensive. With structural properties ranging from soft to semirigid, these closed-cell materials are inert and easy to work with. Some, such as Plastazote and UCOlite*, are cross-linked, whereas others, such as Aliplast*, are cross-irradiated. Cross-linking and cross-irradiating polyethylene contributes to the material's acquired memory for a new shape. Almost all the polyethylene foams are inert and do not react with human tissue.

The density of these foams varies from less

than 2 lb/ft³ to almost 12 lb/ft³, with the surface durometer* varying in a similar pattern. Typically, a 2-lb foam would be soft, so it would have a low durometer. As the density approaches 7 lb/ft³, the material becomes more rigid and the surface durometer increases.

Copolymer Foam and Combinations. A new family of materials has been introduced. These are basically copolymer foams, combining polyethylene, ethyl vinyl acetate (EVA), and rubber. In some cases these copolymer foams have other materials, such as cork, blown into them to enhance their qualities. These materials are usually denser than polyethylene foams and should be used as the base for a multidensity system. It is not uncommon to find surface durometers ranging from 30° to 60° shore A. Materials such as UCOkork are workable and vacuum-formable at approximately 325° F (163° C). They are also easy to sand. The rigidity of the material depends on its thickness after sanding.

A novel approach, with both firmness and softness, involves the combination of a material such as 1/4-inch Plastazote 2 on top with 8-mm UCOkork as the base. This combination provides accommodation with some degree of control without presenting the hazards of a rigid material.

Viscoelastics. Another relatively new area of materials is the viscoelastics. Designed primarily for shock absorption and force dissipation, viscoelastics tend to be in the form of a molded unit or a sheet material that has certain characteristics of a thick fluid.

Primary viscoelastics in use today are usually blends of silicon polymers or a mixture of silicon and rubber. Although this family of viscoelastics is superior at force dispersion and accommodation, it has certain drawbacks. When mixing silicon polymers, weight and temperature must be carefully monitored. Attempting to use these mixed polymers without the proper equipment frequently results in a poor-quality

---

*UCOlite is a registered trademark of UCO International; and Aliplast is a registered trademark of Ali Med, Inc.

---

*A durometer is a measure of surface hardness. Typically measured on a shore A scale, durometer ranges from 1 to 100°: A low durometer material is more accommodative, while a high durometer material is more supportive.

product. When combined and fused to a material such as Plastazote 1, the result is an accommodative foot orthosis that tends not to bottom out. Excellent results in relieving pressure on ulcers have been reported,[2] but there is a tendency to provide a less than stable base for the weaker foot. It is difficult to make changes or modifications after the silicon has set, because it is not thermoplastic, is difficult to sand, and does not readily adhere to other materials using conventional adhesives.

Urethane Polymers and Composite Plastics. A variation from the silicon viscoelastics is the family of urethane polymers. Although not possessing all the viscoelastic properties of the silicon-based materials, polymers in the urethane group are somewhat easier to work with. These materials can adhere to a thermoplastic foam using a neoprene-based, heat-reactivated adhesive, such as Superbond. This feature allows the urethane sheet and the foam sheet to be coated with adhesive, which is allowed to dry completely. The thermoplastic foam is then heated until it is formable, at which point the adhesive sides of the sheets are put together and hand- or vacuum-formed over a mold of the foot. The result is a stable orthosis with shock-absorbent and accommodative properties and a resistance to pack out. Although the urethanes are not generally thermoplastic they easily follow the shape of a hot thermoplastic, and can retain the new shape if the thermoplastic is allowed to cool thoroughly before removing pressure from the mold.

A final area of materials to consider is the new composite plastics. These materials are generally rigid to semirigid and are extremely strong. Caution must be exercised when considering use of these materials for the diabetic foot, because they tend to be difficult to modify after the mold is finished.

ANKLE-FOOT ORTHOSIS

An ankle-foot orthosis can be constructed of various materials, all of which serve a particular purpose in the need for stabilizing the lower limb. Typically, metal or plastic or a combination of the two materials is used.

Metal Systems. Metal systems can be used for those patients who present with a condition requiring the need for stabilization and a high degree of adjustability. Plastic systems generally do not provide an easily adjustable orthosis, but do allow more intimate total contact and potentially better control over the skeletal prominences of the lower limb. Hybrid systems consisting of metal and plastic combine the desirable effects of each and are commonly used in lower limb management today.

A metal ankle-foot orthosis can be attached to the patient's shoe using a stirrup, which is riveted to the sole. This provides a stable attachment point and, when used in conjunction with an extended shank, limits foot and ankle motion considerably.

Attached to the stirrup are mechanical ankle joints that control the range of motion allowed at the anatomic ankle. These joints are easily adjustable and have considerable strength and durability. The most commonly used type is the double-action ankle joint, which provides all the adjustments necessary for ankle joint control in the sagittal plane. This ankle joint is an excellent clinical tool because of the ease of adjustment permitted by adjustment screws.

Attached to the ankle joints are the sidebars, which extend proximally to the calf band. The calf band is the area at which force is applied to control the tibia as it progresses forward over the foot during the stance phase of gait. Care must be taken to distribute these forces over a large enough area to distribute pressure properly on the tibia at that point.

A potential problem with the use of a metal system attached to the shoe can be caused by the stirrup attachment. Rivets might protrude into the inner surface of the shoe. These irregular bumps against the plantar surface of the foot can create pressure if not carefully evaluated at the time of fitting and throughout the duration of the patient's care.

Steel and aluminum alloys are the metals of choice for most orthotic systems requiring a high degree of adjustability. They are lightweight and easily formed to the contours of the patient's leg. The steel stirrups and shank material, when used in association with shoe modifications such as rocker soles, can be heavy and not cosmetically acceptable. These factors have an effect on patient acceptance.

Plastic Systems. Plastic systems have the

advantage of being lightweight, yet strong and durable. Polypropylene has been used for some time in orthotic management, but in some cases has been found to be too brittle. Copolymers such as polypropylene and polyethylene combinations are now being used more frequently, reducing the problems of breakage and fatigue of the plastic (Figs. 14-5 and 14-6).

The advantage of plastic systems is that they can be intimately formed over a cast (model) of the patient's leg and foot. This provides the orthotist with the ability to provide an orthosis that is close to the functional characteristics of a total contact cast.

Disadvantages of the plastic systems are that they are difficult to modify and, depending on the clinical requirements, do not lend themselves easily to adjustments for limiting variable amounts of ankle joint control.

Another advantage of the plastic system is that the outer shell of plastic can be formed around a foot insert. In addition, an extra-deep shoe can be fitted to accommodate the orthosis or a custom-made shoe built around it.

Hybrid Systems. Hybrid systems are available that combine plastic leg and foot sections with metal ankle joints. These hybrid systems are the systems of choice, allowing the clinician to combine the advantages of total contact plastic with the

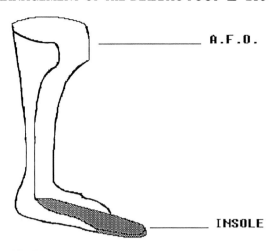

FIGURE 14–6 ■ Ankle-foot orthosis (A.F.O.) of plastic copolymer material, with insole.

characteristics of the ease of adjustment provided by the metal ankle joint system.

PEDORTHIC MANAGEMENT

Selection of Footwear

Footwear tends to be a forgotten area when discussing techniques of management of foot problems. Fewer high-quality shoe factories remain in the United States because of the influx of inexpensive low-grade shoes from other countries, a situation that bodes ill for the person such as the diabetic, with foot neuropathy. Attempting to manage diabetic neurotrophic feet with regular shoes, which often are only available in one or two widths, becomes a difficult if not impossible task. It is important that the diabetic foot, even one that appears not to be at risk, be fitted carefully in a shoe that does not bind or cause excessive pressure.

The rather recent introduction of extra-deep shoes has provided a more utilitarian vehicle for the relief of foot problems, and can be used along with foot orthoses. Initially available from a limited number of factories, more shoes are becoming available that have removable inserts and nominal extra depth. The major drawbacks of most commercial or athletic-type shoes with extra-deep features are lack of width selec-

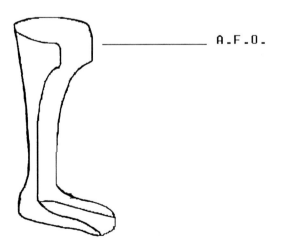

FIGURE 14–5 ■ Ankle-foot orthosis (A.F.O.) of plastic copolymer material.

tion and lack of structural support. Prescription-type extra-deep shoes* tend to have more toe room, depth, and strength and better-quality construction than other commercially available shoes (Fig. 14-7). In addition, it is more likely that shoes of this nature are fitted by an experienced professional than shoes available at the local shoe store. Quality footwear fitted by professionals represents a cost-effective method of reducing the risk of diabetic foot complications.

One feature that is available primarily in prescription-type extra-deep shoes is the contour or anatomic shaped toe. Although not a hallmark of fashion, this broad, deep toe in a shoe is the best combination of toe room and firm heel fit.

Several factories have introduced heat-moldable or easily reshaped extra-deep shoes for use in feet with moderate deformities. Names such as Thermold are indicative of heat-moldable construction. These deerskin shoes are lined with a layer of polyethylene foam, which provides stability at room temperature. The shape, however, is easily deformed at a higher temperature. The layer of polyethylene foam also provides a protective inert surface against the problem foot.

---

*Available from such factories as P. W. Minor and Son, Inc., Batavia, NY, Drew Shoe Corporation, Lancaster, OH, and the Musebeck Shoe Company, Oconomowoc, WI.

These shoes can also be relasted to provide a quick solution when fitting the foot with moderate deformity. The technique requires considerable skill, but, relasting techniques can be carried out by qualified personnel after appropriate training.

When the combination of extra-deep footwear and a foot orthosis is not a workable solution and the facility does not have customizing capabilities, the next consideration is the custom-molded shoe. To start the process of fabrication the clinician must first make a negative mold of the foot. This is generally done with the patient's foot and leg aligned with the hip and with right angles at the hip, knee, and ankle.

The mold is usually made using extra fast setting plaster bandages or splints, using a "clamshell" molding technique. This process consists of making a plantar mold first, then applying a dorsal mold to complete the shape of the foot.

The negative mold is then sent to a factory specializing in the fabrication of custom-molded shoes. A positive plaster model is completed from the mold of the patient's foot and is further modified to provide balance and accommodation, with the result being a plaster last. The shoe is molded over this last, theoretically according to the instructions of the clinician. Often the instructions are interpreted differently by the manufacturer than they were intended by

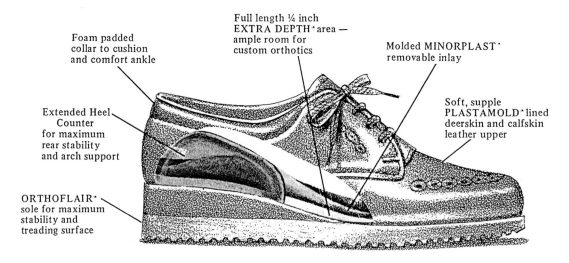

Foam padded
collar to cushion
and comfort ankle

Full length ¼ inch
EXTRA DEPTH* area —
ample room for
custom orthotics

Molded MINORPLAST*
removable inlay

Extended Heel
Counter
for maximum
rear stability
and arch support

Soft, supple
PLASTAMOLD* lined
deerskin and calfskin
leather upper

ORTHOFLAIR*
sole for maximum
stability and
treading surface

FIGURE 14–7 ■ Extra-deep high-quality shoe with more toe room and greater strength than an ordinary shoe. (Courtesy of H. Minor III, P.W. Minor & Son, Inc., Batavia, NY.)

the clinician and this is one of the disadvantages of the custom-molded shoe. Because the plaster last is usually broken when being extracted from the molded shoe, any major modification required when fitting the patient involves recasting and delay while the shoe is being remade. It is sometimes difficult, therefore, to carry out modifications to the shape or fit of the molded shoe.

When ordering a custom-molded shoe, a removable insert is generally desirable. This allows the clinician some leeway in adjusting the fit of the shoe and, more importantly, in making modifications to the way in which the foot reacts with the floor. Although a soft, accommodative insert is helpful with the fragile foot, a firmer insert is necessary for the Charcot foot. Charcot feet with deformity seem to do well in this type of shoe. The patient is informed that it usually takes 8 to 12 weeks for delivery of custom-molded shoes.

When all else fails, or when style is a major consideration, custom-made shoes might be the only solution. Orthopedic custom-made shoes are readily available in Europe, but domestic manufacturers are uncommon. This is a rather complicated process and accordingly an expensive one. Access to this technique is based on the local availability of a skilled craftsman or contact with a specialized facility and close cooperation between the physician, pedorthist, and manufacturer.

Footwear Modifications

Footwear modifications helpful in the management of diabetic feet are generally of four basic types—stabilizing or supporting, rocking, shock-reducing, and pressure-reducing.

STABILIZING OR SUPPORTING MODIFICATIONS

Stabilizing or supporting modifications are used primarily when an instability, such as a Charcot joint or severe pronation, exists or when a deformity creates an unstable foot. Commonly used modifications such as heel or sole wedges are not generally recommended for those with neurotrophic feet. Sole wedges tend to increase floor reaction under the first or fifth metatarsal head and can lead to excessive pressure, with resultant tissue breakdown and ulceration. Heel wedges are seldom adequate to manage the degree of varus or valgus associated with neurotrophic instability or deformity.

Some of the most successful variations in footwear modification are the flared and offset or buttressed heels and soles. In certain cases the vertical force vector against the sole cannot be returned as floor reaction at the point of maximum effectiveness, because varus or valgus deformity has altered force distribution. By extending or flaring the heel or sole medially or laterally, or both, the base of support is broadened (Fig. 14-8). By proper positioning of the flare a lever arm can be created to limit the deforming forces. A medial heel flare helps to limit the moment-producing eversion about the subtalar axis that is created by a valgus deformity. When a flare is not adequate to control motion about such an axis, it might be helpful to use an offset. For instance, if the patient with heel valgus overrides a medial heel flare it is helpful to use a medial offset heel, which combines the effect of a medial flare and reinforcement of the medial shoe counter. When an offset heel is made of a firm, lightweight crepe, the result is a strong modification with only minimal weight increase (Fig. 14-9).

ROCKER BOTTOM SHOES

Rocker soles and heels are especially effective when seeking to relieve the strain on a Charcot ankle or a fused ankle or when it is desirable to reduce floor reaction at a specific point on the sole. To visualize the concept behind the rocker sole one must drop

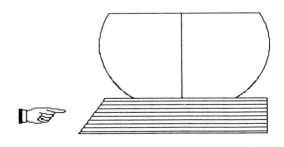

FIGURE 14–8 ■ Medial heel flare, right shoe.

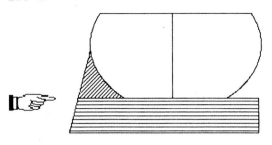

FIGURE 14–9 ■ Medial offset heel, right shoe.

a vertical line from the hip to the floor. This line then becomes the radius of a circle, with the hip at the center (Fig. 14-10). By establishing an arc based on the length of the leg with a shoe on, the rationale for the basic shape of a rocker sole is determined. This contributes to a smooth gait. To make changes in floor reaction or in the patient's gait, alternatives can be made to vary the shape of the rocker.

For instance, to achieve a fast rocker to avoid pressure on the forefoot, the height of the rocker and contour of the base are increased to cause the forepart of the arc to drop away quickly.

If the patient has difficulty with balance, or is uncomfortable with a continuously rocking surface, a flat stance phase is made in the midportion of the rocker. The length of this stance phase affects the amount of time spent reacting with the floor at a specific point on the plantar surface of the foot (Fig. 14-11).

To reduce the stress on a fused or Charcot ankle further, it might also be necessary to fabricate a rocker heel. This modification is designed to move the heel strike point forward and so reduce the plantar flexion moment exerted about the ankle axis. A rocker heel is made by grinding the posterior aspect of the heel at an angle that moves the strike point in closer alignment with the ankle joint (Fig. 14-12).

To further enhance this rocker heel, a solid ankle cushion heel (SACH) type of construction is used. By inserting a posterior wedge of a softer material combined with the firmer outsole-heel material for floor contact, shock into the heel and ankle is reduced. A SACH heel combined with a rocker provides the optimal reduction of shock and plantar flexion stress on the involved ankle complex.

Another pressure-reducing technique is excavation. By removing firm insole material from under a plantar lesion and replacing it with material of substantially lower density and more resilience, direct pressure on the lesion is reduced.

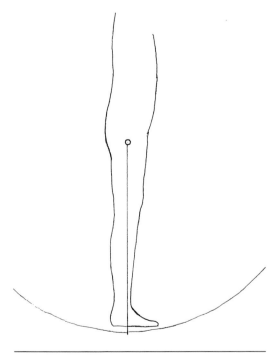

FIGURE 14–10 ■ Schematic representation of rationale behind development and use of rocker sole. See text for details.

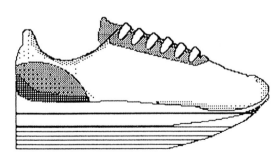

FIGURE 14–11 ■ High rocker sole—straight heel, long stance.

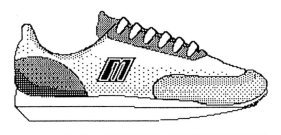

FIGURE 14–12 ■ Rocker sole with slight heel rock.

MANAGEMENT OF SPECIFIC PATHOLOGIC CONDITIONS

One excavation technique removes outsole material directly under a lesion or along a zone of high pressure. This technique combined with a rocker sole is one of the few that has been found useful in relieving plantar pressure under a Charcot foot.

Most diabetic foot ulcers are neurotrophic. It is necessary to differentiate between ischemic lesions and lesions resulting from repetitive stress. Actual treatment for these problems has little variation, because the goal must always be the relief of pressure. Fine tuning of a technique, however, is determined by the true etiology of the lesion.

When treating an ischemic lesion, blood flow at the surface is an important consideration. It is necessary to ensure that no constriction or excessive pressure occurs at the affected area. This can influence the shaping of an orthosis or might require hollowing of an area to create a negative pressure zone relative to that of the surrounding tissue.

Lesions caused by repetitive stress are frequently the result of a bony prominence striking tissue continuously, with additional forces being imparted by floor reaction. If, for instance, a metatarsal head presses against the skin of the sole from the inside, with no contact outside the skin, it is unlikely that repeating this impact would result in tissue breakdown. When the foot makes contact with the floor, the action of the metatarsal head pressing down and the reaction of the floor pressing up creates pressure on the skin. Constant repetition of this action, even if the forces are minimal, places the tissue under increased pressure.

This cannot be relieved without surgery, but certain measures can be carried out.

The pedorthotic solution to treatment of neuropathic ulcer is varied. To organize treatment based on degree of involvement, Wagner's scale can be modified for a classification of foot lesions based on mechanical management. Because pain is seldom the incentive for compliance of the patient, fear of ulcers is helpful. It is necessary to educate the patient by proceeding with conservative management using the acronym, "SCALE":

S—no lesions; patient should wear sensible footwear with soft insoles

C—prelesion, conservative management; patient should wear proper footwear and contoured foot orthosis

A—active lesion, no infection, active management; patient should always wear extra-deep shoes, molded orthosis, with modifications at this stage (be aggressive!)

L—lesion with infection, risk of loss of limb; redistribute load and change lever arm; learn more "A" (above)

E—deep lesion with osteitis; everything possible should be done to relieve pressure and enhance medical management in an effort to retain the limb

No Lesions. This is the most important time for the physician, orthotist, or pedorthist to direct the patient in health care. Education of the importance of proper footwear, correctly fitted and with soft resilient insoles, is necessary. Many shoes of this type are available, but the patient should be instructed to look for the following hazards:

1. Thick seams across the vamp or toes and along the sides
2. Low toe box
3. Constriction at throat of shoe, common in slip-on shoes
4. Shoes made of plastic or hard leather; plastic or hard leather does not give and can contribute to high pressure at prominence
5. Shoes that are fitted too tightly or too loosely—tight shoes present greater risk, especially if tightness is at one specific site
6. Inside of shoe should have no lasting tacks, unseated nails, or other potential perforation problems

Generally, neoprene crepe soles tend to distribute floor reaction forces and reduce impact better than leather. High-quality footwear should be bought and fitted by retail professionals with experience.

Prelesion. Typically, a preulcerous condition, one in which color changes are present with callus formation, cracking of epidermis, or blistering are treated by fitting the patient in shoes with ample depth and a molded polyethylene foam foot orthosis. The orthosis must be molded to allow total contact with the contours of the foot. This technique redistributes pressure to allow the involved area to quiet down. When combined with proper medical management to reduce callosities and recondition skin, this results in resilient, healthier, tissue that has a reduced tendency for breakdown. At this stage of the "SCALE" intervention can be carried out. Management here is more cost-effective and the results are more successful when compared to that in later stages.

Some believe that everything necessary should be done at this stage to avoid progression to an ulcerous condition. It is difficult, however, to convince the patient that significant steps should be taken at this stage, because often patients think that nothing is wrong. In addition, many physicians unfortunately fail to recognize the risk at this point, and these two factors make patient compliance difficult.

Patients must be motivated properly. They might be "angry at God for giving them diabetes," angry at the physician for revealing the problem, or angry because they must buy "ugly" shoes.

Active Lesions, No Infection. Active management is essential at this point. Once the skin has been opened, the risk of infection and other complications increases dramatically. The minimum level of management requires extra-deep shoes, a molded foot orthosis, and appropriate modifications to the orthosis, shoes, or both.

The most effective footwear has at least a removable 3/16-inch insole to allow for placement of the foot orthosis. Broad-toed shoes with a combination last (heel smaller than forefoot) provide the most usable space with the least risk.

Orthotic management of ulceration is relatively straightforward. Polyethylene foams are the best materials with which to start, whereas single-density orthoses are relatively easy to make and fit. Disadvantages of this approach, however, make this only a short-term solution.

An alternative choice is a dual-density or multidensity system with synergistic qualities unavailable in single-density inserts. Although single-density inserts made from Plastazote 1 (soft) are effective, this density packs out in a short time. A dual-density orthosis using Plastazote 1 as a top layer, combined with Plastazote 2 (medium) or UCOlite as the bottom layer, provides a soft, accommodative, contact layer, an interface to deflect floor reaction force vectors, and a base that, although accommodative, resists quick pack out.

Dual-density systems can be directly molded to the foot, but are more versatile when vacuum-formed over a modified model of the foot. The key when using dual-density or multidensity systems is selection of materials; these should accommodate, dissipate forces on the foot, be easily modified or adjusted, and be inert.

A shoe should be used that correctly fits both the foot and orthosis. The patient with impaired sensation might be unable to determine whether the shoe is correct or comfortable.

If the ulcer is recalcitrant, without infection present, pressure has probably not been adequately relieved beneath the ulcer. The orthosis and outsole of the shoe should be examined to determine the wear pattern and to decide on further treatment.

If the orthosis is compressed under a metatarsal lesion, it is best to apply a modification proximal to the metatarsal head. It is preferable to apply modifications to the underside of accommodative orthoses in diabetics.

ASSESSMENT OF TREATMENT

Short-Term Evaluation

In monitoring treatment, the orthosis, shoes, or both are observed for signs of excessive pressure:

1. Is the lesion noticeably reduced in size and severity after the first 3 to 6 weeks of management? If not, look for the

source of pressure, infection, or noncompliance.

2. Note the physical characteristics of the orthosis after initial use. Is excessive compression or deformation present? Look for discoloration or signs of abrasion on the orthosis.
3. Check the wear pattern inside and outside the shoes. The outsole and heel can reveal evidence of excessive pressure or misalignment. The inside can reveal areas of pressure on the toes or pressure from seams.
4. Is a change in gait pattern present? Gait changes are to be expected when the patient first starts to use the new orthosis or footwear (or both). Is the change favorable, and does a review after 3 to 6 weeks' use indicate sustained improvement or deterioration?
5. Is the patient experiencing side effects? Aching in the feet or legs is normal after the first several days. Does the patient experience unreasonable discomfort, loss of balance, or other symptoms not previously experienced? Is a skin reaction present?
6. Is the patient actually using the orthosis and footwear?

Long-Term Evaluation

Evaluation includes not only a short-term review, but additional considerations of long-term use.

1. The most obvious positive indication is freedom from lesions. If not, why not?
2. If good results were present initially, but the patient now has a recurrence of tissue breakdown at the original site or nearby, look carefully at the orthotic-footwear system. Has the system been maintained or is it now starting to break down? It is not unusual for a polyethylene foam foot orthotic system to look as if it is in good condition, only to find excessive compression under one site.
3. Remember that the shoe is the vehicle for the orthosis. An ankle-foot orthosis or a foot orthosis might appear to be in good condition but, if the shoe is worn out or the heel run over, the orthosis cannot work as it did at the beginning.

4. Have structural changes occurred in the foot and ankle? Are they favorable? If not, are they major changes, such as Charcot joints? If the changes are major, should the design of the system be changed?
5. If structural changes have occurred, check carefully for neurotrophic or arthropathic processes.

Follow-up and Long-Term Maintenance

"The hole is closed, I'm cured!" "I finally got rid of the diabetes in my right foot." These announcements are common after a lesion has healed. It is important that the patient be followed closely.

Contrary to popular belief, the healing of a lesion does not mean that the problem is solved. It is critical that all concerned be aware that the problem will last the rest of the patient's life. Constant vigilance, continued evaluation, and careful maintenance of footwear and orthoses help the patient to walk with reduced risk.

References

1. Wagner FW Jr. A classification and treatment program for diabetic neuropathic and dysvascular foot problems. Inst. Course Lecture. 1979; 28:1–47.
2. Boulton AJM, Franks CI, et al. Reduction of abnormal foot pressures in diabetic neuropathy using a new polymer insoling material. Diabetes Care. 1984; 7:42–46.

Bibliography

1. Baroni G. et al. Hyperbaric oxygen in diabetic gangrene treatment. Diabetes Care. 1987; 10:81–86.
2. Black J. Orthopedic biomaterials in research and practice. New York: Churchill Livingstone; 1988.
3. Brand PW. Repetitive stress on insensitive feet. Carville, LA: US Public Health Service; 1975.
4. Coleman WC, Brand PW, Birke JA. The total contact cast: a therapy for plantar ulceration on insensitive feet. J Am Podiatry Assoc. 1983; 74:548–549.
5. Dillon RS. Successful treatment of osteomyelitis of soft tissue infections in ischemic diabetic legs by local antibiotic injections and the end diastolic pneumatic compression boot. Ann Surg. 1986; 204:643–649.

6. Edmonds ME. Improved survival of the diabetic foot: the role of a specialized foot clinic. Q J Med. 1986; 60:763–771.

7. Holstein P. Decompression with the aid of insoles in treatment of diabetic neuropathic ulcers. Acta Orthop Scand. 1976; 47:463–468.

8. Levin ME, O'Neal LW, eds. The diabetic foot. St. Louis: CV Mosby; 1988.

9. Mulder GD. Synthetic membranes. Use in diabetic ulcers. Clin Podiatr Med Surg. 1987; 4:419–427.

10. Pollard JP. Method of healing diabetic forefoot ulcers. Brussels Med J. 1983; 286:436–437.

11. Tan JS, Flanagan PJ. Team approach in the management of diabetic foot infections. J Foot Surg. 1987; 26:512–516.

12. Wagner FW Jr. Treatment of the diabetic foot. Compr. Ther. 1984; 10:29.

13. Wagner FW Jr. The insensitive foot. In: Symposium on the foot and ankle. Kiene, RH and Johnson KA, eds. St. Louis: CV Mosby; 1983; 140–150.

14. Wagner FW Jr. A classification and treatment program for diabetic neuropathic and dysvascular foot problems. Instr. Course Lect. 1979; 28:1–47.

15. Wagner FW Jr. The dysvascular foot: a system for diagnosis and treatment. Foot Ankle. 1981; 2:64–122.

This handout sheet is for patients.

This instruction sheet is for patients with foot orthoses.

APPENDIX 14-1. CARE OF FEET WITH IMPAIRED SENSATION

It is important that you prevent any injury to your feet and follow a careful plan of foot hygiene.

1. *Inspect your feet daily.*
   a. Check visually for sores or changes in skin color.
   b. Use the back of your hand to find any areas of high temperature on the bottom of your foot.
   c. Any major change in skin temperature, or the appearance of a sore, should be reported to your doctor, *at once.*
2. *Wear clean socks*—change them daily and discard them when they have holes in them.
3. *Wear shoes that fit properly.* To help ensure dryness, change to a different pair each day. Keep the heels and soles in good repair.
4. *Break in new shoes gradually.* Wear a new pair no more than 2 hours at a time for the first few days. Inspect your feet after each usage. If no changes occur, gradually increase the time of usage.
5. *Do not attempt to trim your own corns or calluses* or to use commercial corn remedies. Get professional advice regarding corns, calluses, and toenail trimming.
6. *Do not walk barefoot.* Bare feet invite injury.
7. *Avoid extremes of heat or cold.* If your feet are cold, wear warm socks. Never use hot water bottles or heating pads. Protect your feet from sunburn.
8. *Avoid wearing anything tight* around your legs or ankles that might reduce the blood supply to your feet in any way.
9. *Bathe your feet daily* in lukewarm (not hot!) soapy water and rinse thoroughly. Carefully and gently, with a soft towel, pat (don't rub!) your feet dry, especially between the toes.
10. Inspect your feet daily!!

APPENDIX 14-2. USE OF YOUR FOOT ORTHOSIS

1. *Break-in period:*
   a. You might experience some side effects from your new orthosis, especially if *OVERUSED.*
   b. You might experience aching in the feet or legs because of muscle fatigue and the change in foot function and position. *This is normal and expected.*
   c. Your break-in period normally lasts 1 to 3 weeks.
2. *Recommended usage during break-in period:*
   a. *Do not* exceed 1 to 2 hours the first time you wear your orthoses. This includes sitting and standing.
   b. *Do* limit your usage if you experience aching in the feet or legs or skin discoloration.
   c. *Do* increase your usage slowly (add 1 to 2 hours more each day) if you do *not* experience side effects.
   d. *Do not* get discouraged if it takes more time to adjust than you expected.
   e. *Do not* attempt to wear your orthosis all day at the beginning. *Overuse* is the most frequent problem encountered.
3. *After break-in period:*
   a. Please call your physician after 3 weeks!!
   b. If you are doing fine, and receiving the expected results, this needs to be recorded on your file.
   c. If you are having problems, or continued symptoms, please advise your physician at this time. An appointment will be set up to evaluate the problem and make the necessary modifications.

Please note: An appointment is required to make any changes or adjustments to your orthosis.

4. *Plaster cast:*
   a. This should be allowed to dry thoroughly and stored in a dry place.
   b. It might be needed to make an adjustment to your orthosis.

5. *Care of your orthosis*—most of the materials used in the fabrication of your orthosis are inert and easily cleaned. Please check with your physician regarding specific instructions for your orthosis.

Index

Page numbers in italics indicate illustrations; numbers followed by "t" indicate tables.